e Hemlock.

VERS.

parine.

uth Groton, Ms.

lb *Extract of*

PEACH,

Amygdalus persicaria,
D. M.
Prepared in the United Society,
New-Lebanon, N. Y.

Jar *lb* *oz.*

COMPOUND CONCENTRATED

SYRUP of SARSAPARILLA,

CONTAINS 10 PER CENT. ALCOHOL.

PREPARED BY
CANTERBURY SHAKERS,
East Canterbury, N. H., U. S. A.

This medicine has proved to be most valuable in the following diseases :—

Chronic Inflammation of the Digestive Organs ; Dyspepsia, or Indigestion ; Weakness and Sourness of the Stomach ; Rheumatism ; Salt Rheum ; Secondary Syphilis ; Functional Disorders of the Liver ; Chronic Eruptions of the Skin, and all Scrofulous diseases and disorders arising from impurities of the blood. It is also an excellent remedy for the Erysipelas, Asthma, Dropsy, Dysentery, and Diarrhœa, and for the complicated diseases of females, so apt to end in consumption.

DOSE.—For an adult, a teaspoonful four or five times a day, with or without a little water, which may be increased to a tablespoonful, as best suits the patient.

To guard against counterfeits, observe the signature of the inventor on each label and on each wrapper.

Thos Corbett.

Serial No. 6261. Guaranteed under the Food and Drugs Act, June 30, 1906.

MARJORAM.

ULV.

O BE DIRECTED TO
TON, United Society,
GROTON, MASS.

BONESET,
Eupatorium perfoliatum.
D. M. & Co,
Watervliet, N. Y.

BORAGE.
Borago officinalis.
D. M. & Co.
Watervliet, N. Y.

Prepared at the Labaratory of the
United Society of Shakers.
For MEYER BROTHERS & Co
at St Louis & Fort Wayne.

Essence Pennyroyal.

HARDHACK.

Spiræa Tomentosa.

United Society, South Groton, Ms.

LB *EXTRACT OF*

SARSAPARILLA,

Aralia Nudicaulis,

D. M.
Prepared in the United Society,
NEW-LEBANON, N. Y.

Jar *lb* *oz.*

ROSE WATER.

D. M.

Prepared in the united Society
of SHAKERS,
New Lebanon, N. Y.

DANDELION ROOT.

Taraxacum Dens-leonis.

United Society, South Groton, Mass.

Essence SPEARMINT.

SCULL CAP BLUE.

Scutellaria Lateriflora.

United Society, South Groton, Mass.

Shaker Herbs

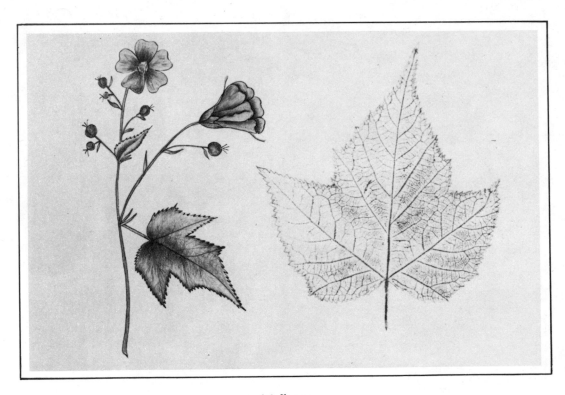

Mulberry

AMY BESS MILLER

Shaker Herbs

A
HISTORY
AND A
COMPENDIUM

Clarkson N. Potter, Inc./Publisher NEW YORK

DISTRIBUTED BY CROWN PUBLISHERS, INC.

To
LAWRENCE KELTON MILLER

Published simultaneously in Canada
by General Publishing Company Limited

FIRST EDITION

Printed in the United States of America

Designed by Shari de Miskey

Library of Congress Cataloging in Publication Data

Miller, Amy Bess Williams.
Shaker herbs.

Bibliography: p.
Includes index.

1. Shakers. 2. Herbs—Therapeutic use. 3. Botany,
Medical. I. Title.
BX9785.M4M54   289.8   76-40485
ISBN   0-517-52494-5

The text of this book is printed on Bergstrom Text, which is totally recycled paper.

Go work with ardent courage,
　　and sow with willing hand
The seed o'er barren deserts
　　and o'er the fertile land.

And, lo! earth yet shall blossom
　　Though the brighter morn delays;
For God perfects the harvest,
　　Yea, "after many days."

The Life and Gospel Experience of Mother Ann Lee
(East Canterbury, New Hampshire: Shakers, 1901)

CONTENTS

THE HERBAL COMPENDIUM

vii

ACKNOWLEDGMENTS

Most of my work on this book was done in libraries and while my great esteem for these institutions needs no reinforcement, an inside view of how they operate impels even more appreciation.

At first hand I experienced the efficiency of such systems as state interlibrary loan and interstate loan. Their swift operation belies the notion some people have that all tax-supported institutions are wasteful and inefficient. The ready availability of Xerox machines and microfilm equipment saved hours of writing and searching. The linchpin was sometimes a member of the staff, sometimes the director or head librarian, who with cheerful support from a number of departments made hours of work stimulating and refreshing.

I am deeply indebted to the members of the staffs of these institutions for their patience, helpful suggestions and encouragement:

The American Antiquarian Society, Worcester, Massachusetts

The Berkshire Athenaeum, Pittsfield, Massachusetts

Cleveland Public Library, Cleveland, Ohio

The Filson Club, Louisville, Kentucky

Fruitlands, Harvard, Massachusetts

Kentucky Library and Museum, Western Kentucky University, Bowling Green, Kentucky

The Emma B. King Library of the Shaker Museum, Old Chatham, New York

Library of Congress, Washington, D.C.

Library of the Francis H. du Pont Museum, Winterthur, Delaware

Library at Shaker Community, Inc., Hancock, Massachusetts

New York Botanical Garden, New York City

New York Public Library, New York City

Pleasant Hill, Shakertown, Kentucky

The United Society of Shakers, Sabbathday Lake, Maine
University of Kentucky, Lexington, Kentucky
Western Reserve Historical Society, Cleveland, Ohio
Williams College Library, Williamstown, Massachusetts

Eldress Gertrude M. Soule, now residing at Canterbury, New Hampshire, encouraged and inspired me as did Eldress Bertha Lindsay and Sister Miriam Wall, also of the Canterbury Society. I am indebted to them and Charles E. Thompson for permission to use the beautiful colored drawings by Cora Helena Sarle.

Mr. and Mrs. Donald E. Richmond, Julia Neal, and Elmer R. Pearson were most generous in sharing their research with me. Mr. and Mrs. William Henry Harrison at Fruitlands were most helpful, too, with source material and boarded me in great luxury, as well. Robert F. W. Meader of the Shaker Museum also was a source of information and generous help.

Douglas Bogart, Persis Wellington Fuller, Veola Lederer, and John Ott supported me in every way. Nancy Epley, Joelle Caulkins and Phyllis Rubenstein typed the manuscript efficiently and without a word of complaint. Philip L. Clark, who since 1960 has grown herbs and tended the Hancock Shaker gardens with devotion and style, was an almost daily reminder that I was working with and annotating facts about living material.

PREFACE

An anonymous Shaker editor of the medicinal herb catalog published by the New Lebanon society gave his readers a bonus—a "supplementary" in 1851 which today would be termed a preface. This was the first time such a statement appeared in a Shaker medicinal marketing publication. It reflects the reasons the Shakers felt so much care and effort should go into the production of medicinal products:

> Perhaps no study contributes more to the length, utility, and pleasure of existence—which adds to health, cheerfulness and enlarged views of creative wisdom and power, and which improves the morals, tastes and judgment, more than the science of botany.

During the 14 years Hancock Shaker Village has been opened to the public we have witnessed with pleasure the increasing interest in herbs and have therefore been greatly encouraged in our efforts to restore the herb gardens originally planted by the Shakers.

It is my purpose in this work to provide the historical background of the Shaker herb industry, to answer questions about the growing and use of herbs by the Shakers, and in enlarging the knowledge in this area to encourage the interest in this field of botany.

Edward Fowler observed that "the majority of persons, even in cultivated society" were ignorant not only of botany as a science but of the "character and nutritive properties of the most distinguished products of vegetable nature."

Would that this brother could observe the return to nature, the widespread interest in organic foods, and the growing of herbs. We agree with him that it is strange so inviting a subject has been so long generally neglected and we rejoice that whatever turned the tide has made the renewed interest in and use of herbs a notable part of today's mode of living for a great many people of all ages.

I have also tried to show how an industry was founded and how the Shakers with a sophistication not supposed to be a part of the Shaker tradition marketed their products in a very competitive field. The largest communities in New York State, Ohio, and Kentucky had their own printing presses for labels, leaflets, and catalogs, as did the Eastern societies at Hancock and Harvard, Massachusetts, Canterbury, New Hampshire, and Sabbathday Lake, Maine. They chose their agents in the large cities carefully and less than 70 years after the first true hospital was established in Philadelphia were trusted suppliers to these medical institutions. They advertised their products systematically and with studied appeal. Nothing was left to chance.

This book is focused on the medicinal aspect of the herb business of the Shakers and only briefly mentions the use of herbs in cooking, in dyeing, and in housekeeping procedures. Like all early country people the Shakers used barks from trees, roots, and nuts, berries, and flowers to make their colored dyes. They resorted to certain herbs to control moths, and perfume their linens; of course, they created delicious dishes flavored with herbs.

The Shakers took the time to develop an awareness of the needs of the members of their communities to maintain their health, and of others, and they studied the best ways of meeting those needs. They especially were committed to maintaining the good health of their communities, for they were few in number and, furthermore, did not bear their own children to assure the perpetuity of their society. They also were committed to making the surplus of their manufactures and products available to the world's people.

One of the world's people, although hardly totally committed to the world, was Henry David Thoreau. In August and September of 1839 he made a voyage on the Concord and Merrimack rivers, and from this "river-party" the twenty-two-year-old naturalist condensed his excursion into one volume, assertedly a week on the two rivers. It is much more than a mere reproduction of his journal kept during the period under consideration and one digression is of particular interest as it discusses the useful herbs of his day. This is coincidental in time with the most fruitful era in the medicinal herb business of the Shakers.

Thoreau had gazed upon Uncannunuc Mountain in Goffstown from Amoskeag, New Hampshire, and then he said:

A little south of Uncannunuc, about sixty years ago, as the story goes, an old woman who went out to gather pennyroyal tripped her foot in the bail of a small brass kettle in the dead grass and bushes. Some say that flints and charcoal and some traces of a camp were also found. This kettle, holding about four quarts, is still preserved and used to dye thread in. It is supposed to have belonged to some old French or Indian hunter, who was killed in one of his hunting or scouting excursions, and so never returned to look after his kettle.

But we were most interested to hear of the pennyroyal; it is soothing to be reminded that wild nature produces anything ready for the use of man. Men know that *something* is good. One says that it is yellow-dock, another that it is bitter-sweet, another that it is slippery-elm bark, burdock, catnip, calamint, elecampane, thoroughwort, or pennyroyal. A man may esteem himself happy when that which is his food is also his medicine. There is no kind of herb, but somebody or other says that it is good. I am very glad to hear it. It reminds me of the first chapter of Genesis. But how should they know that it is good? That is the mystery to me. I am always agreeably disappointed; it is incredible that they should have found it out. Since all things are good, men fail at last to distinguish which is the bane and which the antidote. There are sure to be two prescriptions diametrically opposite. Stuff a cold and starve a cold are but two ways. They are the two practices both always in full blast. Yet you must take advice of the one school as if there was no other. In respect to religion and the healing art, all nations are still in a state of barbarism. In the most civilized countries the priest is still but a Powwow, and the physician a Great Medicine. Consider the deference which is everywhere paid to a doctor's opinion. Nothing more strikingly betrays the credulity of mankind than medicine. Quackery is a thing universal, and universally successful. In this case it becomes literally true that no imposition is too great for the credulity of men. Priests and physicians should never look one another in the face. They have no common ground, nor is there any to mediate between them. When the one comes, the other goes. They could not come together without laughter, or a significant silence, for the one's profession is a satire on the other's, and either's success would be the other's failure. It is wonderful that the physician should ever die, and that the priest should ever live. Why is it that the priest is never called to consult with the physician? Is it because men believe practically that matter is independent of spirit? But what is quackery? It is commonly an attempt to cure the diseases of a man by addressing his body alone. There is need of a physician who shall minister to both soul and body at once, that is to man. Now he falls between two stools.[1]

The early Shakers also professed to healing by spirit touch and mental control. Physicians from the world sometimes were employed after 1813 when there was more medical freedom within the societies. The answer to Thoreau's question as to why the priest is never called to consult with the physician may not be found precisely in Shaker practice. However, it was a precept of the Shakers that their religion was their way of life and most often their religious leader fulfilled the function of the family physician. For the Believers this was an anodyne as readily effective as any of the healing herbs, and they said with characteristic honesty: "Duty is our's; results, God's."[2]

NOTES

1. Henry D. Thoreau, *A Week on the Concord and Merrimack Rivers* (Boston: Houghton Mifflin Co., 1893), p. 337.
2. *The Shaker Manifesto,* July 1899, p. 112.

SHAKER SOCIETIES

For the convenience of the reader a list of Shaker societies is given:

	ESTABLISHED	DISSOLVED*
1. Watervliet (Niskeyuna), New York	1787	1938
2. New Lebanon (Mt. Lebanon after 1861, when the first Federal post office was installed), New York	1787	1947
3. Hancock, Massachusetts (Shaker Community, Inc., was established as a nonprofit organization to operate Hancock Shaker Village in 1960 as a museum open to the public)	1790	1960
4. Enfield, Connecticut	1792	1917
5. Canterbury, New Hampshire	1792	Still active
6. Tyringham, Massachusetts	1792	1875
7. Alfred, Maine	1793	1931
8. Enfield, New Hampshire	1793	1918
9. Harvard, Massachusetts	1791	1919
10. Shirley, Massachusetts	1793	1909
11. Sabbathday Lake (New Gloucester), Maine	1794	Still active
12. Union Village, Ohio	1812	1910
13. Watervliet (Beulah), in Dayton, Ohio	1813	1900

* Where date is known.

	ESTABLISHED	DISSOLVED
14. Pleasant Hill, Kentucky (an independent, nonprofit corporation was organized to operate Pleasant Hill in 1968 as a museum open to the public)	1814	1910
15. South Union, Kentucky (an independent, nonprofit corporation was organized to operate South Union in 1972 as a museum open to the public)	1811	1922
16. West Union (Busro), Indiana	1810	1827
17. Whitewater, Ohio	1824	1907
18. Groveland, New York	1836	1892
19. North Union, Cleveland, Ohio	1826	1889

Group Meetings, Missions, Branches, "Out Families," and Short-lived Communities:

	ESTABLISHED	DISSOLVED
Cheshire, Richmond, and Ashfield, Massachusetts. Group meetings in the 1780s were absorbed into the organized communities.	1780	
Gorham, Maine. Members moved to New Gloucester, Maine.	1808	1819
Straight Creek, Ohio	1808	
Canaan, New York: Lower Family 1813–1884; Upper Family 1813–1897	1813	1897
Savoy, Massachusetts. Members moved to New Lebanon, Canaan, and Watervliet, New York	1817	1825
Darby, Ohio	1822	1823
Sodus Bay (Sodus Point, or Port Bay), New York	1826	1836
Philadelphia, Pennsylvania. Members moved to Watervliet after a few years. Revived temporarily in 1860.	1846	
Narcoossee, Florida. A branch of the community of Mt. Lebanon, New York.	1896	1913
White Oak, Georgia.	1898	1902

The History

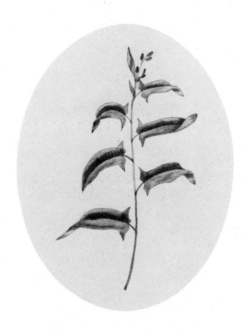

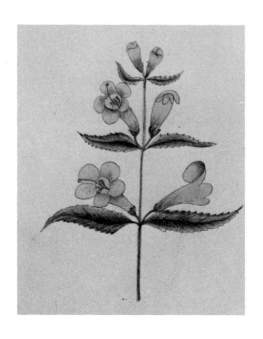

INTRODUCTION

In the Midlands of England during the 1740s a girl was growing up whose force of character and selfless efforts on behalf of a religious ideal might in an earlier era have made her a sainted martyr. In circumstances least likely to provide her with good health or even the luck to live to middle age, she grew up in a community where only one in every twenty-eight children lived to see a fortieth birthday and where childhood in many cases was over almost before it started.

Ann Lee, the founder of the Shaker movement, was born in Manchester, England, February 29, 1736. A few years earlier this town was described by another nonconformist and dissenter, Daniel Defoe:

> One of the greatest, if not really the greatest mere village in England. It is neither a wall'd town, city or corporation; they send no member to Parliament; and the highest magistrate they have is a Constable, or Head-borough; and yet it takes up a large space of ground, and including the suburb, it is said to contain about fifty thousand people.[1]

The chaotic state of such rapidly growing towns as Manchester during the eighteenth century has also been luridly depicted by Sidney and Beatrice Webb:

> The narrow ways left to foot and wheeled traffic were unpaved, uneven and full of holes in which the water and garbage accumulated. . . . Public provision for street cleaning or the removal of refuse, there was none, so that garbage and horse dung accumulated in places even a yard deep. There were, of course, no sewers and no water closets. . . . At night when there was no moon, the streets were in pitch darkness, except for an occasional lantern swinging over the door of an energetic shopkeeper or a rich householder.[2]

Manchester is described by John Clayton as teeming with filth and crime. Writing his "Friendly Advice To The Poor" in 1755, he declared: "We cannot walk the streets without being annoyed with such filth as a public nuisance . . . our streets are no better than a common dunghill."[3] This publication was written at the request of "the late and present officers of the Town of Manchester" who, it seems, were trying to improve the situation and who emphasized that Manchester did indeed have sewers, their deficiency being that they were uncovered.

Although it has been generally agreed by both earlier and later historians that the

1

local government remained grotesquely inadequate to the needs of the town until after the middle of the nineteenth century, we do know that during Ann Lee's residency there was policing of a sort as she was more than once abused by the "street-keepers." These descendants of the early warders were appointed to "keep the peace." The street-keepers also on occasion acted as informers, and two of them (in 1773) were paid for "assisting the Deputy to make distress upon twenty Quakers for refusing to pay their small tithes."[4]

Manchester, at the time of Ann Lee's birth, was called "The Black Country." Its houses, built of brick made from the nearby clay beds, were thick with soot. Charles Dickens called it "Coketown," and said it was a town of red brick that would have been red "if the smoke and ashes had allowed it; but as matters stood it was a town of unnatural red and black, like the painted face of a savage."[5] The rivers Irwell, Medlock, the Irk, and the Tib became mere dirty ditches as they ran through the central part of the city. Treeless cobblestone streets were dark, narrow lanes, lit only by an occasional street-corner flare or the light from a grimy window seen through a narrow gap between two buildings. These conditions were the same for rich and poor alike.

The England of the Georges was at this time distressed by war and heavy taxation. Popular discontent was met with repression and cruelty, often at the hands of drunken cavalry turned loose upon unresisting masses. Manchester, a cotton manufacturing community, was not unlike other large factory cities. It had its royal infirmary, its churches, a handsome cathedral and its pride, the great Memorial Hall, where scientific meetings and musical performances were held. For in that day there were many educational facilities, the oldest being the grammar school founded in 1519, but these institutions were not for the poor until well into the nineteenth century.

The greatest of all travel commentators, Alexis de Tocqueville, visited Manchester in 1835, 99 years after Ann Lee's birth. His summation and evaluation a century later leaves one with an even more vivid picture. He thought that Manchester compared very unfavorably with Birmingham. The people looked less healthy, less well-off, were "more preoccupied," and "less moral." The police were less efficient, and there was a terrible contrast between the sights of "civilization" and the scenes of "barbarism." "Fine stone buildings" with Corinthian columns suggested that Manchester "might be a medieval town with the marvels of the nineteenth century in it. But who could describe the interiors of these quarters set apart, homes of vice and poverty, which surround the huge palaces of industry and clasp them in their hideous folds?" In Manchester "humanity attains its most complete development and its most brutish; here civilization works its miracles, and civilized man is turned back almost into a savage." With no love of revolution, nevertheless, Tocqueville wrote: "The respect paid to wealth in England is enough to make one despair" and about the same time the American Henry Colman, in his *European Life and Manners* (1845), wrote:

> Wretched, defrauded, oppressed, crushed human nature, lying in bleeding fragments all over the face of society, every day I live I thank Heaven that I am not a poor man with a family in England.[6]

He went on a tour of the black spots of Manchester with Dr. Lyon Playfair and two police officers and saw "exhibitions of the most disgusting and loathsome forms of destitution, and utter vice and profligacy." He told a friend that he could not describe the visits in detail for "the paper would, I fear, be absolutely offensive to the touch." The visits had left such a mark on him that "it will make my life hereafter an incessant thanksgiving that my children have not in the inscrutable dispensation of Heaven been cast destitute, helpless, and orphans in such a country as this." It also was fortunate for

Mother Ann and her followers that another "inscrutable dispensation of Heaven" guided her way from the misery she endured for 38 years to the promise and hope of a better life in the New Land.

There are many accounts, written by Shaker historians, of the life and work of Ann Lee in England. They tell of her humble birth in 1736 in a "lowly" cottage on Toad Lane. She was the daughter of an honest and industrious blacksmith and an affectionate, sensible, and pious mother. There were other children in the family, five boys and two girls. As there were no free schools for the poor, Ann, like so many in that day, soon went to work in the mills and is supposed never to have learned to read or write.

At an early age Ann revealed a remarkable spiritual force, the kind of force which in that time sent some to the witch's gallows. The little factory girl told her mother about her visions of angels, but this God-fearing woman dared not repeat such things. We are told that an "intense desire for purity and holy living filled the girl's heart, and as she grew older she was deeply impressed by the depravity of human nature and showed a strong repugnance to marriage."[7] Nevertheless, much against her will, she was married to Abraham Stanley on January 5, 1762, and by him bore four children, all of whom died at birth or in infancy.

During Ann Lee's lifetime in Manchester, between 1736 and 1774, there was hardly a year in which the threat of food scarcity or death did not color her life. In the autumn of 1756, when Ann went to work as a cook in the royal infirmary, food riots broke out in many parts of England, especially in the manufacturing districts. More riots took place in Manchester during early summer the next year. Mobs plundered, stole, and burned, disrupting the life of the town for days.

There were frequent outbreaks of epidemic disease, and, once a pestilence descended, it tended to hang on for years, being carried from town to town by infected vagrants. Even so, Manchester was better off than most. Since 1752 it had its public hospital, and, such was the growth of medical science, it soon became one of the most important medical centers in the Midlands. Before the end of the eighteenth century the town also had a lunatic asylum, "lock hospital," special fever wards, and, very important, a local board of health.

It is doubtful if Ann Lee, as a cook in the infirmary, learned anything much about medical procedures, but she was exposed to the dismal conditions and the endless suffering of the poor, who were primarily there to die. Her determination to find a better quality of life somewhere else was mounting. However, it was to be 18 years before she left England to find that better life in America, and while her life, remarkable in its accomplishments, was also to be full of sorrow and persecution, she never ceased in urging her followers to heal the sick, succor the poor, and provide plentifully for all Believers. She also joined the society of the Wardleys in 1758. It was a religious group founded by James Wardley, a tailor, and his wife, Jane, of Bolton-le-Moors in Lancashire, both of whom had dropped out of the Quaker society which they had belonged to for several years. Some years later Ann became frustrated in her marriage, and was troubled by qualms of conscience and a deep feeling of sin and shame. In her own simple language, as repeated to her followers, she said:

> Soon after I set out to travel in the way of God, I labored anights in the work of God. Sometimes I labored all night, continually crying to God for my own redemption; sometimes I went to bed and slept; but in the morning I could not feel that sense of the work of God which I had before I slept. This brought me into great tribulation. Then I cried to God and promised Him that if He would give me the same sense that I had before I slept, I would labor all night. This I did many nights; and in the day time I put my hands to work and my heart to God.[8]

Someone who knew her well testified that during the periods of mental suffering Ann
wasted away like one with consumption and became so weak and emaciated that her
friends had to feed and care for her as if she were a child. Eldresses White and Taylor of
the Mt. Lebanon society* ask the question: "Why was Ann Lee so unlike all the other
poor women in Manchester, her neighbors on Toad Lane?" And they give this answer:
"Because she was called of God and obeyed the call, and thus became the Chosen, the
Daughter of God, of whom it may be said, 'Many daughters have done virtuously, but
thou excellest them all.' "

The life of a religious leader is not easy at any time or place, and one whose ideas
were so radically at variance with the established ways of life in eighteenth-century
England met with especially great hostility. Ann also met with hostility, and twice she
was thrown in jail for disturbing the peace, "profaning the Sabbath." It was when she
was in prison the second time that a vision came to her that she should go to America:
"She received a divine promise that the work of God would greatly increase, and the
Millennial Church would be established in that country."[9] Permission to accompany her
was given by the Wardleys and other members of their society to "all those of the society
. . . who were able and who felt any special impressions in their own minds so to do."[10]
On May 19, 1774, she sailed from Liverpool with eight of her followers aboard the ship
Mariah (under the command of Captain Smith from New York). They arrived in New
York harbor after a dangerous and stormy trip on August 6, 1774.

Judging from pictures of New York in 1774,[11] there was a bright and charming air
about the city which must have been encouraging. The streets were paved with cobble-
stones and in many places they were shaded by trees and hedges. The air was clear and
in the section of the town where Mother Ann worked as a laundress the houses were
brick and white-painted clapboard. A neighborhood pump gushed forth clear, clean
water.

The Believers had no friends or relatives in America, yet their lot seemed to be
better than the life they had left behind. And so, with a faith that never diminished in
its intensity, and a drive that never faltered, the little group held together.

The men in the party traveled north up the Hudson to Niskeyuna, or Niskayuna,
later named Watervliet, about seven miles northwest of Albany. This was to become the
first home of the Shakers in America. In the spring of 1775 Mother Ann and the women
joined them, and throughout the summer they worked hard clearing the land, often
working all night, cultivating the soil, and building houses to prepare a permanent
home. The community was finally settled in September 1776. These two years were
primarily concerned with survival. Then the Shakers turned to recruiting new members,
and they successfully did so as the result of holding a series of religious revivals. The
Believers worked ceaselessly to convert people, for they were few in number, and, being
celibate, they had no other means to enlarge their communities. But the faithful did
encounter intolerance and violence in many communities. Ann Lee, accordingly, spent
much time traveling among her followers to comfort them: "It is good to watch," said
Mother, "and you should always watch and, always pray."[12]

Mother Ann died in 1784 at Watervliet and the leadership passed into the hands of
Joseph Meecham and Lucy Wright. By 1800 11 Shaker communities had been organized
in the northeastern states and thereafter they expanded into the west. And by the
mid-1800s the Shakers attained their largest number of members, variously given as
"6,000," "more than 7,000," and "perhaps 8,000." A card file, first started in the 1920s by
the director of the Western Reserve Historical Society, Willard Cathcart, now contains
somewhat over 30,000 names of people who were covenant Shakers or who lived a

---

*New Lebanon was renamed Mt. Lebanon in 1861.

lifetime and died in the Shaker society and many others who lived long enough as Shakers to be so recorded.

Watervliet was the Shakers' first settled home. New Lebanon, New York, was the first in the society to be fully and formally organized and for many years was to be the most influential. It had the largest population and greatest acreage. The community grew in the 1780s from a few small farmhouses, surrounded by neighbors who were sympathetic to the Shakers and who eventually formed the first "order with them." It became a property of about 3,000 acres and 125 buildings in 1839. In later years its holdings increased to 6,000 acres. The population of the Mt. Lebanon society, at its height in the 1870s, reached 600 members.

This community was the home of the central ministry and for decades the rules and regulations governing all aspects of Shaker life, spiritual and material, emanated from this source, and, among the material aspects, the drug industry was started there and developed rapidly. Other Shaker communities at Watervliet, New York; Harvard, Massachusetts; and Canterbury, New Hampshire; soon took up this trade as well. Of the western societies the one to carry on the largest medicinal herb business was the Society of Believers at Union Village, near Lebanon, Ohio. At the height of its population this village numbered 600 members with some 4,500 acres of land.[13]

As millennialists, the Shakers were dedicated to making a society which would be free of crime, poverty, and misery. Their purpose was to be as self-sufficient as possible and to establish and preserve a quality of life which would support their growing membership and attract many to it. They spoke of "consecrated industry," and none of their industries was more consecrated than that of the medicinal herb business. How could it not have become so important when it was directed by men and women who said:

> We believed we were debtors to God in relation to Each other, and all men, to improve our time and tallents in this life, in that manner in which we might be most useful.[14]

The Shakers are their own best historians. We know as much as we do about their life in this country during the past two centuries because of what they have told us in their journals and letters, the printed testimonies of their disciples, their monthly publications, their own literature. This is not by chance. Their Millennial Laws very clearly set forth orders concerning "Books, Pamphlets and Writings in General" and state that "two family journals should be kept by, or by the order of the Deacons and Deaconesses, in which all important occurrences, or business transactions should be registered."[15] Therefore a vast amount of manuscript material exists which covers every aspect of Shaker life dating from the earliest records written in the late 1700s. Sometimes to ensure perfect communication, journals were duplicated and sent from family to family within a society or from society to society. This occasionally causes confusion for the researcher, especially if there were some variance in the material, but such procedures guaranteed complete coverage.

Without fail, the state of a community's health was given in some detail, as well as the weather and the success or failure of crops. These were obviously the important concerns of the community, and it was especially important to protect the health of every individual. There were few Shakers, and an epidemic disease could cause a disastrous setback. The Millennial Laws accordingly provided for the care of Believers by physicians and nurses: "As the natural body is prone to sickness and disease, it is proper that there should be suitable persons appointed to attend to necessary duties in administering medical aid to those in need."[16] Those appointed were required to give to the Elders a full account of their proceedings regarding the administration of medicine and it was definitely "forbidden to employ Doctors of the world, except in some extreme cases, or the case of a sick child, whose parents are among the world and desire such aid."[17] Even in this event it was left to the Elders to decide whether the step was necessary or proper. Well-appointed, efficiently managed infirmaries were organized in each community, and, of course, extensive records were kept of medicines given, the course of treatment which was followed, and whether or not it was effective.

Medicines for large numbers of people required immense amounts of herbal material and its careful preparation. At first, the Shakers gathered plants in the fields and woodlands and then grew certain varieties in "physic gardens" to supply the family. If they harvested more than they needed themselves, they sold the herbs or preparations to buy other medicines which a family could not produce itself. In a very short time, outside demand for the herbs grew. From this modest beginning, born of necessity, the Shakers became the first people in this country to produce herbs on a scale large enough to supply the pharmaceutical market, netting many thousands of dollars annually.

Charles Nordhoff was the first to give a detailed account of the communitarian societies in the United States. He wrote at length about the Shakers in 1875 after a visit to the Mt. Lebanon society and was greatly impressed with Elder Frederick Evans as a person of enthusiastic and aggressive temperament with "a hobby for science as applied to health, comfort and the prolongation of life."[18]

> He gave me a file of the *Shaker*, a monthly paper, in which the deaths in all the societies are recorded; and I judge from its reports that the death rate is low, and the people mostly long-lived. In nine numbers of the *Shaker*, in 1873, twenty-seven deaths are recorded. Of these, Abigail Munson died at Mount Lebanon, aged 101 years, 11 months and 12 days. The ages of the remainder were 97, 93, 88, 86, 82, six above 75, four above 70, 69, 65, 64, 55, 54, 49, 37, 31, and two whose ages were not given.
>
> We look for a testimony against disease [Evans said] and even now I hold that no man who lives as we do has a right to be ill before he is sixty; if he suffer from disease before that, he is in fault. My life has been devoted to introducing among our people a knowledge of true physiological laws; and this knowledge is spreading among all our societies. We are not perfect yet in these respects; but we grow. Formerly fevers were prevalent in our houses, but now we scarcely ever have a case; and the cholera has never yet touched a Shaker village.

The concern for the good health and the well-being of her followers was passed on from Mother Ann to those who immediately succeeded her and thereafter from "lot to lot" of the ministry. She knew from bitter experience of the utter misery of the sick and poor, and it was to create a new and better life that her heavenly visions had led her to a new country.

NOTES

1.   Arthur Redford, *The History of Local Government in Manchester, England,* 3 vols. (New York: Longmans, Green and Co., 1939) 1:79, 2:670–675.

2.   Redford, *History of Local Government,* 1:80.

3.   Ibid., p. 85.

4.   Asa Briggs, *Victorian Cities* (New York: Harper and Row, 1963), p. 112.

5. Ibid.

6. Ibid., pp. 111, 112.

7. Anna White and Leila S. Taylor, *Shakerism Its Meaning and Message* (Columbus, Ohio: Press of Fred J. Heer, 1904) p. 15.

8. White and Taylor, *Shakerism*, pp. 16, 17.

9. *A Summary View of the Millennial Church* (Albany, N.Y.: 1823), p. 5.

10. Ibid., p. 13.

11. For example, a watercolor by the Baroness Hyde de Neuville, painted in 1765 and in the New York Public Library.

12. Henry Clay Blinn, *The Life and Gospel Experiences of Mother Ann Lee* (East Canterbury, N.H., Shaker Society, 1901) p. 109.

13. Charles Nordhoff, *The Communistic Societies of the United States* (New York: Harper & Brothers, 1875). Nordhoff also totals the land owned by the Shakers in 1875 to be 49,335 acres and says this is incomplete because of real estate in distant states, for which he could get no precise returns. If Shaker holdings in mills, wood lots, and "out farms" were added, the figure would certainly well exceed 60,000 acres. One farm in Kentucky owned by the Watervliet, New York, society was 30,000 acres in size and was operated by tenants.

14. Shaker Covenant, recorded at New Lebanon, New York, 1795, unpaged.

15. Millennial Laws, recorded at New Lebanon, New York, August 7, 1781.

16. Ibid., pt 1:5, p. 30.

17. Ibid., p. 31.

18. Nordhoff, *Communistic Societies*, p. 160. Frederick W. Evans, an Englishman by birth, came to America in 1820. He joined the Shakers in 1830 and was in the Elders Order from 1836 to his death in 1893 at the age of eighty-five.

1. WATERVLIET, NEW YORK

Near Albany they settled,
and waited for a while,
Until a mighty shaking
Made all the desert smile.
At length a gentle whisper,
The tidings did convey,
And many flock'd to Mother,
To learn the living way.

Millennial Praises, 1813[1]

Elder John Hocknell, who came to America with Mother Ann when he was well over 70 years of age, told one of his contemporaries that he started out one day from Albany to purchase land for the Shakers to settle on and that during the course of his search his hand was forcibly stretched out in the direction of Watervliet. It remained in that position, resisting all efforts to draw it in, until at the spot afterward called by Believers "Wisdom's Valley," his hand fell to his side and he knew it was the place appointed for the work to begin.[2] Elder John bought the land and settled the small Shaker colony in 1776.

This was the only community settled by the Shakers under Mother Ann's leadership, and it was her first home in America. It became a covenanted society in 1787 after Mother Ann's death in 1784 and after New Lebanon was founded. There has been some confusion over this point; Watervliet was the oldest of the communities, but it was second in order of formal organization. All of the early colonists to America brought with them a dependable knowledge of herbs from their homelands, but they were unfamiliar with many of the plants of the New World. This was true of the Shakers, too, many of whom were not country people. They discovered and sampled the flora of their new habitats in their search for food. They learned also from the Indians, from earlier settlers, and from their own converts who generally were natives and knew what grew locally. Many plants were known or discovered to have medicinal properties, but there are accounts of frightening experiences from those who experimented carelessly with

8

certain plants that were poisonous. Actually many plants later employed by the Shakers were deadly in all but small doses.

At first, wild herbs were gathered and others cultivated for the use of the physicians within the community. Only a very few were sold except for the purpose of purchasing other medicine the Shakers could not or did not prepare. This was a procedure followed by the Watervliet society whose herb business became a brisk and lucrative one even if it were not to grow as large nor last as long as the one at New Lebanon.

There were exact rules vigorously enforced governing the gathering of herbs:

1. One variety only was picked at a time. One herb in the morning, another in the afternoon, but not both at the same time.

2. Tow sheets 15 feet square were used to collect the more fragile plants, and baskets were used for roots.

3. Material was collected "in season" when it was dry and ripe, before the sun had hit it, but after the dew had evaporated. If flowers or seeds were to be gathered, "in season" meant in full flower with leaves fully developed.

4. Tree bark was collected during the spring when the sap was rising and the bark peeled off easily. Bark was generally brought in as needed and orders were permitted to accumulate and then filled as soon as the material was processed.

5. Roots were dug up when the plants had matured and finished growing. They had to be clean, free of all extraneous matter, and then dried.

Although the Shakers of Watervliet did not offer their first printed catalog of medicinal plants and vegetable medicines until 1830, account books exist that record the sale of herbs and extracts to dealers, agents, drug firms, and doctors as early as 1827. In this year Brother Harvey Copley listed 129 herbs and roots, and 7 extracts: *Hyoscyamus niger* (black henbane), *Solanum nigrum* (garden nightshade), *Datura stramonium* (thorn apple or jimson weed which was discovered at Jamestown in 1620), *Taraxacum officianale* (dandelion), *Atropa belladonna* (belladonna), *Conium maculatum* (cicuta, poison hemlock), and *Trifolium pratense* (red clover).[3] Oil of pumpkin seed, oil of juniper, and bottles of sarsaparilla syrup were sold in addition to the extracts, as was moss by the box, metheglin by the gallon, and gallons of peach and rose water.

Several journals from 1827 and 1830, in addition to Brother Harvey's, record the increasing diversity of the business in herbs, roots, barks, and seeds.[4] One kept in 1848 by William Charles Brackett listed orders for the following: motherwort, peppermint, spearmint, thoroughwort, catnip, pennyroyal, thyme, butternut, henbane, saffron, boneset, white root, dandelion, bloodroot, spikenard root, belladonna, elder flower, lobelia, wintergreen, solomon seal, scullcap, comfrey root, blackberry bark and root, sage, wormwood, southernwood, blue cardinal flower, bittersweet, marshmallow, tansy, thyme, hyssop, lemon balm, slipper elm, horehound, foxglove, summer savory, sweet bugle, sweet marjoram, lettuce, sweet fern, rue, ground ivy, chamomile flower, double tansy, dwarf elderroot, liverwort, skunk cabbage root, angelica seed, burdock root, pleurisy root, mugwort, coltsfoot, male fern root, buckthorn berries, bayberry bark, smallage, cranesbill, stramonium, frostwort, sweet flagroot, moldavian balm, goldthread, poppy flowers, poppy seed, poppy capsules, mullin, cleavers, cohosh root, yarrow, thorn apple, mayweed, coriander seed, elecampane, hemlock and oak barks, mandrake root, cranberry bark, caraway seed, indigo root, balm of Gilead buds, hickory ash bark, wild turnip, snakehead, gold seal root, bethroot, crawley root, cicuta, calamus root, sweet basil, rose willow bark, rose leaves, celadine, marygold flowers, garden and wild lettuce, datura, garget, ladies slipper, marsh rosemary root, princess pine, Oak of Jerusalem, avens root, larkspur seed, vervain, yellow dock, life everlasting, white lily root, fever-few, queen of the meadow, horseradish, prickley ash, savin, *Lactuca virosa* (poison lettuce), scabish, maidenhair fern, scurvy grass, bladderroot, John's-wort, and elderberry wine.

The big orders were placed in the fall between October and December and again in the spring from March to the end of May.[5] Smaller orders came in and were filled monthly during the year. Two catalogs had been issued by 1835, and there now was as much business as the Shakers could handle. One hundred and thirty herbs and 25 other items were sold to 22 agents, 10 doctors, and 14 "individual purchasers." A Dr. Mary Entwistle was a regular customer, the only woman doctor listed. Those orders went to Albany, Utica, Hudson, New York City, several hospitals in Philadelphia, and some even further afield. Two hundred pounds of material was shipped to an agent, A. Thompson, in San Francisco, California. The bill was $184.36 and $6.00 for freight. On November 4, 1857, one of the largest orders to be filled from Watervliet went to Butler and McCullock, Liverpool, England. It was comprised of garden seeds and herbs, and the total cost including "freight, carriage and custom house charges" amounted to $175.46. The herbs sent were basil, sage, lavender, rue, mandrake, lobelia, mint, lemon and Moldavian balm, vervain, and poppy seed. The garden seeds were short top scushot radish, scarlet turnip, white winter Spanish onion, black Spanish onion, white flat Dutch turnip, rutabaga, round spinach, Richley spinach, early oxheart cabbage, early York cabbage, cauliflowers, and "purple" eggplant.

Very often the order book also recorded observations about the plant being sent. When filling a large order in 1832 for "Hemlock plant" (*Conium maculatum*), the clerk noted: "Grows high, 6 feet."[6] The brother keeping the book, William C. Brackett, also noted of *Conium maculatum*: "Good to ease pain in open cancer which it does more powerfully than opium. Produces sweat and urine, but this plant is so very poisonous that it is imprudent to eat. It ought not to be administered by those unskilled in medicine." He also gives the "dose of the leaves in powder and extract" and concludes, "great care ought to be taken to distinguish this plant from water hemlock for the latter is a deadly poison." The account books throughout show a constant concern for accuracy and a professional knowledge of the material being handled. On March 22, 1852, "lobelia sent to Geo. Belay, Crown Chambers Red Cross at Liverpool, England. $83.10, lobelia is too dangerous for internal use by unskilled. 408 pounds at $.20; $81.60 and boxes, $1.50."

A much later order went to Hopper and Company, Central Avenue, Covent Garden Market, London, England, on October 20, 1860. "One hundred forty-one and a half pounds of sweet basil; $29.00 including box." The total amount of herbs processed, pressed, and delivered as recorded in this particular account book for 1859 and 1860 was 15,100 pounds. Several books for the previous year indicated a very good season, but only one gives a total. The Trustee who kept the account writes: "Several new plants this year, ozier, boxwood flowers, red cardinal, peony flower and blue violet. End of fiscal year 1859 for this one [meaning himself] 2,825 pounds, a tidy sum."

The Shakers offered the first discount, of 6 percent, in 1832 and thereafter offered discounts of from 25 to 50 percent to the larger and older accounts. But, at the same time, a charge for packing was instituted. By 1847 most bills were discounted, but still this was not allowed consistently, as an entry of November 1846 indicates: "to Hibbard: Vervain, sculcap, comfrey root, elder-flowers, marshmallow root, foxglove, and rue, less 50%, hyssop and lobelia in bulk no %." As in all businesses, there were complaints; material was returned and much bookkeeping had to be adjusted. "November 26, 1846, Cutler returned herbs, roots and extracts: $152.58 with sharp letter."

The Shakers bought products from many of the companies they dealt with in herbs, as many of those sold hardware and other commodities. Among them was R. F. Hibbard Co. A journal entry in October 1846 noted: "Bought from Hibbard and Co., Mollases, rice, raisins, 1 gross ivory buttons, 2 gross brown buttons, 1 dozen fine scissors, 1 gross steel pins, brown shirting, 1 dozen silk handkerchiefs, 1 dozen cotton handkerchiefs, black pepper and hops, quite a lot."

CATALOGS

The Shakers published catalogs, advertising flyers, and broadsides of medicinal plants and vegetable medicines, and herb and garden seeds from 1830 to sometime after 1880. These publications, covering more than 50 years of the industry, give a complete picture of its growth and also of the medical needs of that time. The first of these catalogs was printed in Albany by Packard and Van Benthuysen and dated 1830. Printed on its cover it asked:

> Why send to Europe's bloody shores
> For plants which grow by our own doors?[7]

It was eight pages in length and listed 120 varieties of wild herbs, which, with the roots, barks, berries, and seeds of many plants, brought the total items offered to 142. The common name, botanical name, and the price per pound were given. A note said that the common names in the catalog "are such as are in general use in the cities of New York, Albany and Troy, etc. The Botanical names are from Eaton's *Manual of Botany*, last editions," and further informed that "orders for samples should be forwarded early in the season, as this will give an opportunity for their collection in their proper season. Orders for such indigenous plants or vegetable preparations as are not in the catalogue, will be attended to with care and fidelity."

In addition to listing herbs for sale in bulk, the Shakers offered 12 medicinal preparations, giving the disorders they were supposed to cure, and the price per box or by the dozen.

VEGETABLE BILIOUS PILLS

Prepared from Vegetables only, and contain no unsafe nor deleterious property whatever.

That medicine which goes slowly along the intestines, permitting the nutriment to be taken up by the absorbents, and gently stimulating the intestines, is the one to which we should have recourse in all bilious disorders. That this is the operation of the above Pills, has been abundantly proved by experience. They are a safe and valuable medicine in all bilious complaints, diseased liver, stomach and bowels, loss of appetite, foetid breath, piles and costiveness.

Their use as a cathartic, prevents or removes bilious fevers and inflammations in their forming stages. As an alternative, they can be taken without regard to diet or hindrance of business. Price 33 cents a box, or $3. a dozen.

CEPHALIC PILLS

For periodical and nervous headache, chronic lameness and nervous debility.

These pills are prepared from vegetables only, and contain no mineral, nor narcotic substance whatever. They have been in use in our society for more than thirty years, and from a practical knowledge of their virtues, are confidentially recommended as a safe and efficacious remedy, in the above complaints. Price 50 cents a Box, or $4 a dozen.

DIGESTIVE PILLS

For indigestion or dyspepsia, sourness of the stomach, loss of appetite and liver complaints.

These pills are made of the extracts of our indigenous plants, and have proved very useful in curing the above complaints, even after the failure of various approved remedies. Price 50 cents a Box, or $4 a dozen.

VEGETABLE BALSAM

Prepared from Pterospora and Populus balsamifera. (*Balmsam. Tacmahac.* Balm of Gilead)

This medicine is found by experience to be a safe and excellent remedy for pain in the breast, coughs, and a faintness of the stomach, attended with debility and partial sweats. [No price given.]

CONCENTRATED SYRUP OF LIVERWORT

(*Hepatica triloba*)

A new safe, and valuable medicine for cough spitting of blood and consumption. [No price given.]

COMPOUND CONCENTRATED SYRUP OF SARSAPARILLA

(*Aralia nudicaulis*)[8]

This medicine, taken in doses of an ounce, four or five times a day will fulfil every indication that the boasted panaceas and catholicons can perform; is free from the mercureal poisons such nostrums contain; and is much more safe and efficient as a medicine for cleansing and purifying the blood. [No price given.]

COMPOUND SYRUP OF BLACK COHOSH

(*Acteardcemosa*)

[*Cimicifuga racemosa*]

The black cohosh is one of the most powerful deobstruents and alternatives in the vegetable kingdom; and as such has proved an effectual remedy in rheumatism, gout, chronic lameness; and in scrofulous, glandular and eruptive diseases.

N. B. The formulae and preparation of the above medicine is known and approved by the first physicians in our country. [No price given.]

LAURUS EYE WATER

A valuable remedy for chronic and acute inflammation of the eyes, weakness of sight, and morbid dryness of the eyes.

In inflammation of the eye, the motions of the eye are rendered painful, by an unnatural roughness of the parts; arising from an enlargement of the cutaneous vessels of the eye, or from small granulations on the inner surface of the eye-lids.

This eye-water contains a most delicate vegetable mucilage, which lubricates the eye and renders its motions easy and natural, while its tonic properties restore the vessels of the eye to healthy action.

Price 25 Cents a Bottle, or $2. a Dozen.

OIL OF WORMSEED

The Oil of Wormseed is considered as the most innocent as well as the most powerful vermifuge yet known: If properly managed and genuine (as this is warranted to be) it scarcely ever fails.

N. B. The Oil of Wormseed is a powerful antispasmodic, and may be given with perfect safety and advantage, in most cases of fits and convulsions in children. In such cases, the doses should be one-third larger than the above. [No price given.]

ROSE WATER

Double distilled, very fragrant, equalling the English. [No price given. No description.]

SUPERFINE FLOUR OF SLIPPERY ELM

(Ulmus fulva)

This flour is applicable to a variety of important uses. Experience, and the concurret testimony of the most eminent physicians, prove it to be a valuable medicine, in all inflammations of the mucous membranes; such as colds, influenza, pleurisy, quinsy, dysentary, stranguary [slow and painful urination], and inflammation of the stomach or bowels. It is also a pleasant, salutary medicine and diet in consumption. [No price given.]

POWDER OF WHITEROOT

(Asclepias tuberosa)

Also called Pleurisy root, and Cholic root, from its use in these disorders.

This root is highly recommended by the first physicians in our country, as a safe and valuable remedy in pleurisy, and diseased lungs attended with cough and a dryness of the mucous membranes. Also in fevers, where a sudorific is required; and in diseases of the digestive organs, flatulency, etc. See Barton, Bigelow, Thacher; Rafinesque's Medical Flora, and various Materia Medicas.

N. B. Plain directions for using accompany the medicines; and also various formulae for their preparation. [No price given.]

These preparations were curatives for the basic ailments and were carried in nearly every edition of Watervliet catalogs with additions and improvements sometimes. Seldom, however, were any of the 12 dropped.

Another eight-page catalog was issued in 1833 (printed date) carrying 137 herbs, most of the same pills and compounds, but adding PEACH WATER, "Very valuable as a perfume, and in eruptive diseases."[9] A vegetable cough drop was also included and the manual proclaimed that it was "a safe and approved remedy for pulmonary complaints, asthma and for the prevention of consumption." Extracts of boneset, butternut, cicuta, cow parsnip, dandelion, henbane, hop, lettuce, both garden and wild, nightshade, both garden and deadly, and thorn apple appeared for the first time as did four ointments: elder, marshmallow, savin, and thorn apple.

The market in which the Shakers competed to sell their herbs was flooded with exotic elixirs and extracts, "remedies for every malady," and there were few, if any, controls over them. The situation became so serious that the House of Representatives made a report to the Second Session of the 30th Congress in 1849 which stated that "the increase of impiricism and of patent medicines within the 19th century is an evil over which the friends of science and humanity can never cease to mourne."[10] However, the Shakers built up a confidence in their business in many ways. First of all they emphasized the purity of their herbs, which became well known, and reliance on *Eaton's Manual of Botany* and *Rafinesque's Medical Flora* for identification of the wild herbs must have been most reassuring.

The catalogs became increasingly more useful, for the Shakers included more material and information in each new edition. In the issue for 1837, on page one, 25 properties were listed and then ascribed to the 119 herbs within its eight pages.[11] Terms were stated for the first time, although we have seen that they were noted in the account books. "A discount of twenty-five per cent from the catalog or retail prices, is made to those who purchase 25 dollars worth or more. Payments to be made once or twice a year, generally in the fall."

The 1837 catalog continued to offer the same extracts, but prince's pine, sarsaparilla, wormwood, and "inspissated juices generally double the price of Extracts" were added. The same four ointments were listed, "And any other kinds made to order, and strictly according to the Pharmacopaeia." Taraxacum Blue Pills, having "nearly double the effect upon the liver and its secretions as the common blue pill," was added and also Alterative Syrup for Purifying the Blood, and Tooth Wash and Cosmetic, "a superior article for cleansing and preserving the teeth and gums, and removing diseases of the skin." Cephalic Snuff, "a powerful remedy for pain and dizziness in the head, palsy, etc." was a new item and five double-distilled and fragrant waters were added to rose and peach. They were "cherry, sassafras, peppermint, spearmint, and elder flower."

For the first time the Shakers made an appeal directly to the medical profession in the catalog.

Notice to Physicians—The foregoing compounds are recommended with confidence, as being selected from the best remedial agents that our knowledge of medical science can produce. The names of the active or leading articles of which they are composed accompany the medicines, and also plain directions for using, so that every person who understands the materia medica, can judge of their fitness for fulfilling the indications intended.

The attention of medical men is also particularly invited to the following samples:

BUGLE [BUGLE WEED]. *Lycopus virginicus.*

In spitting of blood and similar diseases, it is, perhaps, the best remedy known. It is a sedative, and tonic, and appears to equalize the circulation of the blood. It is an active ingredient in the comp. syp. of Liverwort, and in cough and diseases of the lungs, should be taken along with that medicine, in cold infusion. The strength of an ounce of the bugle may be taken in one pint of infusion daily.

BUTTON SNAKE-ROOT. *Liatris spicata.*

A powerful diuretic, well adapted to cases of stranguary, in cases of partial paralysis of the secreting vessels. Dose, 1 gill of the decoction made by boiling 1 oz. of the bruised root in 1 pint of water, 15 minutes. Saturated tincture, dose half an ounce.

GOLDEN SEAL. *Hydrastis canadensis.*

Tonic and gently laxative. Promotes the biliary secretions and removes jaundice. Dose of the powder, 10 to 20 grains three times a day. For dyspepsia combine ginger one quarter, and take as above.

GRAVEL PLANT. *Epigaea repens.*

Diuretic. Infuse an ounce in 1 quart of boiling water. Drink freely. Has often cured where the catheter had to be habitually used.

INDIAN HEMP. *Apocynum* and *Rosaemifolium.*

[*Apocynum androsaemifolium*]

Diuretic, tonic and vermifuge. Is a powerful remedy in dropsy. Dose, 1 ounce of the infusion every four hours, or as often as the stomach will bear without nausea. A vinous tincture is also proper, where there is attendant debility. The extract is excellent in dyspepsia. Dose, 5 grains three times a day.

PLEURISY ROOT. *Asclepias tuberosa.*

In all inflammations of the chest this is an invaluable medicine. It is sudorific, anodyne and expectorant. Dose of the powder, 10 to 15 grains. Decoction, 1 oz. Combined with a tea of Skunk Cabbage, it is given in pleurisy with great relief.

SWEET GALE. *Myrica gale.*

Schirrous tumors have been removed by the use of this medicine. The strength of an ounce of it should be taken daily as a tea, and the patient rigidly confined to a diet of water biscuit or crackers. No other food or drink is allowed for 40 or 50 days. A compress of silk, or a mild discutient plaster is to be worn on the tumor. The Myrica seems to promote absorption and keep up the strength.

THIMBLE WEED. *Rudbeckia lacinata.*

In wasting diseases of the kidneys, this plant has proved an excellent medicine. It is diuretic and balsamic. Its properties were first learned by noticing its effects on a sheep that had lost the use of its hind legs. This animal daily dragged itself to this plant, and eat of it, when to the astonishment of all who noticed its situation, it recovered. By shepherds and herdsmen it has since been used in happy effects in stranguary and similar diseases. It is given in decoction, without much nicety as to dose.

There are many other kinds worthy of trial of physicians, such as Bellwort, for curing the poison of rhus, and removing apthous sore throat; Cohosh, for rheumatism; Flea Bane, essential oil in haemorrhage; Ladies' Slipper and Skunk Cabbage, as antispasmodics; Snakehead, in jaundice, etc. etc. For a full description of the properties of these and many other active medicinal plants indigenous to our country, see Rafinesque's *Medical Flora*, Bigelow's and Barton's *Medical Botanies, American Dispensatories*, etc. etc. where it will be found that the use of many of our foreign drugs may be advantageously superseded by our own native remedies.

The catalogs for 1843, 1845, and 1857 carried additional varieties of herbs, several new extracts and pills, but held to the same 25 properties and terms.[12] In 1843, sage, summer savory, sweet marjoram, and thyme were offered for the first time, pulverized "for culinary and other use," and a journal entry for September 1846 recorded that the Hibbard Co. printed 1,000 eight-page medicinal catalogs for the society for $30.00.

In 1845, in addition to 166 herbs, 73 garden seeds were included toward the end of the book. The Shakers included another notice to physicians:

> The foregoing compounds are recommended with confidence, as being selected from the best remedial agents that our knowledge of medical science can produce. The names of the active or leading articles of which they are composed accompany the medicines, and also plain directions for using, so that every person who understands the materia medica can judge of their fitness for fulfilling the indications intended.

Again, the Shakers were well aware of the fiercely competitive patent medicine industry. They remained convinced of the purity of what they offered and did not hesitate to promote it.

The Shakers offered the same items for sale in the 1847 catalog that they had in preceding years, but there were advertisements for four different products sold by R. F. Hibbard and Company, 98 John Street, New York, on the last two pages, and on the back cover the names of 15 agents were listed; distributors in New York City, Albany, Utica, and Troy, and agents in the cities of Syracuse, Rochester, Buffalo, Watertown, Ogdensburg, and Rome were also included. This is an interesting publication, as it is a real selling piece for the R. F. Hibbard Co., who nevertheless indicate that the herbal materials they use in the four medicines offered are "Raised, Prepared and put up in the most careful manner by the United Society of Shakers, Watervliet." The medicines advertised under the Hibbard label were: Wild Cherry Bitters, Carminative Salve, Vegetable Family Pills, and Circassian Balm.

Compound concentrated syrup of sarsaparilla was made and sold in the Watervliet society even before the Shakers listed it in the catalogs. The product was described in one or two sentences, and usually priced at $1.00 a bottle, $9.00 a dozen, until 1847, when the Shakers included a paragraph extolling its merits and successes. As a skillful example of selling appeal it is included here:

COMPOUND CONCENTRATED SYRUP OF SARSAPARILLA
Price 75 cents a bottle.

We are aware that the public are not only burdened, but in many instances have been imposed upon, with the almost endless variety of compound Medicines, whose virtues only exist in their boasted name.

But the Compound Syrup of Sarsaparilla having been used with peculiar success in our community for many years, as a restorative, laxative, tonic, diuretic, and alternative, we are able to present to the public a medicine possessing real merit, and one which has been used with universal success in cases of Chronic, Inflammation of the digestive organs, Saltrheum, Diarrhoea, Cutaneous Eruptions, Acute and Chronic Rheumatism, Dropsy, Dyspepsia, Scrofula, Erysipelas, Headaches of every kind,

General Debility, Mercurial Diseases, and all diseases arising from an impure state of the Blood, and in the first stages of the consumption.

This medicine is also a Preventive against diseases, as it strengthens and cleanses the system, and has given general satisfaction to those who have used it in the cure of the above and many other complaints; and from the observation of competent medical judges, not of our community, it is found to be fully equal to any medical preparation offered to the public for the Syphillis.

It is not our aim to rate a thing above or below its merits, or to rival or monopolize in the presentment of this medicine. But as we desire the happiness of our fellow mortals, we solicit the afflicted to prove for themselves the trust of the above.

The 1850 catalog differed from earlier ones in that 18 new herbs and their properties were listed bringing the total to 43.[13] Again the printer was Charles Van Benthuysen. One hundred and eighty-six herbs were listed, 27 extracts, four ointments, five pulverized herbs for cooking, and composition powders. Also, the Shakers offered the same 73 garden seeds, and one snuff.

The Shakers printed and distributed many flyers and broadsides during the years when the catalogs were published. These advertised medicines for the relief of nervous headaches, chronic lameness, piles, dimness of vision, inflammation of the eyes and morbid weakness of sight, and medicines for coughs and consumption. They also made broadsides relative to garden seeds, brooms, brushes, and other products.

Chauncey Miller issued the 1860 catalog which is one of the most comprehensive and interesting in this category of Shaker literature.[14] He greatly enlarged it, in comparison to earlier catalogs, in content and information; it was 22 pages in length. Trustee Miller entitled the new catalog "Catalogue of MEDICINAL PLANTS, Barks, Roots, Seeds and Flowers, with their therapeutic qualities and botanical names, also, PURE VEGETABLE EXTRACTS, and Shaker Garden Seeds, Raised, prepared, and put up in the most careful manner, by the UNITED SOCIETY OF SHAKERS, Watervliet, (near Albany) N.Y." All orders were to be directed to Chauncey Miller, Shaker Village (Albany Post Office), New York. This was the first new catalog to be printed in ten years as was referred to in a statement which preceded the list of 44 properties of the herbs he offered for sale. This was one more than in previous years, the new one being "Antlithlic (A-lith) which was to be used to prevent the formation of calculus matter."

TO OUR PATRONS

In presenting a new edition of our Catalogue, we embrace the opportunity to inform the public that we have made, and are now making, heavy expenditures in buildings, machinery, and very complete accommodations and fixtures for drying and preparing the various articles in the following Catalogue, and hope to be able, in answer to our rapidly increasing calls, to supply articles of superior excellence with the utmost promptitude.

Our society having been actively engaged in the business over thirty years, we claim the advantage of experience; and the rapidly increasing demands for "SHAKER HERBS" and botanic preparations—notwithstanding the influence and supplies from rival establishments—is a satisfactory evidence of public approval and esteem.

The following list comprises nearly *the whole vegetable Materia Medica* now in use; and physicians and druggists may depend on receiving the GENUINE ARTICLES according to their order. For the generic and specific names, we have relied on Gray's *Botany of the Northern United States*—adopting those common names best known among druggists, herbalists and botanic physicians. Gray's, we believe, is now considered the standard.

Any of the following Herbs, Roots, Seeds, Barks, Extracts, or Botanic preparations sold in bulk at satisfactory prices, or neatly prepared in assorted packages for the convenience of purchasers.

We pledge ourselves to furnish articles of superior excellency and are determined not to be surpassed in the *quality* or neatness of our preparations.

Orders attended to at all seasons. Parties ordering will please state whether they wish articles in bulk or otherwise, and the size packages they would prefer.

The catalog listed 292 herbs, 25 extracts, 73 garden seeds, and for the first time a list of 168 synonyms by which the herbs were commonly known. The extracts were boneset, burdock, butternut, cicuta, clover (red), dandelion, dock (yellow), fleabane, foxglove, gentian, henbane, horehound, hop, lettuce (garden), lobelia, mandrake, nightshade (deadly), poke, poppy, princess pine, sarsaparilla, savin, thorn apple, tomato, and wormwood. They were introduced by this statement signed by Chauncey Miller:

PURE VEGETABLE EXTRACTS

It is a matter of eminent importance to the interested and benevolent physician, to be able to calculate with certainty, on the effect of any drug or medicine he may administer. This he cannot do, unless he be able to judge of its purity, condition, and carefulness of preparation. Perhaps no class of medicines present so many difficulties, and certainly none which have given such universal dissatisfaction on this point, as vegetable extracts; and some of our best physicians have nearly abandoned their use on this account.

This is not surprising, when we consider the rude and imperfect means generally employed for evaporating, and the want of suitable knowledge and carefulness in the whole process of manufacture. Indeed, it requires much experience and consummate skill, in addition to the most perfect apparatus, to produce extracts that will be uniform and certain in their effects,—as much depends on the freshness of the vegetable operated upon, maturity, season of collection, and influence of climate.

To remedy the difficulties complained of, and furnish the profession with the article they so earnestly requested of us—*pure and reliable extracts*—we have directed our attention to this end, and spared no expense to procure the best information and conveniences for the purpose. Our former experience and observations, of thirty years, have been of value; and the possession of large botanic gardens gives us important advantages in the collection and freshness of the vegetables.

Having built a new laboratory, and furnished it with very complete fixtures for the various manipulations, among which is a vacuum pan for evaporation, embracing the late improvements of Benson and Day, and others peculiarly our own, built expressly for the purpose, we have succeeded in producing extracts which meet the approval of the faculty, from whom we are receiving very flattering encomiums of praise.

Thankful for past favors, and soliciting a continuance of the same, we subscribe in behalf of the Society,

Chauncey Miller.

This was the last of the complete formal catalogs issued by the society.

In 1860 Chauncey Miller also began to merchandise what farmers considered "the greatest acquisition to our small fruits." It was "The Great Austin Shaker Seedling Strawberry, The Largest Strawberry in the World," and the *Gardener's Monthly* of September 1, 1860, carried a testimonial signed by three men who said that they had visited Watervliet, and found the Austin strawberry growing "in the most common way, in masses and not in hills, without any particular care. . . . We found the fruit to average nearly twice as large as any now in cultivation."

The Austin strawberry had been developed by Brother Austin in 1855, but it was Chauncey Miller who promoted it. In 1859, 8,984 plants were given away to introduce it and the next year $1,979.24 was realized from its sales. The Albany newspaper reported this new variety in 1860 and announced that "it is very prolific and the fruit is the largest we have ever seen, some of the berries measuring five inches. It is also rich and luscious, being as remarkable for flavor as for size and thrift." In 1863 "the sum total of the Austin strawberry, plants and fruits, sold at different prices amounted to $3,722.37.," according to Brother Chauncey's notes, and he added, "Doctors use it for syrup in medicine."[15]

Wines were made at Watervliet and the Northern Muscadine grape was raised and widely advertised for "all interested in the growing of the grape either for wine or for the table." A recipe for making fruit wines "such as cherry, grape, plum, elderberry and blackberry for medicinal purposes or otherwise" appeared at the end of an account book and seemed to be a simple operation:[16]

> To each gallon of fruit allow 2 gallons boiling water poured on the fruit in a large pan. Let stand for one week (cover with muslin cloth) stirring every day. Then strain once through a sieve, then through muslin. Measure and add 3 lbs. sugar to each gallon of liquid and if partial ½ lb. whole ginger bruised. Boil with the bruised ginger for 20 minutes. When made in large quantities for sale, prepare in vats and increase quantities of material.

Gradually the community at Watervliet declined, and its herb and medicine business gave way to those of the commercial enterprises of the world. In 1938 the one remaining family of the oldest community of Shakers gave up the hopeless struggle. The "wilderness tract" that was John Hocknell's gift to the Believers, the fulfillment of Mother Ann's visions, the answer to the prayers of the earliest Shakers for a home of their own, passed into other hands. Margaret Melcher says: "The last survivors turned their backs sorrowfully on the buildings and the grounds they had known so well and so long, and went to Mt. Lebanon."[17] There were only three of them left, all women. The occasion for their departure was the death of Sister Anna Case, an outstanding personality who had been promised that she should live her life out at Watervliet. The West family lot had been sold to farmers years before. The Church family had been bought by the county of Albany in 1828 to found a home for the poor and infirm—the Ann Lee Home. (The Church family was the founding unit of any Shaker community; the West, East, Second, etc., families were added later.)

NOTES

1. *Millennial Praises* (Hancock, Mass.: 1813). This was the first hymnbook the Shakers published exclusively for themselves. Library at Shaker Community, Inc., Hancock, Massachusetts.

2. Anna White and Leila S. Taylor, *Shakerism Its Message and Meaning* (Columbus, Ohio: Press of J. Heer, 1904), p. 82.

3. Journal, Brother Harvey Copley, 1830, Cleveland, Western Reserve Historical Society.

4. Herb journals, 1830–1848, by William Charles Brackett, Cleveland, Western Reserve Historical Society.

5. Herb catalog issued by Watervliet Society, 1835, Cleveland, Western Reserve Historical Society.

6. Account book kept by Shakers at Watervliet, 1832, Cleveland, Western Reserve Historical Society.

7. Catalog of medicinal plants and vegetable medicines, 1830, Cleveland, Western Reserve Historical Society.

8. The Shakers used the variety *Aralia nudicaulis* as sarsaparilla, rather than *Similax officinalis,* the true sarsaparilla of South America.

9. Catalog of medicinal plants and vegetable medicines, 1833, Cleveland, Western Reserve Historical Society.

10. Margaret B. Keig, *Green Medicine* (Chicago: Apollo, 1971), p. 93.

11. Catalog of medicinal plants and vegetable medicines, 1837, Cleveland, Western Reserve Historical Society.

12. Three herb catalogs, 1843, 1845, 1847, Cleveland, Western Reserve Historical Society.

13. Catalog of herbs, medicinal plants, and vegetable medicines, 1850, Cleveland, Western Reserve Historical Society.

14. Catalog of medicinal plants, barks, roots, seeds, and flowers, 1860, Cleveland, Western Reserve Historical Society.

15. Daybook and letter of Chauncey Miller, 1863, Cleveland, Western Reserve Historical Society.

16. Account book with wine recipe, 1850, Cleveland, Western Reserve Historical Society.

17. Margaret F. Melcher, *The Shaker Adventure* (Cleveland: The Press of Case Western Reserve University, 1968), p. 262.

2. GROVELAND, NEW YORK

The Shakers established a small community in 1826 on Sodus Bay.[1] The land was sold ten years later when a canal terminus was projected there, and the Shakers moved to Groveland, New York. Then in 1892 this community of about 200 members, in two families, was sold, and the Shakers moved to Watervliet.

Although the Shakers apparently did not offer herbs for sale from Groveland, a little book, "Receipts of Materia Medica, written at Groveland, May 1842," contains several herbal remedies.[2] Five of the recipes containing 26 different herbs are given here.

PURIFYING TEA

TAKE

1 tablespoon Spanish pins [pines]	2 tablespoons Princes pine
2 tablespoons Bittersweet	2 tablespoons Mountain lettuce
2 tablespoons Green Ozier bark	2 tablespoons Sarsaparilla
2 tablespoons Black Birch bark	½ tablespoon Saffron. Pulv. &
3 tablespoons Black Cohosh	Mix.

1 lb. to be in a gallon of water and boiled down to two quarts. Strain and add three lbs. of sugar and one pint Spirits. This medicine purifies the blood and excites the secretions, in general, it should be taken for a considerable time as much as the stomach will bear. A dose of Billious pills should be taken once or twice a week while taking this syrup.

PECTORAL SYRRUP

TAKE

2 tablespoons Wa-a-hoo bark   1 tablespoon Princes pine
1 tablespoon Boneset   1 tablespoon Bittersweet bark
1 tablespoon Waterpepper   1 tablespoon Black Cohosh

To be boiled in an iron kettle with soft water, when the strength is out, to be strained off then boiled down to the consistency of thin Molasses, to which add one fourth West India Molasses. This should be scalded an hour over a slow fire and it is fit for use. Dose a tablespoon full to be taken three or four times a day before eating. To be used in consumption, Coughs, affections of the liver, spleen, etc.

INDIAN CONSUMPTIVE SYRRUP

TAKE

4 ounces Wild Turnip   1 ounce Rum
1 ounce Skunk Cabbage seed   1 ounce Honey
1 ounce White root

To be put in a stone jug unstopped and boiled in a kettle of water for an hour. Dose ¼ of a wine glass three or four times a day before eating.

COUGH DROPS
---

2 ounces Liquorice root   1 ounce Skunk Cabbage
1 ounce Blood root   1 ounce Elecampane
1 ounce Senica Snake root   1 ounce Crawley root

Infuse in a quart of soft water until the strength is extracted, strain, then add two ounces of Tint. Lobelia two ounces Tinct. Bloodroot and four ounces Loaf Sugar. Strain and it is fit for use. Dose a teaspoon full thrice or four times a day half an hour before eating.

SYRRUP FOR PAIN IN THE STOMACH AND SIDE

T A K E

4 ounces White root   ¼ ounce Angelica seed
4 ounces Skunk Cabbage   ¼ ounce Coriander
2 ounces Boneset   ½ ounce Ginger
2 ounces Prickley Ash bark

To be put in a stone jug unstopped and boild in a kettle of water for an hour. Dose ¼ of a wine glass three or four times a day before eating. From two to three pills should be taken in 24 hours while using this syrrup composed of equal parts of Extracts of Butternut and Dandelion worked in White root, Ipecac and ginger of equal parts.

The little book carried other remedies which used the following herbs:

Black alder, avens root, lemon balm, sweet basil, borage, buckthorn, catnip, caraway seed, chamomile, cicuta, cleavers, fleabane, white hellebore, liverwort, marshmallow, rue, saffron, squawroot, thyme, wintergreen, wormwood.

A second book, dated 1858–1859 and kept by Susan Love, is called *The Cheap Family Dyer, containing a full and complete list of receipts for making various colors and dyes used in this country for coloring yarn or cloth.*[3] Some of the ingredients are yellow oak bark, indigo, hemlock bark, swamp maple bark, nutgalls, butternuts, peachwood, and brazilwood.

There is no known printed catalog from this society.

NOTES

1.   Anna White and Leila S. Taylor, *Shakerism Its Message and Meaning* (Columbus, Ohio: Press of Fred J. Heer, 1904), p. 155.

2.   ''Receipts of Materia Medica written at Groveland, May 1842,'' Cleveland, Western Reserve Historical Society.

3.   *The Cheap Family Dyer,* 1858–1859, Cleveland, Western Reserve Historical Society.

3. NEW LEBANON, NEW YORK (1787–1860)

MT. LEBANON, NEW YORK (1861–1947)

Years before any written acknowledgment, it was known that the Shaker brothers engaged in the business of preparing and selling herbs "to the world." The first actual mention of the activity, however, was in a diary kept by "Jethro" between 1789 and 1812.[1]

The Great House was built. The Church began to gather last year—gardens plowed—houses built—Bake house built. . . . Feb. 1809 decide to reprint Believers Publication—The Testimony of Christ 2nd Appearance. Sept. 1810 we have built a new hog pen this season. . . . Apr. 28, 1811 a company of Negroes to Calvin's [Wells] after Betty's daughters but fail of seeing them. . . . June 1812. A violent storm did much damage in herb garden. 283 pains of glass broken in the 1st family's buildings.

The herb business soon was to equal another enterprise of the New Lebanon society, growing crops for garden seeds. This business grew sufficiently large and became so well known that the Shakers of New Lebanon made a pact with their brethren in Watervliet, New York, and Hancock, Massachusetts:[2]

AN ANCIENT WITNESS

We, the undersigned, having for sometime past felt a concern, lest there should come loss upon the joint interest, and dishonor upon the gospel, by purchasing seeds of the world, and mixing them with ours for sale; and having duly considered the matter, we are confident that it is best to leave off the practice, and we do hereby covenant and agree that we will not, hereafter, put up, or sell, any seeds to the world which are not raised among believers (excepting melon seeds).

New Lebanon, April 13, 1819.

DEACONS

Richard Spier	Stephen Munson
Israel Hammond	Jonathan Wood
Daniel Goodrich	John Wright
Hancock, N.H. [Mass.]	Hancock, N.H. [Mass.]

24

Eventually other societies would sign the pact. The Shakers felt that such an agreement was necessary to guarantee and maintain the quality of their seeds and herbs and to facilitate improving their methods in a time when the demand for pure and unadulterated products had increased greatly. They resolved this problem by planting "physic gardens," rather than relying completely on wild herbs as a source. In several years the gardens were made so productive that the Shakers grew a surplus that could be marketed.

All of this prosperity had been gained only after the Shakers had first suffered through lean times. They still remembered 1788 when the brethren in Watervliet had nearly starved. It was a year of famine in the region around Lake George, New York. The principal food was rice and milk, with an occasional fish from the Hudson River even though they tried to plant vegetables, grain, and hay. "We were so weak we could not have run twenty rods, but we could work!" For breakfast and supper they had small bowls of porridge; for dinner, "a bit of cake about 2½ inches square which Aaron Wood cut up and gave to us." On Sundays they sometimes omitted dinner, as that was not a working day. In the fall when the crops began to ripen and potatoes were eatable they lived better.[3]

Other communities had lived through lean days, too. When Rebecca Clark came to live at Hancock in 1791, 14 slept in one room, and she wrote about their meals: "For breakfast and supper we lived mostly upon bean porridge and water porridge. Monday morning we had a little weak tea and once in a while a small piece of cheese. Wheat bread was very scarce; and when we had butter it was spread on our rye and Indian meal bread before we came to the table. Our dinners were generally boiled. Once in a while we had a little milk, but this was a great rarity. . . ."[4]

At New Lebanon, too, the diet was scant for a time. The brethren there often had only broth and bread to eat. Bread was "allowanced" for three years; a small piece was placed by each one's dish, with a piece of pie on special occasions. After a while potatoes and bean porridge became the staple, and a typical breakfast consisted of bread, sometimes a little butter, fried potatoes, fried gammon (a kind of bacon), and sage, celandine, or root tea. For coffee the root of water avens was used, or burnt rye, or barley. Then, pork, beef, mutton, eggs, turnips, and cabbage appeared about 1800.

The hungry days were easier to bear than repeated assaults by hostile mobs. An account of events early in the day of September 2, 1783, the year the New Lebanon community was being established, is reported by Rachel Spencer and is typical of the abuse the Shakers suffered for their unusual religious beliefs:

I was very early in the morning employed in the kitchen, with a number of the sisters, in preparing breakfast and putting the house in order; and we had nearly finished our work when the mob came. The house was at that time clean and decent, and all was still and quiet, when suddenly we were beset on every side by a large gang of unprincipled wretches in mob array. The principal rooms below were nearly filled with the brethren and sisters, who endeavored to keep the mob out; but regardless of remonstances or entreaties, they

rushed in like furious tigers. A number of them burst into the kitchen and furiously as-
saulted the sisters who were collected there. We strove with all our strength to keep them
back, but in vain. They seized and hurled us out of doors, one after another, with the utmost
violence. I was thrown out and beaten so that my flesh was black and blue in spots all over
me. Many others of the brethren and sisters shared the same fate. Several doors were broken
to pieces; the ceiled partition of the little room where Mother had retired, was torn down flat
to the floor; and she was hauled out and thrown into the carriage without any ceremony.
Two of the young sisters followed her and sprung into the carriage.[5]

More violence followed but the resilient Shakers never gave up and finally their
persistence and their hard work brought them just rewards. Outsiders were hostile to
the Shakers because they refused to bear arms, often broke up families when they
recruited new members, and because they upheld celibacy. However, people outside of
the sect began to feel that the Shakers were good and generous neighbors after all and
conscientious businessmen.

The Shakers had come to this country when the wilderness seemed inexhaustible
and when large sites for potential farming operations were easily available. Therefore,
the Shakers would not start a community unless an adequate supply of pure water was
found nearby and there were sufficient woodlands to provide timber for building dwellings and shops. The virgin forest also produced vast amounts of botanical herbs. These
natural resources, combined with wise planning and the ability to attract converts, many
of whom had good properties which they donated to the society, enabled the leaders
to build up profitable farms on rich and productive land. The Shakers estimated that it
cost $100.00 to clear each acre, if hired hands were needed, although the land was
acquired for very little in the early days.

New Lebanon was no exception, and many travelers have given us accounts of this
dramatically placed village whose spiritual name was appropriately "Holy Mount."
Benjamin Silliman in the autumn of 1819 traveled from Hartford, Connecticut, to
Quebec, Canada, and passed through New Lebanon. He recorded that:

. . . we were indeed not clear of the mountain, before we found ourselves in the midst of
their singular community. Their buildings are thickly planted, along a street of a mile in
length. All of them are comfortable and a considerable proportion are large. They are, almost
without an exception, painted of an ochre yellow, and, although plain, they make a handsome appearance. The utmost neatness is conspicuous in their fields, gardens, court yards,
out houses, and in the very road; not a weed, not a spot of filth, or any nuisance is suffered to
exist. Their wood is cut and piled, in the most exact order; their fences are perfect; even their
stone walls are constructed with great regularity, and of materials so massy [sic], and so
well arranged, that unless overthrown by force, they may stand for centuries; instead of
wooden posts for their gates, they have pillars of stone of one solid piece, and every thing
bears the impress of labour, vigilance and skill, with such a share of taste, as is consistent
with the austerities of their sect. Their orchards are beautiful, and probably no part of our
country presents finer examples of agricultural excellence. They are said to possess nearly
three thousand acres of land, in this vicinity. Such neatness and order I have not seen any
where, on so large a scale, except in Holland, where the very necessities of existence impose
order and neatness upon the whole population; but here it is voluntary.[6]

Charles Nordhoff writing about Lebanon when he visited it in 1874 said:

Mount Lebanon lies beautifully among the hills of Berkshire, two and a half miles from
Lebanon Springs, and seven miles from Pittsfield. The settlement is admirably placed on the
hillside to which it clings, securing it good drainage, abundant water, sunshine, and the
easy command of water-power. Whoever selected the spot had an excellent eye for beauty
and utility in a country site. The views are lovely, broad, and varied; the air is pure and

bracing; and in short, a company of people desiring to seclude themselves from the world could hardly have chosen a more delightful spot.[7]

Charles Dickens, writing a few years before this, had visited the Village in 1842 and found everything about it "grim, grim, grim," but said:

> They are good farmers, and all their produce is eagerly purchased and highly esteemed. "Shaker seeds," "Shaker herbs," and "Shaker distilled waters" are commonly announced for sale in the shops of towns and cities. They are good breeders of cattle and are kind and merciful to the brute creation. Consequently Shaker beasts seldom fail to find a ready market.[8]

Another writer, Evert A. Duyckinck, editor of *The Literary World*, visited the Shakers at Lebanon and wrote:

> It was a cool and bright Sunday morning among the hills of the Taconic, as we rode across the Hancock mountain, from Pittsfield to the Shaker settlement of that name. Heavy summer rains on the previous day had refreshed the vegetation and hardened the usually excellent roads of the region. The cleanly shaved edges of the upland meadows, as they touched the woodland, gave token of the approach to the Hancock Village, for the Shakers are excellent farmers and their fields are nicely groomed. By neat fences and through avenues of shady roadside trees, you approach the variegated houses, red and yellow, rising many stories in height and not unpicturesquely gathered together at regular angles. There is the great circular stone barn, with the huge haymow in the centre, and the numerous stalls where the cattle, each with head toward the great king post, are fed through the cold months of winter. A stone pathway on which you pass a simple dial plate, leads between two groups of houses. Near by, on the opposite side of the road, is the religious house where the services are held of the several families. We found it closed, the brethren, it was said, being off to a meeting on the mountain.
> . . . .Three miles farther on is the scattered settlement at Lebanon. Descending upon it from a hill side, groups of carriages were drawn up at the great meeting house, stage coaches, light wagons, rockaways and others of the neighboring watering place. With the light airy building before them shining with its rounded tin roof in the pure atmosphere, the whole had the gay appearance, with the bustle of the grooms and horses, of a fair or race course.[9]

But Mr. Duyckinck also attended the religious meeting and unkindly criticized "the preacher, a grim, spectral, cold-eyed piece of human timber, boarded up to the ears in a long unwrinckled drab coat." He found the ceremony "ludicrous," the dancing "monotonous," the older people "pitiable," and "but for the young and the few beautiful persons in the company, the exhibition was profoundly melancholy."

> . . . The Shakers form a community of associated industry where, at least, the first rude wants of life—pure air, cleanliness, and a sufficiency of food are provided for. Their homes are, to this extent, a refuge for the harassed and destitute. Many disappointed broken down men turn in thither from the buffets of the world and the irresolution of their uncontrolled passions—a safe haven and anchorage for the wreck of a troubled life. The more obvious moralities of life seem to be observed by them with faithfulness. They are honest, sober and industrious. There is a thoroughness of labor in many of their works which commands respect. Slovenly workmanship is a gross practical lie running through the world. The Shakers, limited in the extent of their manufactures, offer the best of the kind. The covers of their boxes fit, their brooms sweep, their packets of herbs are approved by the physicians, the products of their farms and dairies are sound and wholesome. This, with the fair and exact culture of their land, is a virtue before the world. Dealing simply with nature in their

relations as agriculturists, in spite of constraint and their barren culture, beauty waits upon them. Their brimming water fountains by the roadside, for man and beast, the cleanliness and order of their farmyards and meadows, a certain grandeur (of a limited character) in their huge dwellings, the mountain simplicity of their retirement, are tributes to the spirit of Art.[10]

On this lovely mountainside the largest, the most prosperous, and most influential of all the Shaker communities, if not the longest lived, was settled and considered in complete "order" by 1798. The early days of hunger and persecution were behind the Shakers, although there were still harassment and ridicule ahead.

Journals, daybooks, diaries, and printed catalogs give a picture of the enormous botanical medicine business the New Lebanon Shakers developed. The sisters made numerous and continuous excursions into the woods, swamps, and fields to gather thousands of pounds of wild herbs. Later, "botanic gardens" were begun in which transplanted wild herbs and acres of herbs from seed were grown within the village for easier harvest.

"A Journal of Domestic events and transactions; In a brief and conclusive form; Commenced January 1st, 1843; Kept by The Deaconesses, Church 2nd Order" was written for 21 years, until June 23, 1864. The activities of one family in supplying and preparing herbs were recorded:

> June 14th. George C. James L. Samuel W. go after meddow [sic] sweet, have good luck.
> June 27th. This morning a company of sisters start for Richmond swamp to gather tea. [Meadowsweet tea is steeplebush; *Spiraea tomentosa,* an astringent tonic in diarrhea] George L. starts with the one horse waggon and James Gilbert takes the covered waggon. We start from home immediately after breakfast and arrived at 7 o'clock in the evening with a good load of meadow sweet tea. June 30th. Sisters go again after tea and have good luck. Get a meal of strawberrys for supper this is the first we have this year.
> July 1st. This morning Abigail S. Lea, Phebe S. Elinor B. and James start on the mountain after Crosswort. [Crosswort is boneset; *Eupatorium perfoliatum;* this and meadowsweet were gathered in enormous quantities.] July 4th. Have pease for dinner, the first time. James L. prepares tea to the dry house. July 6th. Go after Elderflowers. Hannah A. and I go a strawburying [sic], got a few, too. July 7. Their [sic] are 9 start to the sage place to cut sage, done about noon. . . . July 19th, Finishing preparing and pressing tea. July 20th. Go to empty the press and clean up. Have 307 lbs. of tea.[11]

This is a lot of tea, picked in a month.

It is tempting to quote voluminously from the deaconess's entries, and they shall be referred to again, but the fact remains that from many such records we know this was a large-scale operation, and it is not surprising that less than ten years later an article appeared in the *American Journal of Pharmacy* describing a visit to the Shakers. The writer tells about his tour of the gardens, the "arrangements for drying and packing herbs and for making extracts," and says that during the short visit a very hearty welcome was extended by "chief Trustee, Edward Fowler" whom he quotes regarding the history of the business:

> It is about fifty years since our Society first originated as a trade in this country and business of cultivating and preparing medicinal plants for the supply and convenience of apothecaries and druggists, and for about twenty years conducted it on a limited scale. Some thirty years since Drs. E. Harlow and G. K. Lawrence, of our Society, the latter an excellent botanist, gave their attention to the business, and induced a more systematic arrangement, and scientific manner of conducting it, especially as to the seasons for collection, varieties, and method of preparation. Since their time, the business has rapidly in-

creased, and especially so within the last ten years. We believe the quantity of botanical remedies used in this country, particularly of indigenous plants, has doubled in less than that time.

There are now probably occupied as physic gardens in the different branches of our Society, nearly two hundred acres, of which about fifty are at our village. [This number includes the settlements of Shakers in New England, Kentucky, Ohio, and New York.] As we find a variety of soils are necessary to the perfect production of the different plants, we have taken advantage of our farms and distributed our gardens accordingly. Hyoscyamus, belladonna, tarazacum, aconite, poppies, lettuce, sage, summer savory, marjorum, dock, burdock, valerian, and horehound, occupy a large portion of the ground; and about fifty minor varieties are cultivated in addition, as rue, borage, carduus (Benedictus), hyssop, marsh-mallow, feverfew, pennyroyal, etc. Of indiginous plants we collect about two hundred varieties, and purchase from the South, and West, and from Europe, some thirty or forty others, many of which are not recognized in the Pharmacopoeia, or the dispensatories, but which are called for in domestic practice and abundantly used.[12]

The article continues to describe the herb house, storage rooms, and methods of drying various types of plant material before they were removed for pressing. The writer, obviously knowledgeable about these procedures, says: "Some plants which are very succulent or viscid, and which are difficult to properly cure, as conium, hyoscyamus, and garden celandine are desiccated in a drying room, constructed for the purpose where a temperature of about 115° Fahr. is maintained. Most of the roots are dried in this way, after being sliced." He approved of the double presses, each of which could press one hundred pounds daily and were in constant operation. Then he discusses the vacuum apparatus in the evaporating room and whether the Shakers or the Tilden Company of New Lebanon had it first.

In our last communication we stated, what we believe to be true, that the "Society" had adopted the vacuum pan in their manufacture to compete with their neighbors Messrs. Tilden, who we believe, preceded them in its employment, not intending to infer that they would not have adopted it, had the idea been suggested in any other way, as appears to have been understood by Mr. Fowler and his friends, who feel themselves called upon to "deny the insinuation that *no other* motive was sufficient to induce the improvement; as not a member of our community had the least knowledge that medical extracts had ever been manufactured in America by that process at the time our apparatus was built. We know that the imported extracts were generally esteemed as superior to many if not all the American, and feeling desirous of having *our* articles *right* we adopted the vacuum pan as a necessary item by the recommendation of several members of the New York College of Pharmacy, whom we consulted on the occasion."

The article goes on to say:

Mr. Fowler informs us that the amount of extracts manufactured at their establishment annually was about six or eight thousand pounds, but since their improvements in apparatus and manipulations, this amount has been greatly increased, and the quality improved. Extract of tarazacum [dandelion] is in the greatest demand, their product in this article amounting the past year to 3700 pounds. Conium, hyoseyamus [henbane], and belladonna class next. They do not cultivate conium [poison hemlock], but collect that of spontaneous [wild] growth, believing it to be more active. Belladonna and hyseyamus, especially the latter, require a rich deep soil and abundance of strong animal manure. They find henbane a very precarious crop, as when young it is almost impossible to keep it from being destroyed by insects, and some years they have entirely lost it, notwithstanding their best endeavors to protect it. The biennial variety of henbane is alone cultivated, and when not destroyed by insects, etc., has under the most favorable circumstances yielded at the rate of 1300 pounds of good extract from an acre of plants.

The article also indicated that the Shakers had competition. A circular was issued in 1849 by the Tilden Company which offered "Shaker Garden Seeds" on its front page with its own list of roots, herbs, extracts, barks, ointments, and black and blue writing ink.[13] Elam Tilden founded the company in 1824 and it was once hailed as the oldest pharmaceutical house in the nation. In a newspaper article written in 1969, six years after the company closed its doors, it was noted that "Industrious, intelligent Elam Tilden discovered that the many beneficial poultices and brews made by the herb-growing Shakers on Mount Lebanon were truly beneficial to man, so he undertook their manufacture and sale."[14]

In 1815, some unknown Shaker wrote in a small leather-bound notebook seventy medical recipes[15] and "cures" for the "Nurse Shop" for the Church family at New Lebanon: "The Strengthening Sirrups [sic] and Cordials; the Elixirs; the Cleansing Bitters; concoctions for The Nerves' Consumption, for The Salt Rume, for The Rumatism, for The Gravel, For the Lungs, For Faintness, For the Use of the blue Violet Root; To Make Clove Water, To Make Liquid Landemon; A Beer to Cleanse the Blood." These brews, with directions for making the many kinds of wines that presumably rendered the dose more palatable, were the forerunners of the dozens of preparations put out commercially by the Medical Department. This notebook for the infirmary was followed by printed catalogs, some of which carried recipes for medicines.

The society issued its first dated catalog in 1836.[16] It offered medicinal plants and vegetable medicines. One hundred sixty-four herbs were listed as well as 12 extracts, 4 ointments, 7 double-distilled and fragrant waters and 4 pills, a cough drop and 2 cough syrups, the compound concentrated syrup of sarsaparilla, offered by all the Shaker medical departments, a syrup of black cohosh for rheumatism and gout, a blood purifier, a "tooth wash and cosmetic," and "Laurus Eye Water."

The 1837 catalog was similar in many ways to that distributed in the previous year and identical to the one the Watervliet Shakers had issued the same year.[17] In 1838 the Shakers of New Lebanon added a few more herbs, bringing the list to 170.[18] One hundred seventy-two herbs, "and various other kinds indigenous to our country," were offered by the New Lebanon Shakers in 1841 with price per pound and the botanical name.[19] Four culinary herbs, pulverized, and 21 extracts, 4 ointments, the same ones as in previous years, and the same listed pills, syrups, other medicines, and fragrant waters were included.

The catalogs of 1848 and 1850 were essentially the same as the earlier ones,[20] but the content of the next four catalogs to be issued under the New Lebanon imprint was greatly increased (and became increasingly useful as botanical manuals as well). There were many changes in the issue of 1851.[21] The cover gave much more information as to the contents of the book: *A Catalogue of Medicinal Plants, Barks, Roots, Seeds, Flowers and Select Powders with their Therapeutic Qualities and Botanical names; also Pure Vegetable Extracts, prepared in vacuo; Ointments, Inspissated Juices, Essential Oils, Double Distilled and Fragrant Waters, etc. etc., Raised, prepared, and put up in the most careful manner by the United Society of Shakers at New Lebanon, N.Y.* Orders, it said, should be addressed to Edward Fowler—and there was a new little verse:

> A blade of grass—a simple flower,
>   Cull'd from the dewy lea;
> These, these shall speak with touching power,
>   Of change and health to thee.

The Shakers now described 44 properties for 356 herbs which was 184 more than ever offered before. The same pulverized culinary herbs were listed as well as a list of 181 fluid extracts. Another list gave "pure inspissated alcoholic and hydro-alcoholic solid extracts, sixty-one in number as well as forty-eight ordinary extracts," 22 alkaloids and resins, 10 ointments, and 7 double-distilled and fragrant waters. "Also waters distilled *in vacuo*, from the expressed juice of Cicuta, Belladonna, Henbane, Sarsaparilla, Dandelion, Thorn Apple; and various others can be had by giving NOTICE in time of preparation, and are recommended to Physicians for trial, especially Cicuta, Dandelion, and Sarsaparilla for the cleansing of foul ulcers, etc." Nine essential oils and 84 powdered articles completed the list.

The society completed the book for the first time with a list of synonyms. Two hundred sixty-four of them were included. It was noted as well that "Difficulties have sometimes arisen from the use of the common name being applied to different plants in different localities, and also from the fact that druggists are frequently called upon for some article which they have, by a name distinct from that by which it is sold under, which they are not aware of, we have appended a list of synonyms, which the seller will please refer to before turning a customer away." The usual pills, snuff, and syrups, and, for the first time, 74 garden seeds, were listed.

This catalog also for the first time carried the endorsement of Professor C. S. Rafinesque who said:

> The best medical gardens in the United States are those established by the communities of the Shakers, or modern Essenians, who cultivate and collect a great variety of medical plants. They sell them cheap, fresh and genuine.

This was indeed high praise from a botanist of acknowledged national repute. There were also complimentary statements from H. H. Childs and Willard Clough, neighboring physicians in Pittsfield, Massachusetts.

The catalogs of 1860 and 1866[22] were identical to the 1851 issue and contained no new or additional material. But in 1867 a three-page list of fluid extracts manufactured by the Lebanon Shakers was issued announcing 182 fluid and 60 solid extracts of herbs, barks, roots, among other things, with the common names followed by botanical names. Prices were stated for one-pound and five-pound bottles.[23] The Shakers issued a second little booklet in the 1870s, listing 132 fluid extracts, along with pearls of ether, pearls of chloroform, and pearls of turpentine with a liberal discount to the trade,[24] and in 1872 they issued a wholesale price list of Medicinal Herbs and Roots giving the common names and prices of 358 herbs.[25]

In 1874 a *Price List of Medicinal Preparations*[26] was issued listing 405 herbs, roots, seeds, and barks with botanical names and the prices for preparations in pulverized, fluid, or solid form. Six ointments, four pulverized culinary herbs, and three syrups were included. The syrups remained the best sellers: bitter bugle, "A new and valuable medicine for coughs, spitting of blood and consumption"; sarsaparilla compound and genuine syrup of buckthorn, used in rheumatism, gout, and dropsy. This number of herbs, exceeding 400, was the most offered for sale by this society or any of the others. It was extraordinary in view of the fact that in 1874 there were many commercial houses "in the world" giving the Shakers considerable competition.

The 1873 *Druggist's Handbook* was the last of the large catalogs, but the Shakers continued to publish price lists, broadsides, testimonials advertising specific medicines, some several pages in length, for many years and a few into the twentieth century. These will be examined in connection with the remedies they promoted, and the men who conceived them.

The Shaker families cared for the sick and maintained large efficient "nurse houses" or infirmaries as well as the botanic gardens and vegetable medicines necessary in the care of the ill and aged, and according to a New Lebanon journal for 1789, the entry for

May 23 establishes an apothecary in residence: "To dressing a hat for the apothecary 2 shillings, 3 pence."[27]

An early physician was "Dr." Eliab Harlow who with Brother Garrett Keatin Lawrence was credited with establishing scientific standards for the medical gardens which gave them such quality and a good reputation.

Benjamin Gates kept a diary starting October 1, 1827, when he was working in the "new taylers shop," in which he describes how varied the chores were in the community and in Brother Garrett's medical department.[28] On the 8th, he goes

> a chestnutting with Joseph Fearey and finish Amos Jewetts drawers. On the 15-16-17th, pick apples, work with Issac Youngs on the Meeting house. May 1828 the 13th through the 21st, I work in the medical garden with Garrett Lawrence. 22nd, work in seed garden. 23rd, work Issac Young's drawers. June 7th help cut slippery elm bark. 9th medical garden with G.K.L. 11th, 12th. work in seed garden. 23rd. to strawberrying. July 1 and 2 work in physic garden with Gideon. October 10th helped about culling tobacco. Broken time [different kinds of chores all mixed up] from now on.

In 1829 he starts his diary on April 8 digging horse "raddish." He then records miscellaneous chores until

> July 14, 15th working in physic garden, here a little, and there a little, but don't fail. August-gathering herbs here and there—go on west hills after lobelia. 26 and 27th work in medical garden. 30 and 31st gathering bugle here and there. Sept. 1830 spend this month gathering herbs and roots here and there, up hill and down. 2nd, 23, 24th. down to Sheffield after blue cohosh. 28th on the mountain after maidenhair.

Another diary was kept by Milton Homer Robinson of the South Union, Kentucky, society.[29] He "went South to New Orleans" for his health. Eventually, after the long journey down the Mississippi, and by slow boat up the coast to Philadelphia, he took passage on a steamboat to New York with some New Lebanon Shakers he met in the City of Brotherly Love. His trip took him up the Hudson to Albany where a wagon was hired for New Lebanon and there he was put in the care of Brother Garrett. These are a few excerpts from his diary that pertain to the Shakers' concern for health:

> May 22, 1831. Pleasant weather. Brother Garrett Lawrence brought me a bottle of syrup to take for my cough. I took a glass and retired to my bed. May 23. Bro. Garrett Lawrence visited me and made some inquires into the state of my health, how long I had been affected with the cough and Elder Brother John visited me again and desired that I would amuse myself by walking in Garrett's garden or to the House. Not to confine myself to close to the rooms. After breakfast Brother Daniel showed me the different gardens. May 26. 10 a.m. Brother Garrett K. Lawrence took me through a good bathing operation. Met John Wright brother of Lucy Wright our last Mother. Isaac also gave me council. Plans to return to New Orleans and then South Union cancelled, will stay now at 2nd Family and see how health improves. Some fears are apprehended that I would not be able to stand the journey home. Visited Garrett's gardens again and went through a sweating operation. May 31, 1831. 90°. I attended to Garrett's bees to watch and give notice when they would swarm. Issac N. Youngs measured me for a new pair of trousers. June 1. Have done a considerable hoeing in Garrett's gardens today. I assisted Eliab Harlow about raising Elmbark. . . . Thurs. June 9th. Moderately warm. Gideon Kibby, Issac Knight and myself hived a swarm of bees this afternoon. Also Charlie Crosman and myself started at ½ after 3 o'clock p.m. with the 2 horse waggon to the mountain directly west of Bro. James Farnums family for a load of dogwood poles for the purpose of getting the bark as a medicine. . . . Received from the sisters a neat and pleasant summer hat and also a genteel and handsome frock for to wear to

meetings at home and Sabbath evenings. June 11th. Went a strawberrying west of the medical garden. June 15th Garrett went with the 2 horse waggon for a load of Elm bark.

June 17, 1831. A group of brothers and sisters took a ride for recreation and health to Lebanon P.O. [post office] thence to town of Hancock a distance of 6 miles—thence to town of Pittsfield—6 miles where we put up at Tussells Tavern and eat supper about 3 o'clock. We return to New Lebanon by way of Hancok [Shaker village] we did not stop there. We arrived at home about 6 o'clock p.m. and I can say that there are few days of my life that I took so much real comfort and satisfaction as I have taken today. The day was uncommon pleasant, the roads good and the company agreeable and interesting.

There were many conferences regarding Milton's health and whether or not he should return to South Union. Brother Garrett attended him with great concern, and Milton records the comings and goings of this greatly admired doctor with fidelity and in detail. He has a tedious day coughing, but is able to go to the Second family to "see them casting stove-plate." Saturday, June 27, he attends Meeting where "they spoke the Gospel in unknown tongues."

Oh that I could give the reader some idea of the beauty and simplicity, the life and the zeal manifested in this meeting. Suffice me to say it was everything that is pretty and good.

June 27th. I attend to keeping the fire rekindles under Garrett's kittles [sic] of liverwort syrup for the purpose of inhaling the steam arising there from for the benefit of my lungs. Mother Lucy Wright died at Watervliet.

June 29, 1831. This morning Elder Bro. Sam Johnson and myself went on a visit to Hancock. [The Shaker village not the town of Hancock.] Sometime after we arrived there we obtained leave to visit their new brick building accompanied by El. Br. William Deming. From there we went to where Comstalk Betts was engaged making the doors for the above mentioned building. While here Elder Nataniel came to the door and beconed to S. Johnson to accompany him to the Ministry shop. Comstalk then accompanied me to a shop where Deacon Daniel Goodrich was employed in pasting paper bags to hold garden seed. I took great comfort with Daniel, he was familiar and pleasant and manifested a great desire for my future happenings and safe return to South Union.

Many words from the next paragraphs of the diary have been deleted by a contemporary editor, but we learn that his health is deteriorating. Nevertheless he watches Benjamin Lyons, "family deacon start to Albany with a barn load of Garrett's medical herbs." On the next day, July 2, he is overjoyed to receive a letter from Elder Benjamin of South Union "and directed to me Milton H. Robinson." He broke the seal and read it in the Elder Sister's room in the presence of the Elder Deacon. It was an early rule that all letters had to be opened and read in the presence of a member of the ministry.

This letter is calculated to give me great releasement in mind. I do feel thankful to El. Benjamin for the kind feelings manifested to me in the letter. Yea, it is calculated to give me peace of mind on a dying bed, and I will treasure up the good council he has given me in this letter. . . . Went to the great house and showed the brethren there the letter and it was read by Issac Youngs and they all expressed themselves as satisfied I had received so comforting a letter.

For a while it seemed as if Milton's health really was improving. At least his diary was not so much concerned with it, and for over a month the entries had to do with the herb industry:

July 12. Clear and moderate. G. K. Lawrence went to Washington for a load of timber and also for the purpose of engaging the digging of 30 or 40 pounds of spikenard roots and to get some other herbs. July 14. This afternoon Issac Knight and myself went up on the mountain and gathered a Dearborn loan of yarrow. Something diverting. July 15. Garrett and company have been cutting and hauling catmint all day. The sisters with my assistance have picked it all over ready for cutting fine. July 18. Bro. Garrett went to Hancock on his professional business [doctoring]. July 19. Clear and warm. This morning Garrett K., Lucy C. Sarah K. and Hannah Ann went in two horse waggon to Whitings pond for the purpose of gathering medical herbs in the lots about home such as yarrow and catmint. Have been engaged this p.m. picking over wormwood. This weather is a great hindrance to the brothers in getting in the hay.

Day after day two horse wagons brought in loads of whortleberries, of wormwood, of catnip, of lobelia, of senna, and of Indian tobacco. The herbs were picked over and dried. Great loads of elm bark were cut up at the machine shop and then he reports: "I am some unwell and take a sweat in the P.M. Aug. 6th. Went to the ministry shop with a letter I have prepared to send to Elder Benjamin [of South Union]. Brother Rufus spared no pains to comfort me and make my way as easy as possible." The handwriting now is very weak, letters small and pale. He is obviously very sick. He writes "THE END" in larger than usual letters. There are two pages accounting for letters written by him and those received by him from South Union. It is a record of his correspondence and the end of the book also.

These excellent journals are only the forerunners of one which is much fuller and gives more information about Brother Garrett. This is Barnabas Hinkley's account written in 1836.[30] He was the physician at the Church family and conducted the herb industry after the deaths of Garrett Lawrence (1837) and Eliab Harlow (1840).

May 16th. I commence working in the medical garden—sow to sage. Sodus Elders arrive here today. [This was the year Sodus Bay, later Groveland, New York, society was organized.] 17th. Scrape up and fix a bed and sow it to whiteroot and summer savory and set out some Butten Snakeroot. Continue plowing East. 19th. Rake and sow a bed—some sweet basil and Foxglove and Moldaven Balm. In the P.M. set out some rose bushes. May 20th. Garrett has a bad turn and I tend upon him beside ploughing the ground for peppermint and for I. Bates' willow slips. I. Bates and Eliab Harlow set out the slips. 21st. We set out the Hyssop bed in the alley and finish fixing the alley. Garrett gets some better so as to ride out with Levi Chauncey. 23rd. We commence setting out catnep. I. B. and E. H. and myself. 24th. We finish setting out catnep and I plough up the tanzy bed and set out some red rose bushes. The Enfield Brethren start for home. Amos Stewart goes with them to help them set up the Machean [sic]. 25th. We transplant some lemon balm and rake and fix a bed and set out some Lobelia Selfelettica [siphilitica]. 26th. Set out the peppermint and tanzy. 27th. Nothing down in the garden today, I put up some extract. 28th. We set out some chamomile and a row of lovage and marshmallow and sow three rows of poppy in the p.m. 31st. Help hoe out horehound.

June 1836. 1st. Sisters clean up the drying house. 3rd. I assist Garret about his alative [alterative] syrup and make some preparations for making a closet in the drying house. 13th. Transplant some horehound. 14th. I hold the plough to brake up east of the herb garden. 15th. I go over to Hancock a visiting with Cinthy Hamblin, Eliza Sharp and Sarrah Fairchild who is here from Watervliet. 18th. We transplant the belladonna and Hysoscyamus and finish setting out horehound. 22nd. Garret and John Dean start out for Hoosic. Cut sage.

July 1st. Powder cicuta. 11th. Weed Foxglove south of the alley. 12th. Weed out the Time [sic]. 14th. Transplant Foxglove. July 16th. Continue pounding Cicuta. G.L. goes after catnep. 28th. It rain today so I set out some sage.

August 23rd. I go with Charles Crossman to Albany. Aug. 24th. I got home about 4 o'clock with 500 and 45 lbs. of horehound from Sodus. 25th. Help Gideon cultivate his sage. 29th. Cut the belladonna and horehound.

Sept. 12th. G. K. Lawrence and John Dean start for New York. I pick over herbs. Elder Brother complains of being sick so I give him an emetic. 13th. Help cut sage. Eliab Harlow goes with N. Bennet[31] out to Kinderhook after fleabane. 14th. Today I take a walk on the mountain with Elder Ruth and Elder Sister Hannah Ann Treadway and I. Bates. We return home in good season and I steam Elder Brother and Gideon Turner who is some sick. 16th. Tend the sick. Help cut Summer Savory. 19th. Go on the mountain after Bugle and sculcap and other herbs.

21st. Do some chores and help the sisters gather Coltsfoot. Sept. 28th [he is on a visit to Watervliet]. Go down to the North farm and back through Deacon Peter's garden then into the big garden from there to the little house, from there to Francis's shop. The shell [bell] sounds for dinner and we return to the house here and find the sisters eating watermellon as big as a cog [keg] Henry and I set down and helpt them eat it. [goes to church meeting] Then we went forth in the square order manner 3 songs, then we march about 3 songs then we face in and sing. Then dance 2 quick songs then we march back and forth about 2 songs. Then Elder Brother spoke some and then opened the way for us to communicate the love which we did and we all spoke some then they sung a farewell song and Elder Brother led Henry and I up and down between the brothers and sisters. Then Elder Sister spoke some of her thankfulness for our coming to see them. Oct. 3. We rise at the sound of the trump [bell] and start for Schenectady. Oct. 5. Back home. I grind some Hellebore and lady-slipper. Oct. 6th. Help pack herbs. snowy today. 11th. Gather garden lettuce stalks for Extract. 24th. I cut some foxglove and tend upon Jonathan Wood who is quite sick at the office. 14th. Measles at the Second House. I get measles and feel sick. 16th. I feel better. My measles have turned and Garret H. Lawrence steam me and I begin to think about getting better. Nov. 21st. G. H. L. bottle up some sarsaparilla syrup. 25th. Garret and I go over to Hancock to see George Wilerson who is sick with dropsey of the heart case. 28th. Garret and I pack some herbs for New York. 29th. Garret goes to the Second House and commence a course of medicine to get prepared for tapping. Takes a dose of senna Jalap and cream a tartar and prepare some pills for Dr. Jonathan's doses. Dec. 19th. Garret H. Lawrence moved into the south west room in the great house. Gideon and I tend upon him til the end. Jan. 1. 1837. I commence again taking care of G. H. L. and continue thru his sickness with help of Dan Wood., after the 9th. 24th. Unwelcome event. Our beloved and useful brother *GARRET H. LAWRENCE* this morning departed this life at 10 mins. past 5 o'clock having passed thru a serious and lengthy sickness and hard sufferings. He has scarcely enjoyed any health since June 1833 at which time he had a severe attack of acute rheumatism. Jan. 5. We tend the funeral at 2 o'clock p.m. 12 of the world, 6 males and 6 females attend.

This record is important for many reasons. It gives a touching account of the love and affection felt for Brother Garrett as well as a real feeling of the activity of the medical herb department which was his business. It describes the business dealings in herbs that were carried on between societies, the visiting back and forth, and some of the medical practices.

Philemon Stewart was an accurate and interesting journalist. In the first of his daybooks quoted here he introduces himself:[32] "April 9, 1826, Philemon Stewart, a young man whose age will be 22 the 20th of the present month takes the business [peddling seeds and herbs] which the above mentioned Benj. Lyon a man of rather more than middle age has left. April 33, 1826 . . . Philemon Stewart relieved of peddling and is appointed to take care of the boys and as the garden is a suitable place for boys to work, he also takes [care of] the garden."

Accordingly, on March 29 of 1831 he writes: "We set some glass in our sashes to cover our hot bed." There are many more entries regarding the hot bed which in the climate at New Lebanon was a great asset to the gardeners and he feels certain that eventually he will have also "a glass house" near and between the "great garden."

April 11th. We are begining to raise some strawberrys and gooseberrys. Graft peach trees. Gather raddish seed at herb house and finish sowing our raddish. We have two kinds here in the garden the scarlet turnip and the salmon. . . . April 20. Gardens too wet to work. . . . April 21. Peter and I sow some early peas. All forces is turned to setting out roots in the Great Garden. . . . May 2, 1831. The boys go after cowslips this forenoon. . . . 5th. We gardners 4 in number go and help rake in the great garden. . . . May 6th. Sow carrawy and parsely. . . . May 9th. It is very cold with repeated snow squalls through the day. We gardners work here and there at this thing and that. . . . May 13th. Have made my alleys with poles for beans and brush for peas, the result pleases my eye. We pretty much finish planting our gardens. The weather is quite warm and pleasant. . . . Elder Calvin [Green] and Brother Seth [Wells] have been compiling the book of extracts.

This book of extracts listed 133 herbs with common and official names in extract form and with prices for one- and five-pound bottles.[33] Doses were given for 29 extracts and three new preparations were advertised: pearls of ether, pearls of chloroform, and pearls of turpentine. This little booklet, published in 1871, stated:

In presenting you a New Edition of our Catalogue, we would call especial notice to our Inspissated Juices and Superior Fluid Extracts, prepared in Vacuo.

Our particular attention has been directed to this branch of business for some years past, and we have Procured very Perfect and Expensive Apparatus and the Instructions and assistance of some of the Best Chemists and Pharmaceutists. We have been able to produce Extracts which we confidently believe are not inferior to any, and for which we have received high encomiums from many of the Medical Faculty and some of our Principal Colleges.

We wish to call the particular attention of the Medical Faculty to our Superior Fluid Extracts, which we Manufacture from the Best Material according to the Established Principles of Pharmaceutical Science. Perfectly Pure—possessing all the Medicinal Properties of the Plant, from which they are manufactured, without the addition of Sugar, or any Saccharine whatever, as in the case with most Fluid Extracts now offered in market.

Our Society having been actively engaged in the business of Manufacturing Extracts over forty years, we claim the advantage of Experience, and the rapidly increasing demands for SHAKER HERBS AND EXTRACTS, with their various Botanic Preparations, is a satisfactory evidence of public approval and esteem.

We pledge ourselves to furnish articles of superior excellence and are determined not to be surpassed in the Quality or Neatness of our Preparations.

New Lebanon Shaker Village.

The travel journal of Eldress Betsy Smith[34] gives us a concise picture of New Lebanon. The company from South Union, Kentucky, and Union Village, Ohio, arrived at "Holy Mount" on August 19, 1854, and stayed ten days:

Aug. 21. . . . Spent the forenoon in company with brothers Jonathan Wood [an herbalist] and Allen Reed, John Dean: They took two carriages & escorted us to the Lebanon springs spent some time looking at the surrounding scenery; The springs are beautiful, the water rises seemingly up out of a solid rock sparkling, and the Pool appeared to be about four feet deep. There did not appear to be anything peculiar in the flavor of the water; only it is quite warm, as it boils up and is said to continue so through the Winter . . . A short distance below where the water rises, they have made beautiful pools for bathing, one for each sex in different appartments. We returned by a different rout. Came by the farm they recently purchased. Halted and went thro the Herb Garden. The lots & farms lying in the township of Lebanon. . . . The Believers carry on the Herb and botanical business quite extensively. Raise a portion of the herbs themselves and buy a great many from the worlds people.

The sales in that business amounts to about $30,000 annually. Garden seed business carried on extensively and perhaps more Lucrative than the Botanic. In the afternoon we visited the second order, had an agreeable time of it with the good souls in that family, and returned to the office about dark, while there we went thro their herb and botanic establishment.

We were taken to bro Barnabas Hinckley medicine shop, saw many nice things & he made us a present of some nice candies of different kinds and gave each one of us a cologne bottle

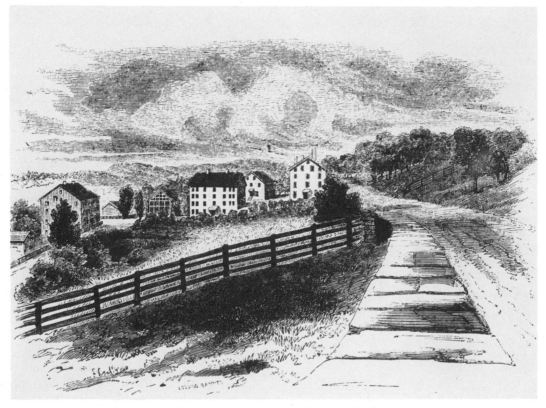

Northern portion of the Shaker village.

filled with cologne of their own manufacture. He conversed some on the subject of medicine. Said he considers water is good in some cases, but dont consider it a specific for all diseases. Uses medicine in some cases, and think's to advantage, and says he would make use in certain cases, any human remedy to mitigate pain. But at the same time he would be cautious about using strong medicines of all kinds, and not use them where one more simple would answer.

Had a visit with bro Henry DeWitt he prints all the herb laybills & seed bags saw him operate on the printing press. He thinks believers ought to avoid unnecessary embellishments in the printing, and instead of gaudy borders, use plain black lines.

Benson J. Lossing gives one the best detailed and illustrated accounts of the Shakers' herb industry. After meeting Elders Bushnell and Evans he had "an excellent supper" and returned to the family at the store where he passed the night. The next day his investigation continued.

The management of the temporal affairs of the community is committed to trustees, who are appointed by the ministry and elders, and these are legally invested with the fee of all the real estate belonging to the Society. They transact all commercial business; and it is the unanimous testimony of those who have had dealings with them, that no men are more just and upright than they. The chief business trustee of the Lebanon community, and whose

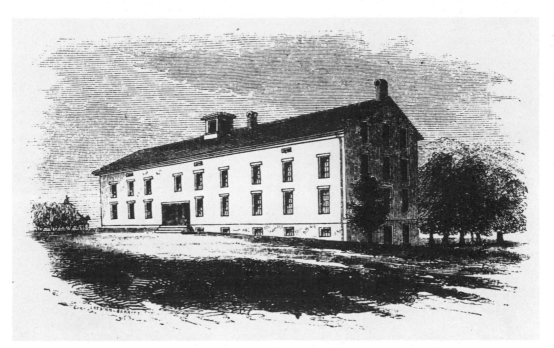

The original herb house of the Church family was destroyed by fire in 1875. It contained all processes necessary to prepare, pack, and ship herbs. In 1870, the Second Order sisters cut more than a million labels.

The powerful hydraulic press, housed in the second story of the herb house, daily turned out 250 pounds of herbs and 600 pounds of roots pressed into solid pound cakes wrapped in dark blue paper.

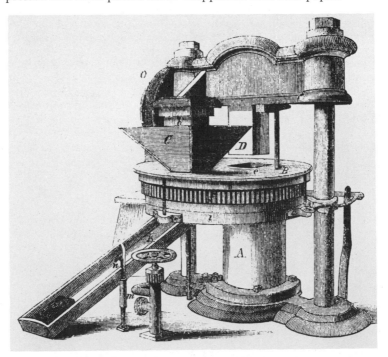

name is best known abroad is Edward Fowler, a middle-sized man, about sixty years of age. With him I visited the various industrial establishments. These are situated in convenient places in various parts of the village. All of them are supplied with the best implements, and are conducted in the most perfect manner. I can do little more, in this paper, than give a bird's-eye view of them.

The Herb House, where the various botanical preparations are put up for market, is a frame building in the centre [sic] of the village, one hundred and twenty feet in length, and forty feet in width, and two stories and an attic in height. There are some spacious out-houses connected with it. The lower part is used for the business office, store-rooms, and for pressing and packing of herbs and roots. The second story and attic are the drying rooms, where the green herbs are laid upon sheets of canvas, about fourteen inches apart, supported by cords. The basement is devoted to heavy storage and the horse-power by which the press in the second story is worked. *That press,* seen in the engraving, is one of the most perfect of the kind. It has a power of three hundred tons, and turns out each day about two hundred and fifty pounds of herbs, or six hundred pounds of roots, pressed for use. This performance will be doubled when steam shall be applied to the press. The herbs and roots come out in solid cakes, an inch thick, and seven and a quarter inches square, weighing a pound each. These are then taken into another room, where they are kept in small presses, arranged in a row, so as to preserve their form until placed in papers and labeled. During the year 1855 about seventy-five tons of roots and herbs were pressed in that establishment. About ten persons are continually employed in this business, and occasionally twice that number are there, engaged in picking over the green herbs and cleansing the roots brought from the medicinal fields and gardens. The extra laborers are generally females. These fields and gardens cover about seventy-five acres, a portion of which is devoted to the cultivation of various herbs and vegetables for their seeds.

The Extract House, in which is the laboratory for the preparation of juices for medical purposes, is a large frame building, thirty-six by one hundred feet. It was erected in 1850. It is supplied with the most perfect apparatus, and managed by James Long, a skillful chemist, and a member of the Society. In the principal room *of the laboratory* the chief operations of cracking, steaming, and pressing the roots and herbs are carried on, together with the boiling of the juices thus extracted. In one corner is a large boiler, into which the herbs or roots are placed and steam introduced. From this boiler, the steamed herbs are conveyed to grated cylinders, and subjected to immense pressure. The juices thus expressed are then put in copper pans, inclosed in iron jackets and the pans, and the liquid boiled down to the proper consistency for use. Some juices, in order to avoid the destruction or modification of their medical properties, are conveyed to an upper room and there boiled in a huge copper *vacuum pan,* from which, as its name implies, the air has been exhausted. This allows the liquid to boil at a much lower temperature than it would in the open air. In a room adjoining the vacuum pan are mills for reducing dried roots to impalpable powder. These roots are first cracked to the size of "samp" [coarse hominy] in the room below, by being *crushed* under two huge discs of Esopus granite, each four feet in diameter, a foot in thickness and a ton in weight. These are made to revolve in a large vessel by steam power. The roots are then carried to the mills above. These are made of two upper and a nether stone of Esopus granite. The upper stones are in the form of truncated cones, and rest upon the nether stone, which is beveled. A shaft in the centre, to which they are attached by arms, makes them revolve, and at the same time they turn upon their own axes. The roots ground under them by this double motion are made into powder almost impalpable [so fine that it cannot be felt].

In a building near the Extract House is the *Finishing Room,* where the preparations, already placed in phials, bottles, and jars, are labeled and packed for market. This service is performed by two women; and from this room those materials, now so extensively used in the materia medica, are sent forth. These extracts are of the purest kind. The water used for the purpose is conveyed through earthen pipes from a pure mountain spring, an eighth of a mile distant, which is singularly free from all earthy matter. This is of infinite importance in the preparation of these medicinal juices. They are, consequently, very popular, and the business is annually increasing. During the year 1855 they prepared at that laboratory and

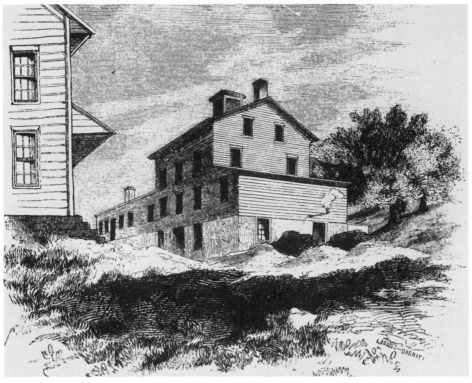

In the extract house, erected in 1850, the laboratory for the preparation of juices for medicinal purposes was housed. By 1855, various extracts were put up by the sisters who prepared more than 75,000 pounds for market during one fifteen-year period.

Roots and herbs were cracked, steamed, and pressed in the laboratory of the extract house. The processes were carefully directed by skilled Shaker chemists. In 1861 and 1862, more than 100 different varieties, both solid and fluid, were manufactured.

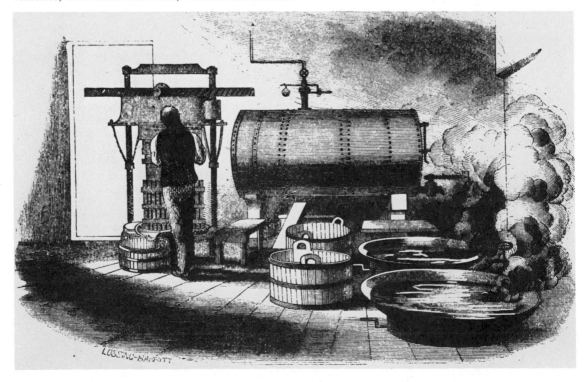

This vacuum pan gave added impetus to the herb industry in 1850. It was airtight and herbal liquids were boiled in it at a low temperature. It was this piece of equipment which attracted Gail Borden and which he perfected in developing his evaporated milk. In 1931, it was purchased for $50.00 from Eldress Emma J. Neale, head of the ministry at Mt. Lebanon, by Borden's Milk Products Company, Inc. It is now in the collection of the Smithsonian Institution, Washington, D.C.

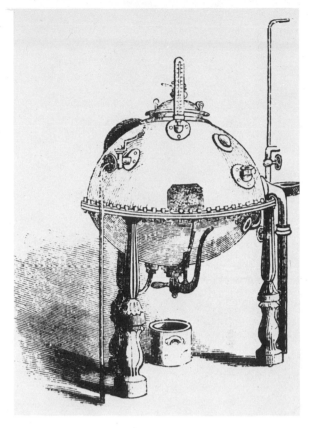

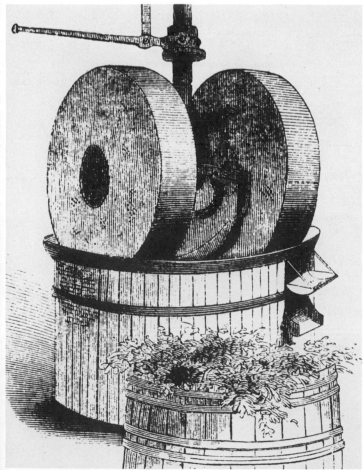

In this crushing mill, the roots and herbs, which were sold in powdered form, were first dried and then cracked and crushed.

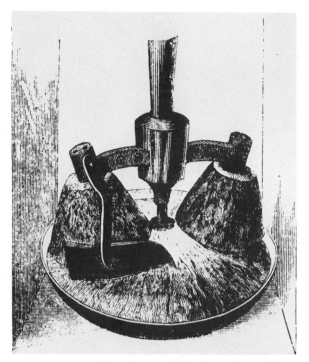

The powdering mill further reduced the crushed roots and herbs to the finest powder.

The sisters worked in the finishing room wrapping and packing herbs. They attached beautiful labels printed on light blue, mint green, salmon, pale pink, nut brown, orange, and yellow paper. The labels for medicines were plainly printed with informative directions that were clear and easy to follow. They were printed on paper made by Crane and Company of Dalton, Massachusetts.

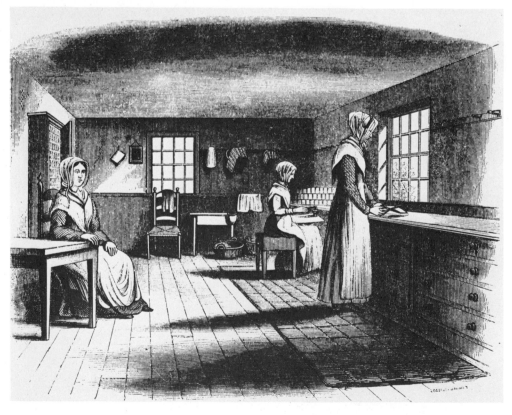

sold about fourteen thousand pounds. The chief products are the extracts of dandelion and butternut. Of the former, during that year, they put up two thousand five hundred pounds; of the latter, three thousand pounds.[35]

Lossing tells about the Seed House and the dairy and workshops where brooms, mats, woodenware, etc. are made. "These, and many useful articles of taste, manufactured in the village, are sold at the store to visitors during the summer. Of the minor

The first church at Mt. Lebanon was raised in 1785 and became the seed house when a larger church was built to accommodate the growing society.

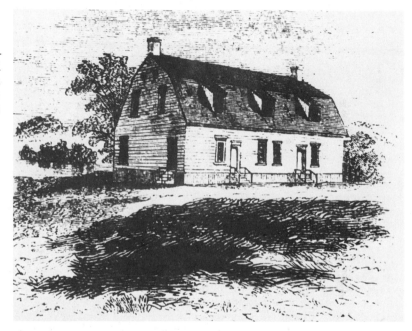

At the village store many Shaker-made articles were sold throughout the year. Business transactions took place here between the Shaker trustees and people of the outside world.

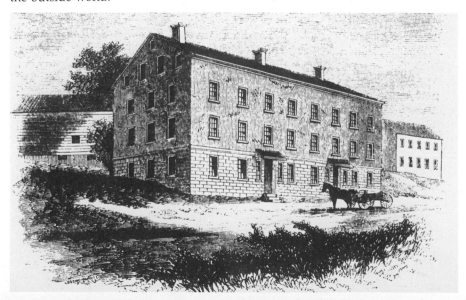

The physician at his desk was Barnabas Hinckley, a well-trained and careful doctor. He came to the Shakers when he was a very young child and became their doctor when he was nineteen years old. Later, after studying at the Berkshire Medical College in Pittsfield, Massachusetts, he received his degree in 1858, only three years before he died at forty-three, young for a Shaker. He left a good medical library to the society.

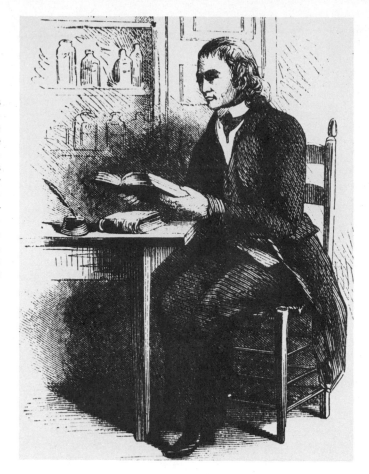

industrial operations of the community I have not space to make a record." He was much impressed with the perfect order and neatness which prevailed. "System is every where observed, and all operations are carried on with exact economy. Every man, woman and child is kept busy. The ministry labor with their hands, like the laity, when not engaged in spiritual and official duties; and no idle hands are seen. Having property in common, the people have no private ambitions nor personal cares; and being governed by the pure principles of their great leading doctrines, they seem perfectly contented and happy. All labor for the general good, and all enjoy the material comforts of life in great abundance."

Lossing also mentions an outstanding Shaker doctor.

> The Medical Department, under the charge of Dr. Hinckley, appears to be perfect in its supplies of surgical instruments, and other necessaries. A large portion of the medicines are prepared by themselves; and Dr. Hinckley applies them with a skillful hand, under the direction of a sound judgment. He has a library of well-selected medical works; and the system which he most approves and practices is known as the Eclectic. [A method of selecting what seemed best from various sources and systems.]

Barnabas Hinckley (1818–1861) joined the Shakers in 1821 and became their medical doctor in 1837. He had received a medical degree from the Berkshire Medical College in Pittsfield, Massachusetts, November 23, 1858. He had a good medical library and was a careful physician.

"They prospered in sales" was frequently said about the Shakers, and indeed their meticulous accounts proved it. One daybook kept by the Church family from 1860 to 1862 records that a prodigious amount of material was processed.[36]

The diary gives an account of the production of extracts from May through December of 1860. The output for May, June, and July totaled over 2,500 fluid pounds, from these herbs:

Quassia, bayberry, lady slipper, common dandelion, stillingia, sarsaparilla, yellow dock, rhubarb, senna, columbo, English valerian, henbane, jalap, belladonna, mandrake, butternut, goldenseal, stramonium, cicuta. Received 9 loads and obtained 8 barrels of juice.

In August the record continues.

1st. James makes 150 lbs. Stramonium ointment. 6th. Spread nine barrels of Golden Seal in kiln. Benj. Gates and Br. Daniel start West. 7th. Press out lobelia tintc. 130 lbs. from 45 lbs of herbs. Press out lady slipper, tintc. 140 lbs. from one bushel of roots. Press out Rhatany tinct., 271 lbs. from 10 lbs. of roots. 10th. Finished Scullcap. Put about 50 lbs. more or less Golden Seal to macerate. James making preparations to go to salt water [on vacation]. 11th. Take up 194 lbs. pulverized Scullcap in 4 days. 24th. Work at the herb shop for Gabriel who goes after Feverbush and Black alder. 28th. Put in a chest full of sarsaparilla. 364 lbs. whole chopped, 92 lbs. chaff leavings off the ground, total 456 lbs. fill chest with water to top of the glass. Put 4 barrels of ground Scullcap in the kiln to pulverize. Receive also 5 bushels of Bayberry for a like purpose and 1 barrel about 98 lbs. yellow dock for fluid extract, 114 gross. 29th. Fire up and cook Sarsaparilla. 30th. Drain off liquor and press the Sarsaparilla. Put into chest 385 lbs. more Sarsaparilla. That being all they have. 31st. Finish evaporating Sarsaparilla, 140 lbs. and cook. SUMMARY 556 lbs. fluid extracts; 140 lbs. solid extracts; 150 lbs. Stramonium ointment; 194 pulverized scullcap.

At this time the Shakers were selling their fluid extracts for $1.25 a pound, but they charged more for pulverized material and ointments. The total output according to this book represents a sales value of at least $4,500.00 for the four months.

The same daybook continuing for September states on September 8 ". . . Press Unicorn [star root, *Aletris farinosa* of the lily family, was widely used for colic]. 11th. James stills cherries and gets between 2 and 3 gallons Brandy. Alonzo and Henry C. [Clough] get 2 bushels of black cherries for S.A. Co."

For some reason October was skipped or perhaps recorded elsewhere. "November 20th. . . . Pulverize with West [family] pair and try the new outlet which works like a charm." And then to start the year's last month:

Dec. 3, 1860. Benjamin [Gates] arrives about noon in company with the State Chemist, Prof. Charles H. Porter, James having reported that he had mislabelled the extracts. Dr. Porter takes a view of matters and gives his advice which amounts to rejecting a few bottles of medicine not adequately designated by their labels, 2 or 3 bottles being distributed. The fact is none of us believe the report to be anything but report, but are confident after a close scrutiny that all is right so far it concerns articles actually labelled. Dr. Porter leaves soon after dinner taking with him a bottle of Veratrum for examination, also some Aconite crystals and Poppy deposites. Three days this week spent putting up extracts, one day spent in unpacking, cleaning and putting away up stairs 200 lbs. white jars. [These beautiful ceramic jars with a fine glaze had snug-fitting lids and held one pound of ointment.]

Dec. 8th. Press Bloodroot. Dec. 10th. Nearly one foot of snow on the ground. Try an experiment making Bloodroot tincture and conclude to resaturate the foot. 12th. Receive a keg of lard containing 90 lbs. hard fat for stramonium ointment. 13th. Alonzo goes to Albany with Benjamin to see the chemist. Find him absent. Take out some of the Quassia above mentioned to have it tested by Dr. Porter's assistant who was unable to detect any copper and gave his opinion that there was not copper enough in it to injure it. Dec. 31st. Pick over Bayberry.

The Shakers of New Lebanon published a booklet in eleven editions from the early 1850s to 1904 which extolled the powerful, but controllable effects of tincture of *Veratrum viride* (hellebore).[37] Preceding the preface in the little booklet was a statement:

ADVERTISEMENT

Having frequently visited the Laboratory and Botanic Gardens of the Shakers, at New Lebanon, Columbia County, New York, I can unhesitatingly recommend their Preparations, as the most pure and reliable Medicines manufactured in the country, as they spare no pains in doing their work on the most scientific and Pharmaceutical principles. Just such articles as the Practitioner wants to ensure him success in his Professional treatment; and as such I recommend them to the Medical Faculty.

Most of the booklet was devoted to specific cases submitted by doctors, the procedure followed in administering hellebore, and the results. Then several pages outlined specific diseases which could be treated effectively by using the medicine, and five pages contained testimonials from doctors.

The last three pages in the book listed 70 botanicals used in: "Pure Vegetable Extracts, solid and fluid, Manufactured by the Shakers." This was preceded by a statement concerning their botanic gardens, the laboratory and its very complete and expensive fixtures and concluded with a point which had created some debate during that period:

> It has been a matter of controversy among Apothecaries and Pharmaceutists, whether it was wise in the Inspissated juices, to retain the Chlorophylle and Albumen, so as to preserve the green color, as an index of its careful preparation; but the well conducted experiments of Mr. Solon have proved them to be nearly inert. Hence their presence only tends to enfeeble the proper extract; and by the recommendation of Professor Proctor of Philadelphia, and others, we shall in most cases reject them, unless otherwise desired by parties so ordering in time for preparing.

The Shakers processed and sold tincture of hellebore under the name of "Norwood's Veratrum" because of the wide distribution and persistent advertising by a Dr. W. C. Norwood, who claimed, "It is nervine, not narcotic." Dr. Norwood had originally produced this medicine, but, as the demand constantly increased, he employed the Shaker society at Lebanon for a number of years to make it under his direction. Before he died he turned the business entirely over to them. It was a powerful drug not to be administered heedlessly or by amateurs.

In March 1934 the Shakers printed the formula for the tincture:[38]

> Take 200 lbs. of White Hellebore Roots put in container & cover with 52 gallons of 85% Alcohol, let stand 16 days in mash, then drain, press & strain. It should be 75% when ready to bottle.
> This medicine prepared by the Shakers, is made from the purest materials obtainable.

(It carried the guarantee of the Food and Drug Act of June 30, 1906, Serial No. 3026.) The manufacturers claimed that it was efficacious in treating "puerperal eclampsia, pneumonia, typhoid fever, hypertrophy of heart, dysmenorrhea, acute rheumatism, aneurism, scarlet fever, measles, etc., yellow fever, and other diseased conditions."

Another Shaker medicine produced at Mt. Lebanon in the eighteen-eighties was Seven Barks, also manufactured exclusively for Dr. Lyman Brown. It contained blue flag, butternut, goldenseal, sassafras, lady's slipper, bloodroot, black cohosh, and mandrake. A second preparation called Pain King is mentioned in an undated letter by Benjamin Gates concerning these preparations: "Lyman Brown goes to Mexico. He has a good supply . . . at present [of Pain King and Seven Barks] so do not distress our good Sisters. Only think they put up in 3 days NINETEEN THOUSAND, TWO HUNDRED BOTTLES." Seven Barks was modified early in 1905 and eventually contained only one of the original barks, powdered sassafras.

Brother Benjamin wrote out the original formula for Pain King.[39]

20 gal. water. 10 lbs. Witch Hazel bark, stir well every-day for one week. 20 gall. strong alcohol—oils Spruce, Sassafras, Peppermint, Camphor gum, dissolve in separate portions of alcohol and mix all together—Opium, reduce to a miscible condition with warm water and Masher till all parts are accessible to alcohol and water, after the former mixture has been put together and well stirred. Or find out by Dispensatory, or by The Pharmaceutical Journal, what is the proper strength of Alcohol to extract the active principle of Opium, and preceed accordingly. Then mix with the rest.

The Shaker Asthma Cure, made at Lebanon, sold very well. The Shakers stated in its promotion that "No disease is harder to cure." And, "We offer the reasonable hope that the preparation will effect a cure, and a still greater possibility exists that it will procure at least so much relief that you can breathe air of heaven without distress and be able to lie down and find rest in sleep."[40]

Shaker Hair Restorer also met with approval from a public which was informed that:

The well-known Society of Shakers . . . has, for a century past been engaged in the cultivation of medicinal herbs and in this preparation of various essences, extracts and compounds, that are largely used in medical practice and by the public at large. The Society takes great pleasure in informing the public that they have added a HAIR RESTORATIVE to their already lengthy list of preparations. GRAY HAIR MAY BE HONORABLE, BUT THE NATURAL COLOR IS PREFERABLE.

Besides their efficacious qualities there was a charm and beauty to the herbal preparations of the Shakers. The labels for Extract of Dandelion, English Valerian, Syrup of Arnikate of Tannin, Shaker Family Cough Syrup, Vegetable Pills, Decoction of Rumex, Vegetable Cough Drops, Taraxacum Blue Pills (for the liver), Concentrated Syrup of Bitter Bugle (for consumption), and Vegetable Aromatic Cephalic Snuff (a powerful remedy for pain and dizziness in the head) were colorful and the products immaculately packaged. Labels for pressed herbs were printed on light blue, mint green, salmon, nut brown, orange, and yellow papers. Medicine labels were plainly printed with informative directions, given in simple English, and were easy to follow.

As so much material was being processed, picked in the green state, and dried, a chart was hung up on the wall of the herb department office and also carried in one of the account books:[41]

May 16th 1829

G. H. gathers 124 pound of green dandelions after dried 18½ lbs.
BUTTERNUT BARK when green weighs 35 lbs. And when dried 17 lbs.
CLEAVERS when green weigh 56 lbs. when dried 15 lbs.
ELDER FLOWERS when green weigh 289 lbs. when dried 56 lbs.
BURDOCK ROOTS when green weigh 50 lbs. when dried 6 lbs.
YARROW when green weighs 21 lbs. when dried 8 lbs.
HOARHOWN [sic] when green weighs 45 lbs. when dried 16 lbs.
BUGLE when green weighs 262 lbs. when dried 76 lbs.
STREMONIUM [sic] when green weighs 15 lbs. when dried 2¾ lbs.
DEERWEED when green weighs 175 lbs. when dried 71¾ lbs.
SASAPRILLA [sic] when green weighs 27¾ lbs. when dried 15 lbs.
BITTERSWEET TOPS when green weighs 25 lbs. when dried 10 lbs.
SPIKNARD [sic] when green weighs 83¾ lbs. when dried 26½ lbs.
COMPHREY [sic] when green weighs 48 lbs. when dried 15½ lbs.
SOUTHERNWOOD when green weighs 32 lbs. when dried 13 lbs.
ELECOMPAIGN [sic] when green weighs 63 lbs. when dried 19¾ lbs.

Although not all those engaged in gathering material would pick the same amounts, it is interesting that "G. H." felt the above amounts were "common" enough to serve as a helpful guide.

As the business grew it was necessary for the Shakers to have help in distribution. In the eighteen-seventies A. J. White of 319 Pearl Street, New York City, served them well, and himself too, no doubt, as it was to be a most lucrative account. Mr. White solicited others to take on the selling and issued a pamphlet outlining the benefits the salesmen would enjoy. The Shakers also made "White's Curative Syrup" for this agent. He advertised that the Shakers had a worldwide reputation for gathering and curing roots, barks, and herbs and had been engaged in the business for "upwards of fifty years." He said that whatever the Shakers manufactured was anxiously sought by the public.

> They are now engaged in making a medical preparation which has been placed in my hands for sale. For the purpose of enlisting your services in selling this Medicine, I send you this Circular, thinking perhaps that you may find it to your interest to take the Agency. The business is respectable, for all goods made by the Shakers are known to possess real merit. It can not be classed with the ordinary patent Medicines of the day, as there is no secret about its composition, the formula from which it is prepared being printed on each bottle.

Some firms, however, found cause to complain that Shaker material was inferior, but this was not the general rule:

Edward Fowler

Friend

The Parsley Rt. and Sage leaves came to hand yesterday and on examination prove very unsatisfactory.

The root seems to be roasted inside and for our use worthless. The sage is all shrivelled up and discolored. We send in this mail samples of each.

We write to have you be more careful of the next lot you put on the kiln.

Send some of each prime quality immediately for we cannot use these. Also chicory and comfrey. The Parsley Leaves are *prime*.

Respectfully yours,

Peek and Velsor

The inferior quality was the result of improper drying in the kiln and not in the choice of material gathered.

The Mt. Lebanon medicine department made a sarsaparilla under its own name as well as preparing quantities of the extract *in vacuo*, which was sold to other manufacturers. It was a medicine made by hundreds of companies and was quite naturally produced by the Lebanon Shakers, but never on as large a scale as that of the Canterbury or Union Village societies.

There were other "best sellers," among them Mother Seigel's Syrup (Extract of Roots), also sold by White, but distributed by other companies as well.

In August, 1884, Benjamin Gates wrote to Henry Clough from the Windsor Hotel in Montreal where he was on a mission of considerable importance to the society. The company making Smith Brothers Cough Drops had, it appeared, been using "Shaker" as a trademark in selling their product. Brother Benjamin and Agent White were trying to settle the problem:

Montreal. August 20th. 1884[43]

Dear Bro. H. Clough. It looks a little like my having to go to Ottawa.

We find Smith Bros. have registered in Ottawa the name Shaker as their trademark. This we must have taken off from the Government records or it will stand for ages. Smith Bro. are poor and want us to purchase their Trademark *"Shakers"*. How funny this looks. How Contemptable. Meaness boiled down!! A. J. White is disgusted and feels determined to uproot this business. I am quite willing to give him a lift in the good work.

Arn't that real Cheeky to ask us to purchase this Trade Mark. A name our Society has used for over one Hundred Years. What will come next?

I need not repeat how much I love thee. Only remember it and think of it often and all is right.

Your Bro. Benjamin G.

The matter was resolved in favor of the Shaker Society according to subsequent references, but we do not know how or if Brother Benjamin had to go to Ottawa. (This was written before Henry Clough left to take employment in New York.)

There is considerable correspondence from Benjamin Gates to Henry during this period. Generally the substance of the letters concerned sales and what firms had placed orders and whether to ship the material by "Express" or "other means." Henry wrote on September 23, 1882: "Now for Witch Hazel. Br. Alonzo [Hollister] said to me there was a good supply on hand. Is he right? Rubber Gloves shall have full attention. The large Corks for Sister Cornelia were shipped long ago. So says our friend Lyman [Brown]. No matter how things go I love THEE still. Your best friend, Benjamin."[44]

Benjamin Gates, on a selling trip in New York City, wrote, on October 31, 1885, to Henry Clough, who was an assistant in the herb department: "Dear Henry, The Prophet, The Wheelman, The Dude. I have secured orders as follows: 4800 Doz. Mother Seigel done in Spanish Labels. 4800 Doz. in English for London. Now is the time to make Hay while the Sun Shines. Don't let them Slumber. Your Br. B.G."[45]

As has been shown the sisters and brothers did most of the picking of the herbs and roots, but on occasions they were helped by others. A letter dated 1807 from "David at New Lebanon, to the World," says: "The Indians are here helping, mostly bringing botanics from the fields and woods."[46]

A journal kept at New Lebanon and dated 1842 has a lot to say about Indians attending meetings and concludes:[47]

> Nov. 30th. All now sat down in a ring and the Indians felt they had a great privilege. Gave baskets of all sizes and showed Elder Sister how to make them. Also blankets, leather pieces and hides and fur skins of animals. Nice large amounts of berries dried very well and wild roots especially prized at this time by our Physicians it being now the beginning of the cold season. We have made an understanding that the wild produce will be coming to us in regular amounts as their picking is clean and material is not cut into or marred. L.G. [Lawrence Garrett] is pleased to have this extra source and will guide them as to the general variety of roots and herbs he needs from their woods which are rich in resources.

There is another entry about the Indians who brought cornmeal ground by them:

> But being of a clean and nice consistency we enjoyed it and gave some fruits in exchange for their children. There were 5 large baskets of roots for the herb house and in a sack many barks all kept apart and easy for us to determine and use. The brothers are very pleased now to have Indians understand and separate properly.

Because the Shakers and other early settlers gathered so many herbs and roots, it is easy to understand why so many wild botanicals have disappeared in certain areas and why so many are still on the protected lists today of wild flower and Audubon societies. The dandelion has never been in danger of extinction even though enormous quantities of its root were used in several Shaker remedies. (Its beneficial properties treated stomach and urinary disorders, and it was easy to gather and readily available.)

The Shakers bought medicinal herbs from the outside whenever they could not gather material themselves. This is indicated by this letter to Edward Fowler from Horace Jennings, a peddler of Searsburg, Vermont, who wrote in August 1860:[48]

> I learnt by a man geathering Hearbs for you you Bought Balmony [snakehead] Sculcap wake Robin etc I am gethering Some of these kinds I have of Balmony 300 Pounds well Sorted & Dried in house on Racks what do you Pey for it Some was gethered in bud Some in blow I cannot make it look as well as Skulcap what is Evens Root worth . . . Dwarf Elder is plenty on my rout wild Latice [lettuce] Pipsisaway Mountain Ash Sassafras etc . . . My Balmony is Dry. . . .

The Shaker Digestive Cordial, however, required rarer varieties of plant material: blue flag, Culver's root (*Leptandra virginica*), stillingia, prince's pine and princess pine, and gentian. (These are all on protected lists in the East today.)[49]

James Vail kept a record of his business in the herb shop at New Lebanon, covering the years from 1841 to 1857. The book was continued by Alonzo Hollister through 1902. According to these records, Vail began pressing herbs in the winter of 1841, and each year he felt constrained to press a greater amount until his activity built up to a production in 1853 of 400 days (he worked some nights all through and included the time as "days"). He gathered and cleaned roots and herbs, made extracts and ointments, and cut labels for the packages, a total of 98,179 pounds for the market, or just over 245 pounds a day.[50]

Continuing his summary Vail says: "1854 covering same material less in pounds and only 160 days worth, but next year 405 days work and about the same pounds as 1853 and in 1857 these new items added: Blue flag, Comfrey, Polewort, Pole Cat Weed, Skunk Cabbage, Hyssop, Nettle blows, Buskbean, Canada Snakeroot, Yarrow, Lovage, Strawberry Leaves, total for 1858, 18,552 pounds. Total for the past 7 years $57,290."

He also wrote that on "January 17, 1851, Herbalists borrowed the printing press from Watervliet from which was dirived [sic] the plans and execution of the press upon which the printing is now done for the Herb Extract and Seed business."

Previous to the year 1841 the "Extracts both Inspissated and Boiled" were made by the Sisters, but the business became more than they could handle and "the Brethren took sole burden of the work." However, the Sisters turned to other activities, as recalled by Sister Marcia Bullard, about the time of the Civil War:

Forty years ago it was contrary to the "orders"[51] which governed our lives to cultivate useless flowers, but fortunately for those of us who loved them, there are many plants which are beautiful as well as useful. We always had extensive poppy beds and early in the morning, before the sun had risen, the white-capped sisters could be seen stooping among the scarlet blossoms to slit those pods from which the petals had just fallen. Again after sundown they came out with little knives to scrape off the dried juice. This crude opium was sold at a large price and its production was one of the most lucrative as well as the most picturesque of our industries.

The rose bushes were planted along the sides of the road which ran through our village and greatly admired by the passersby, but it was strongly impressed upon us that a rose was useful, not ornamental. It was not intended to please us by its color or its odor, its mission was to be made into rose-water, and if we thought of it in any other way we were making an idol of it and thereby imperiling our souls. In order that we might not be tempted to fasten a rose upon our dress or to put it into water to keep the rule was that the flower should be plucked with no stem at all. We had only crimson roses [rosa Gallica officinalis] as they were supposed to make stronger rose water than the paler varieties. The rose water we sold, of course, and we used in the community to flavor apple pies. It was also kept in store at the infirmary, and although in those days no sick person was allowed to have a fresh flower to cheer him, he was welcome to a liberal supply of rose water with which to bathe his aching head.

Then there were the herbs of many kinds. Lobelia, Pennyroyal, Spearmint, Peppermint, Catnip, Wintergreen, Thoroughwort, Sarsaparilla and Dandelion grew wild in the surrounding fields. When it was time to gather them an elderly brother would take a great wagonload of children, armed with tow sheets, to the pastures. Here they would pick the appointed herb [each one had its own day, that there might be no danger of mixing] and, when their sheets were full, drive solemnly home again. In addition to what grew wild we cultivated an immense amount of dandelion, dried the roots and sold it as "chicory." The witch hazel branches were too rough for women and children to handle, so the brethren cut them and brought them into the herb shop where the sisters made them into hamamelis. We had big beds of Sage, Thorn apple, Belladonna, Marigols and Camomile, as well as of yellow Dock of which we raised great quantities to sell to the manufacturers of a well-known "sarsaparilla." We also made a sarsaparilla of our own and various ointments. In the herb shop the herbs were dried and then pressed into packages by machinery, labeled and sold outside. Lovage root we exported both plain and sugared and the wild flagroot we gathered and sugared, too. On the whole there was no pleasanter work than that in the "medical garden" and "herb shop."

During the period of Sister Marcia's reminiscences the sisters made thousands of paper boxes for use in sending out the medicines[52] and were also cutting paper wrappers which they made on a form just large enough to slip around a four-ounce bottle of Norwood's Tincture.

About this same time another preparation became popular and sold on a par with Brother Barnabas Hinckley's Syrup of Sarsaparilla. It was "The Genius of Beauty! Toilet Prize and Sufferer's Panacea or Imperial Rose Balm." It was claimed to be unequaled for cleaning the teeth, healing sore or spongy gums, and the sore mouths of children. It was supposed to cure foul ulcers and pimples, ringworm, salt rheum, chapped hands and face, and could and did soothe burns, scalds, bruised skin and sunburns, and freckles. It was a beautiful and useful toilet soap for ladies and an excellent shaving fluid for gentlemen to rub on their faces immediately after shaving.

On February 6, 1875, eight buildings were burned in New Lebanon. And again, in November 1890, the Church family lost their drying kiln by fire, loss about $4,000. On the eighteenth of September 1894, a midnight blaze destroyed a number of buildings belonging to the same family. One contained a year's store of roots, alone valued at $1,500. These buildings were at the East Farm. Like the previous fires at Mt. Lebanon, it was the work of an incendiary.

In spite of these catastrophic events the medicine department made a strong comeback every time, for the orders continued to pour in and were promptly filled. A typical small order from "Friend W. H. Barnes" dated May 9, the year after the fire of 1875, was filled by Edward Fowler and amounted to seventy-five dollars before discount.[53] It included the following fluid extracts: bugleweed, cherry bark, cleavers, cotton root, hydrangea, motherwort, pleurisy root, Virginia snakeroot, stoneroot, wahoo, witch hazel, yarrow, belladonna, burdock, cinchona, coltsfoot, dandelion, gelsemium, lettuce, mandrake, sarsaparilla, scullcap, *Veratrum viride*, skunk cabbage, and ipecac. Similar orders for extracts and dried herbs and roots at this time indicated the business was good.

A series of Shaker almanacs were printed and distributed by A. J. White, the Shakers' agent in New York, and those issued after the fire of 1875 told of the great loss suffered. But in an editorial, "A Wonderful Success in Business," A. J. White tells how the Shakers got back on their feet in an amazingly short time and continued to produce their medicines ". . . upon which the Shakers had spent much study and labor to bring to perfection."[54]

The Englishman Hepworth Dixon is quoted in the almanac as saying:

> The writer was struck with the excellence of everything they produced. Their butter was of the very best. Their brooms were prime. The chairs easy, comfortable and durable. Their flannels, of an extra quality. Indeed everything they made was of the very best, and commanded an extra price when offered for sale. Each family had some special industry, by means of which a living was made.
>
> One family made a specialty of medicinal herbs and plants and their reputation for this particular branch has become known throughout the world. Going into one large building the writer found thirty or forty women and children putting up medicine, that they said was being sent to all parts of the world.
>
> They had agencies in England, Belgium, Germany, Italy, Spain, Australia, Constantinople, Greece, India, Africa, and in fact in all parts of the world. They said that they had shipped enough to London alone within the last three years to make the enormous number of 5,000,000 bottles. What amazed the writer was that such an enormous trade could be created for a medicinal preparation without the usual newspaper puffing and advertising; and what struck him still more forcibly was that this vast amount of medicine was for the cure of one single disease—Dyspepsia. The Shakers claim that modern civilization and modern cooking produce Dyspepsia in every country and in every climate. That it is not only a national disease with Americans, but it is a prevailing disease everywhere. That nearly all our bodily troubles have their origin in this one case, viz: Indigestion.

When asked how such an enormous demand could be created without the usual puffing, they said the remedy possessed merit, and when once used, the party obtaining relief recommended it to others, so that its good name spread from one to another, as the news spreads in India.

Shaker recipes are included on every page of the almanacs for 1882, 1883, and 1884. These covered a galaxy of dishes such as roast mutton, fried chicken, scalloped oysters, and bread puddings. Also dishes suggested for party fare: okra soup, Spanish cream, lemon cake, and rhubarb pies. They appeared on the same pages with Shaker Family Pills (The Cathartic) and Pain King.

Illustrations portrayed "Mrs. Langtry, said to be the most beautiful lady in England; Arabi Pasha, the Head of the Rebel Army in Egypt; the Khedive of Egypt and William S. O'Brien of Flood and O'Brien, California, the most successful miner in the world."

The "new" Shaker almanacs of 1884 and 1885 gave the history of the Shakers at Mt. Lebanon. The issue for 1884, for the first time, showed the meetinghouse, a group of Shakers, and their dwelling house. In 1885 Dr. White included many more different pictures. The first was of a brother at work crushing the roots for the Shaker Extract or Seigel's Syrup followed by a view of two brothers in the laboratory boiling the roots for the Shaker Extract; then a picture of Alonzo Hollister, "the famous Shaker chemist," concentrating the Shaker Extract of Roots or Seigel's Syrup in a vacuum pan; and five pictures of the Shaker sisters at work in the medical department filling bottles with the extract, from the enormous vats; corking the bottles which were held in wooden, slat-bottomed trays; labeling and wrapping the bottles; sealing the bottles; and the last one of quite an ancient sister pasting the labels on the bottles. A final print shows seven brothers packing and shipping the large wooden boxes containing hundred of bottles of Mother Seigel's Syrup.

Dr. White then concludes the 1885 almanac:

> We confidently recommend this as the most reliable and trustworthy publication of its kind before the public. No care or expense has been spared in its preparation, and the astronomical calculations are the result of many months' untiring labor, both for us and the scientific men whose services we engaged for this purpose. Most of the so-called Almanacs are simply a rehash of the previous years' figures, and are utterly valueless. The Shaker Family Almanac forms a striking contrast when compared with publications of such a class.

And his last pitch:

> The Shakers have sent to London alone 20,000,000 bottles of their Extracts of Roots to cure Dispepsia and Rheumatism.

During this same period seed catalogs were being issued by the Mt. Lebanon society and at least seven carried from 13 to 25 herb seeds, "sweet, pot and medicinal."[55] The Shakers offered the seeds of anise, balm, sweet basil, caraway, castor oil plant, catnip, coriander, dill, fennel seed, hop seed, horehound, hyssop, lavender, sweet marjoram, opium poppy, rosemary, rue, saffron, sage, summer savory, winter savory, broad-leaved sorrel, broad-leaved English thyme, tansy, wormwood, and the medicinal white mustard. Those which included herb seeds were published in 1881, 1884, 1885, 1887, and 1888.

In spite of the advertising, the testimonials, and the known worth of the products, the medicinal herb industry at Mt. Lebanon was slipping badly in the eighteen-nineties. We have referred to Henry Clough leaving the department and a sad letter from his old schoolteacher, Sister Amelia J. Calver, bemoans this fact:[56]

                                                                April 23, 1890

Dear Brother Henry:

When you read this note you doubtless will be far from home and its many friends. It
all seems so strange that I can hardly force myself to realize the truth. . . . It seems
hard to us who have hoped and toiled for so many years, to see one generation after
another of those reared here who are capable of keeping our home buoyed up to a
respectable level, pass out of it and their places filled [by] mendicants, whose only
interest is to find an easy corner and care neither for beauty nor order.

I so regret that you disregarded my advice to you last spring. "It is easier to drop out
of line of duty, than to take it up." Had you pursued the even tenor of your way, your
enemies would have been disarmed, and you triumphant. As it is you and your
friends are the suffering party, while that horrid "I told you so", will do its best to
crowd us back into the shades of long ago.

But we are used to bearing and suffering, and shall still endeavor to bear up; in fact
we shall have to, to save our lives, for the depression we now feel will crush us unless
some new line of thought comes to our relief.

We shall try to keep the things in good shape, over which you have toiled, that *when
you return* you will have no need to go the whole ground over again.

But dear brother, you are going to the city. Beware! Homesick feelings will no doubt
depress you; new acquaintances may excite you; but do for *our sakes* keep a steady
lookout for the little errors which ruin so many. Don't smoke nor chew; nor taste the
social glass. Your nerves your *means* your *happiness;* your *life* will need a safe guard
against every thing which your quiet Shaker life has prohibited. Pardon a sister's
frankness; but be assured we shall still love and earnestly pray for you, that every
blessing of life may be yours. Your sorrow will be our sorrow and your joy our joy and
we shall always think of you as our "Lost Boy".

                                                      Yours sincerely,
                                                      Amelia J. Calver.

In this letter is all the despair of the Shakers as their society began to diminish.

Henry Clough did return 19 years later to direct the medicine department once
again, and a letter went out announcing this fact on February 19, 1909.[57] It was signed by
Timothy D. Rayson for A. G. Hollister and said:

Esteemed Friend:

I write this to introduce to you our friend Henry T. Clough, who is expected from this
time onward, to manage the business in the Shaker medicine department, heretofore
conducted in our name. Any kindness or confidence shown to him, we will regard the
same as shown to us.

                                      With best wishes and kind regards.

But it became more difficult to attract converts and increase the membership in the
society. Keeping the good health of the community thereby became a paramount objec-
tive. The study of dietetics to maintain health had been pursued relentlessly by Frederick Evans in earlier days. These methods were now relied upon more than ever and
guided many of the Shaker leaders in maintaining the health of the Believers. (The
Shakers tried to prevent disease by promoting good living habits, and turned to new
means of curing ailments without drugs.) One sister wrote:[58]

Last note for Mt. Lebanon—Social Life and Vegetarianism, by Martha J. Anderson, Mt.
Lebanon 1893. We are increasing our fruit crop every year. Grapes are especially wholesome
and are much cheaper and more palatable than drugs. We have not had a fever in the family
for 50 years. Judicious water treatment, simple massage and the use of hot herb drinks are
our methods of cure in cases of sickness.

Some must always battle with inherited tendencies to disease but if they live strictly moral lives, and adhere to hygienic laws they will live more comfortably. Great good is attained in this direction by fortifying the mind against the ills of the body, and rising superior to them.

Perhaps it seems contradictory that a society which had used herbs and roots, and had derived such a large income over the years from the manufacture of drugs, should in its waning days change its practice. But the Shakers were confident of their ability to keep up with the times, and they readily accepted modern innovations. Thus, the days when the sisters 15 strong went to gather thyme and saffron, every day for a month, collected sage and stramonium leaves, and cleaned roots all day long for 30 days in October—these days were gone.[59] Gone, too, were the visits recorded so dutifully: "Jan. 13, 1858 Doctor Norwood of New York is here to get some tincture of Hellebore made at our Extract works."[60]

The business, 120 years old, became history at Mt. Lebanon in 1932.

NOTES

1. Diary of "Jethro," New Lebanon, N.Y., 1789–1812, Library of Congress, Washington, D.C.

2. *The Shaker Manifesto,* February 1881, p. 45.

3. Margaret F. Melcher, *The Shaker Adventure* (Cleveland: Press of Western Reserve University, 1960), p. 55.

4. E. D. Andrews, *The People Called Shakers* (New York: Dover, 1963), pp. 199, 200.

5. *Testimonies Concerning the Character and Ministry of Mother Ann Lee* (Albany, N.Y.: 1827), p. 27.

6. Benjamin Silliman, "Remarks Made on a Short Tour between Hartford and Quebec in the Autumn of 1819," *Christian Monthly Spectator* (New Haven, 1820), pp. 41–53.

7. Charles Nordhoff, *The Communistic Societies of the United States* (New York: Harper & Brothers, 1875), pp. 154–55.

8. Charles Dickens, *American Notes for General Circulation Written After His First Visit in 1842* (New York: D. Appleton and Co., 1872), 2:211.

9. Evert A. Duyckinck, *The Literary World,* vol. 9 (September 13, 1851), 11:201, 202.

10. Ibid.

11. Journals of the church deaconesses at New Lebanon, N.Y., January 1, 1843–June 23, 1864, Library at Shaker Community, Inc., Hancock, Mass.

12. *American Journal of Pharmacy,* n.s., vol. 18, no. 24 (1852), American Pharmaceutical Association, Washington, D.C.

13. Advertising circular, Tilden and Company, 1849, Cleveland, Shaker Collection, Western Reserve Historical Society.

14. *Chatham Courier,* January 9, 1969, p. 12. Emma B. King Library, Shaker Museum, Old Chatham, N.Y.

15. Notebook of medical receipts and cures from the nurses' shop, New Lebanon, 1815, Library at Shaker Community, Inc., Hancock, Mass.

16. Catalogue of medicinal plants and vegetable medicines, 1836, Cleveland, Western Reserve Historical Society.

17. Catalogue of herbs, 1837, Cleveland, Western Reserve Historical Society.

18. Catalogue of medicinal plants and vegetable medicines, 1838, Cleveland, Western Reserve Historical Society.

19. Catalogue of medicinal plants and vegetable medicines, 1841, American Antiquarian Society, Worcester, Mass.

20. Catalogues of medicinal plants and vegetable medicines, 1848, 1850, American Antiquarian Society, Worcester, Mass.

21. Catalogue of medicinal plants, barks, roots, seeds, flowers, and select powders, 1851, Cleveland, Western Reserve Historical Society.

22. Catalogues of medicinal plants, barks, roots, seeds, flowers, and select powders, 1860, 1866, Cleveland, Western Reserve Historical Society.

23. "List of Fluid and Solid Extracts," n.d., Cleveland, Western Reserve Historical Society.

24. "List of Fluid Extracts," 1871, Library at Shaker Community, Inc., Hancock, Mass.

25. "Wholesale List for Dealers Only," 1874, American Antiquarian Society, Worcester, Mass.

26. "Price List of Medicinal Preparations," Emma B. King Library, Shaker Museum, Old Chatham, N.Y.

27. Journal kept at New Lebanon, May 23, 1789, Library at Shaker Community, Inc., Hancock, Mass.

28. Diary of Benjamin Gates, New Lebanon, 1827, Andrews Collection, Henry Francis du Pont Museum, Winterthur, Del.

29. Diary of Milton Homer Robinson, New Lebanon, 1832, Library of Congress, Washington, D.C.

30. Journal of Barnabas Hinckley, New Lebanon, 1836, Andrews Collection, Henry Francis du Pont Museum, Winterthur, Del.

31. DeRobigne Mortimer Bennett. Autobiographical sketch in *The World's Sages, Thinkers, and Reformers,* 2nd ed. rev. (New York: Liberal and Scientific Publ. House, 1876), p. 192. "N. Bennett" actually was DeRobigne Mortimer Bennett, who was born on December 23, 1818, died on December 6, 1882, and was received into the New Lebanon Society when he was fourteen years old. He worked in the seed gardens and learned the primitive pharmacy of roots, barks, and herbs. He became the physician of the community fourteen years later and left in 1846. He then became a purveyor of a number of spurious concoctions: Dr. Bennett's Quick Cure, Golden Liniment, Worm Lozenges, and Root and Plant Pills. He was an amalgam of quack, crank, and idealist.

32. Three journals, Philemon Stewart, New Lebanon, 1826–1831, Library of Congress, Washington, D.C.

33. "List of Fluid Extracts," 1871, Library, Shaker Community, Inc., Hancock, Mass.

34. Eldress Betsy Smith's journal, South Union, Ky., 1854, Library of the University of Southern Kentucky.

35. Benson John Lossing, "The Shakers," *Harper's New Monthly Magazine,* vol. 15, no. 86 (1857), 172–75.

36. Account book of the extract herb industry, Church family, New Lebanon, 1860–1862, Andrews Collection, Henry Francis du Pont Museum, Winterthur, Del.

37. Booklet, *Veratrum Viride*, 4th ed. (New York, 1858), Library at Shaker Community, Inc., Hancock, Mass.

38. Formula for tincture of *Veratrum viride*, March 1934. Emma B. King Library, Shaker Museum, Old Chatham, N.Y.

39. Benjamin Gates to "Our Seneca II," and formula for "Pain Killer," n.d., Library at Shaker Community, Inc., Hancock, Mass.

40. Catalogue for Shaker asthma cure, 1886, Cleveland, Western Reserve Historical Society.

41. Chart in account book, n.d., Emma B. King Library, Shaker Collection, Shaker Museum at Old Chatham, N.Y.

42. Peek and Velsor, botanic druggists, to Edward Fowler, Oct. 10, 1877, Williams College Library, Williamstown, Mass.

43. Benjamin Gates to Henry Clough, August 20, 1884, Library at Shaker Community, Inc., Hancock, Mass.

44. Gates to Clough, September 23, 1882.

45. Gates to Clough, October 31, 1885.

46. "David at New Lebanon, to the World" (the people of the world), 1807, Williams College Library, Williamstown, Mass.

47. Journal kept at New Lebanon, anon., 1842, Cleveland, Western Reserve Historical Society.

48. Journal and letters kept at New Lebanon, 1860, Cleveland, Western Reserve Historical Society.

49. Formula for the Shaker digestive cordial, anon., Emma B. King Library, Shaker Museum at Old Chatham, N.Y.

50. Record book kept by James Vail at New Lebanon 1841–1857, Cleveland, Western Reserve Historical Society, Shaker Collection.

51. Sister Marcia Bullard, "Shaker Industries," *Good Housekeeping* (July 1906), 43:33–37.

52. *The Shaker Manifesto*, February 10, 1892, Library at Shaker Community, Inc., Hancock, Mass.

53. Order for herbs, May 9, 1876, Emma B. King Library, Shaker Museum at Old Chatham, N.Y.

54. Almanac, 1882 (New York: A. J. White), Library at Shaker Community, Inc., Hancock, Mass.

55. Vegetable seed catalogues (1881, 1884, 1885, 1887, 1888), Cleveland, Western Reserve Historical Society, Shaker Collection.

56. Amelia J. Calver to Henry Clough, April 23, 1890, Library at Shaker Community, Inc., Hancock, Mass.

57. Alonzo Hollister to "Esteemed Friend," February 19, 1909, Library at Shaker Community, Inc., Hancock, Mass.

58. Martha J. Anderson, "History of Dietetic Reform as Practiced at the North Family, Mt. Lebanon and Canaan, Columbia County, New York," *Food, Home and Garden* (Philadelphia, Jan. 1894), pp. 6–7, Library of Fruitlands Museum, Harvard, Mass.

59. Deaconesses journal, 1843–1864, Library at Shaker Community, Inc., Hancock, Mass.

60. Journal, Church Family (2nd Order), 1858–1867, Library at Shaker Community, Inc., Hancock, Mass.

4. CANAAN, NEW YORK

The Shakers at Canaan, New York, three miles from Mt. Lebanon, originated as the Upper Canaan and Lower Canaan families in 1813 and were fully organized in 1821.

Levi Shaw, a member of the Canaan Upper Family wrote in his journal[1] that he was born November 5, 1818, and came to the Shakers with his father after his mother died when he was six years old. "For the first six years after I came among Believers my occupation was chiefly in the Garden and Garden House, putting up Herbs in the summer season and at school in the winter season. In the fall of 1836 I was apprenticed to take charge of the fruit trees and fruit. In December 1836 I was apprenticed to take charge of the Boys there was then 5 of them in the order."

The South Union ministry traveling in the spring and summer of 1869 record their visit at Canaan on August 4, 1869.[2] "This family is not so well supplied. . . . Has a drying kiln for fruit and sweet corn and a good root cutter run by hand. Cuts roots and pumpkins first rate. . . . The ice cream is fine. . . . Free latitude is granted for sociability without a courtship ever having been started. . . . Dried 89 barrels of sweet corn. They have nearly abandoned the seed and herb business."

Diaries and journals, daybooks and account books kept at Mt. Lebanon indicate that the Canaan families assisted to a considerable extent in the herb department of the larger community. The Deaconesses' journal kept from 1843 to 1864 has numerous entries about gathering herbs at Canaan assisted by that family, and having them help out at Mt. Lebanon.[3]

> May 1846. The 4th. Fruit trees in full bloom. Cherry, Peach, Plum. 5th. Our dinner table today was graced with a noble plate of Pot Herbs, for the first time this season [cowslip greens] 6th. The sisters not other ways engaged commenced cleaning elecompane roots. 13th. The sisters engaged in cleaning roots such as blue flag, angelica. 27th. Rhoda and Fanny go out with Canaan herbing after Squaw Weed.
>
> June 3rd. Three sisters go with Joseph to Canaan after herbs. 10th. We go on the Mountain fishing. 11th. Joseph takes sisters to Canaan after herb and Shoemak [sumac] leaves. July 1846. 3rd. Go after *Johnswort* to Canaan. 6th. To Canaan after Johnswort.
>
> August 1st. 5 sisters spend chief of the day cutting Mayweed. 6th. We have a meeting commemorating our blessed Mother's landing in America. 11th. Go after Shoemake. 13th. Go after *raspberry leaves*. 19th. Sisters all engaged in cleaning roots. Canaan here helping. 20th. Go after laurel leaves. 24th. Clean roots. Canaan helps. 28th. After dinner 15 sisters are

called to cutting sage, balm, etc. 29th. 5 sisters work in the garden picking leaves. 31st. Sisters pick leaves. Canaan here to help.

These and many other records indicate the cooperation that existed between the two societies; when the Canaan Shakers dissolved their communities the remaining members went to Mt. Lebanon.

NOTES

1. Journal of Levi Shaw, n.d., Shaker Collection, Library of Congress, Washington, D.C.

2. Travel record, South Union ministry, 1865–1871, vol. 1, Shaker Collection, Library of University of Southern Kentucky, Bowling Green.

3. A Journal of Domestic Events and Transactions, January 1, 1842, to October 1864, at New Lebanon, N.Y., kept by Deaconesses, Ch[urch]. 2nd order, Library at Shaker Community, Inc., Hancock, Mass.

5. TYRINGHAM AND HANCOCK, MASSACHUSETTS, AND ENFIELD, CONNECTICUT

Charles Nordhoff in his otherwise complete and sensitive account of the Shakers dismisses these two western Massachusetts societies in two short sentences: "The societies at Hancock and Tyringham lie near the New York State line, among the Berkshire hills. They are small and have no noticeable features." The communities at Hancock and Tyringham were established two years apart (1790 and 1792 respectively) and three years after Watervliet and New Lebanon. There was complete and close cooperation, love, and respect among the New York and New England families, and constant business intercourse between them.

The two Shaker communities in Berkshire County, Massachusetts, command beautiful scenic vistas. They lie in fertile valleys separated from New York by the Taconic range and on the east from the rest of Massachusetts by what is commonly called the Berkshire Barrier. Tyringham is 18 miles southeast of Hancock.

TYRINGHAM

In the 83 years the settlement existed at Tyringham, the Believers raised some herbs and gathered many more from the fields and nearby woods for their own use.[1] The square little manuscript of "Hints and Recipes" written by Darias Herrick fills eight numbered pages and includes remedies for every ailment: "For The Thrush. To make one pint. A portion of rattle snake Plantain, A small portion of Fox Glove, A little Crawley, some cloves. A good portion of rose Flowers, The same of Balm Flowers, a portion of Camomile. Steep all together, after straining, add 2 table spoonfuls of Sweet Spirits of nitre [native soda, saltpeter], add a small spoonful of balm Gilliad. Sweeten very Sweet with honey."

Other formulas were given: "For the Jaundice, To take the Mercury out of the Blood, Pills For to Strengthen the System [containing wild turnip, Peruvian bark, whiteroot, burdock seed and button snakeroot, among other ingredients]. Syrups for bleeding at the Longues, For the Gravel, the Disentary, the Erisipelas; How to make Egg Ointment and a poltice for swelled feet." There was a "Tincture of opium and Bl. cohosh for the bite of mad dogs; How to Make a Quick Beer; Powders for a cough and loss of Voice," and a dramatic account of a case of lockjaw and its cure. It concerned a Captain C.

Gardner of Newport who "unfortunately jumped upon a scraggy pointed spike which perforated his boot and foot, and he was taken home in most excrutiating torture. The attending Physician could afford him no relief. Providentially, a woman who heard the above came and caused his foot to be put into the warm Lye. The affect was this, in 15 minutes he was released, went to bed and slept well. The application was made for ten succeeding days when the Capt. could walk abroad."

The Tyringham Shakers raised garden seeds in sufficient quantity to print a catalog in 1826, listing 26 varieties of seeds, priced from 4 to 12 cents per paper.[2] This was issued in broadside form. Another catalog was printed in the 1850s.[3] At the end it advises that all orders for seeds are to be directed to Willard Johnson, Agent, South Lee, Post Office.

At this time the society was very prosperous. There were two settlements, three-quarters of a mile apart, each consisting of two families. The first, or Church, family had the most buildings in it. The largest building was the seed house used for drying and packaging the flower, herb, and vegetable seeds grown in the large gardens. The seed business was their chief source of income, and such was its size that in the seed and herb house a freight elevator ran from the basement to the cupola. A printing press in the same building turned out thousands of herb and seed labels.

HANCOCK

Account books kept by the Hancock Shakers indicate an extremely prosperous seed business. One in particular of 80 pages covers the industry for a period of years starting in 1824 at which time the society had issued its fifth "Catalogue of Garden Seeds."[4] This was a broadside listing 51 seeds and stated: "Merchants and others, who wish to purchase seeds, are requested to forward their orders by the 4th of July preceding the time of sale. Directed to John Wright, agent written in Berkshire County, Mass."[5]

The first of the ten broadsides advertising seeds was issued by the Hancock society in 1813 and listed only four herb seeds: parsley, pepper grass, sage, and summer savory. In subsequent catalogs, only burnet, rue, cayenne pepper, and saffron were listed additionally.[6] A seedman from the world provided some competition from nearby Wethersfield, Conn. (James L. Belden's catalog for 1821 carried 61 varieties of seeds among which were mustard, parsley, cayenne, summer savory, coriander, caraway, sweet fennel, dill, saffron, and sage.[7])

Before the Civil War the herb and seed business at Hancock was averaging a gross annually of more than $7,000, the herb side of this being largely sage which was produced in enormous quantities and sold in leaf and ground. (Most of the sage they sent to New Lebanon for processing.) In 1864 gross receipts for herbs and seeds was $2,922.54 but ten years later income from "seeds, brooms and sage" amounted to only $2,525.

A receipt or formula book kept at Hancock by the Church family from 1828 to 1846 details the making of homemade nostrums and directions for their use.[8] It claimed that they were good for "poor appetite, shortness of breath, pains in all parts of the anatomy, boils, small pox, palpitations, stoppage of water, palsy, diabetes, stones in the bladder, warts and corns, pains of fatality and wounds, not minor, burns and scalds." The botanical material needed to support these concoctions included coriander, bloodroot, mandrake root, Culver's root, boneset, elder, marsh rosemary, Canada thistle, spikenard roots, white pine bark, red clover heads, sarsaparilla, camomile, fleabane, hardhack, wormwood, butternut, elecampane, catnip, roots of wild lettuce, sumac bark, evans'-root, yellow dock, burdock, comfrey, wintergreen, balm of Giliad, smellage, and of course rhubarb.

Mention is made in a history of Berkshire County of seven herbs cultivated in the gardens of the Hancock Shakers.[9] These are Virginia snakeroot, sweet marjoram, foxglove, gayfeather (*Liatris*), angelica, blue cohosh, and *Thea viridis* (green tea). Hancock's economy, like that of other Shaker societies, was based on agriculture and horticulture. According to David Lamson who lived at Hancock during 1847 and 1848 more than 5,000 acres including several outfarms were owned and farmed by the six families.

On November 25, 1867, a journal that was kept in New Lebanon reported that the West family at Hancock was about to break up, "removing to the other families of their village.[10] Hancock . . . was on a mountain side much like the Tyringham community, is a very unprofitable and hard place to support a family, the soil is very cold and wet. The buildings, that is, their foundations, difficult to keep in repair, and they have not able abilities to manage a family there." And so as early as 1867 the community at Hancock began to diminish, but it was probably not very noticeable then to the outside world. The decline until 1960 was gradual. It saddened many of the Shakers' neighbors who had grown to love them.

ENFIELD, CONNECTICUT

When the society at Enfield, Connecticut, dissolved in 1917, many of its members went to live at Hancock. But the community had prospered for most of its 125 years, and, as Eldresses White and Taylor commented, "Enfield has always been rich in men and women of strong character and historic worth." The community had made its living almost entirely by farming its 3,300 acres of land on the east side of the Connecticut River. The members had started a garden-seed business as early as any of the other societies and began to sell herbs in 1825. On its broad sweep of fields the Enfield Shakers also grew tobacco, as did many of their neighbors. This was the large leaf or "wrapper" tobacco and commanded a good price by makers of fine cigars.

A book of "Prescriptions Given by Old Dr. Hamilton, family Physician to the Shakers in Enfield, Conn. in 1825 . . ." included a variety of bitters, pills, elixirs, fever powders, cough pills, and a "Spice Cordial" which combined myrrh, absinthe, nutmeg, oil of peppermint, and pure water.[11] "Shake them well together," the directions read, "this is a tonic for the patient after he leaves the sick room. Take a small glass 3 times a day." "Pills for the head" contained "15 grs. of opium and gum and sapo castilo." The directions were: "Mix to a mass with honey and make into pills, one to be taken 4 times a day, dividing the time." A line filling in the bottom of a page reads: "An infallible worm powder is made mostly of skunk cabbage pulverized and Indian hemproot."

Ten catalogs were published by the Enfield Shakers. One listed "Medicinal Plants, Barks, Roots, Seeds and Flowers, with their Therapeutic Qualities and Botanical Names." Also priced were "Pure Vegetable Extracts and Shaker Garden Seeds, Raised, Prepared and Put Up in the Most Careful Manner. . . . First Established in 1802, being the Oldest Seed Establishment in the United States." Seven broadsides were published in the 1850s listing from 46 items at first to as many as 300 items. The Shakers always carried as many as 17 herb seeds and very often several grass seeds.

Jefferson White was an outstanding seedsman in the society for many years. One broadside carrying his name stated: "Some Seeds such as cannot be raised successfully in this climate are procured from the best sources. Herbs for Medicinal purposes, put up in Pressed packages from the one ounce to the one pound each." He offered herb seeds for caraway, coriander, dandelion, dill, fennel, lavender, lemon balm, rosemary, saffron, sage, clary sage, summer savory, sweet basil, sweet marjoram, sweet thyme, marigold "pot," and rue. White directed this lucrative industry with great enterprise and Enfield became the center for raising and trading in vegetable seeds.

NOTES

1. Darias Herrick, "Hints and Recipes" (1845), pp. 66–67, Cleveland, Western Reserve Historical Society.

2. Seed catalogue, 1826, Emma B. King Library, Shaker Museum at Old Chatham, N.Y.

3. Seed catalogue, 1850, Library of Fruitlands Museum, Harvard, Mass.

4. Account book of the seed business at Hancock, Mass. (1824–1829), 80 pp., Cleveland, Western Reserve Historical Society.

5. Broadside (1813), 1 p., Emma B. King Library, Shaker Museum at Old Chatham, N.Y.

6. Paul W. Gates, Hancock broadside, 1839, *The Farmers' Age, 1815–1860* (New York: Holt, Rinehart & Winston, 1960), facing p. 300.

7. Rudy J. Favretti, *Early New England Gardens* (Meriden, Conn.: Meriden Gravure Co., 1962), p. 14.

8. Receipt book, Church family at Hancock, 1828–1846, Cleveland, Western Reserve Historical Society.

9. Samuel W. Bush, *A History of the County of Berkshire* (Pittsfield, Mass.: 1829), pp. 55, 59, 65, 68, 69, 71, 79.

10. West family journal, New Lebanon, N.Y., 1867, Emma B. King Library, Shaker Collection, Museum at Old Chatham, N.Y.

11. A book of prescriptions given by Dr. Hamilton, family physician to the Shakers, Enfield, Conn., 1825. Cleveland, Western Reserve Historical Society.

6. HARVARD, MASSACHUSETTS

The Shaker community at Harvard had consisted of some 1,800 acres and was located about 30 miles from Boston. High on a hill, it looked due west to Mt. Watchusetts, also in Worcester County, and north to Mt. Monadnock in southern New Hampshire.

Mother Ann went to Harvard in 1781 to preach the gospel, and for two years it remained the center of her religious mission. After the period of severe persecutions had abated and the faithful "gathered," the society was established in 1791 and eventually reached a population of 200. By the time of the early eighteen-forties it was already prosperous from its farming operations and its nursery business. The herb industry was to flourish also and compare favorably with that of Watervliet and New Lebanon, Canterbury and Union Village. An indication of the extent of arboriculture and the nursery business is shown in two journal entries of 1843: "April 28. We take up over five hundred fruit trees to sell" and "May 5. Some of the bretheren set out between three and four thousand small apple and pear trees."[1] A catalog issued some years later by Elijah Myrich listed 21 varieties of apples and 16 varieties of cherries.

The Shakers in Harvard at first, as in other societies, gathered herbs for the preparation of medicine for home use. A journal kept for eight years by the physicians in the society from 1834 to 1842 tells what the medical procedures were and in some cases which herbs were used.[2] It records all the appointments designating nurses and "watchers," those who sat with the very ill 24 hours of the day to nurse and observe any change in condition. It was their duty to give constant care.

> . . . A Statement of the Changes in the Physicians Order from the Gathering of the Church in 1791 to the present time, 1843.
> Sister Sarah Jewett was the first physician. Tabitha Babbit (then a girl) was her assistant. In the autumn of 1810 Salome Barrett succeeded her in the medical dept.

This is the first account of a female physician in the Shaker order.

Vast quantities of material was brought in from woods and swamps. Eventually, as the demand for herbs outside the community increased, fields near the village were cleared and large gardens were planted. But before sufficient quantities could be cultivated, the Shakers made daily excursions for herbs in proper season. In an entry for

January 11, 1824, a journal records searching for herbal material, "mostly for bark."[3]

Sept. 1, 2. 1830. Simon T. A., Mary Babbit, Lucy Clark & Selah Winchester to gather herbs.

June 8, 1831. To Dunstable after herbs.

July 15. To south part of Harvard after herbs.

July 22. To Groton after herbs.

Oct. 31. To Shirley after Uva Ursi, or Bearberry.

Other entries tell of going to Boxborough after herbs and raspberry leaves.

A journal entry for September 16, 1820, is the earliest known reference to the sale of herbs by the Harvard Shakers. From Joseph Hammond's daybook we learn: "Fair, warm and pleasant all day. Wrought preparing herbs to go to Boston. September 21. Fair and pleasant but cool. Wrought with Sisters cutting last of things in Garden such as sweet balm, peppermint, spearmint, and various other small parcels of herbs."[4]

The Harvard Shakers ultimately issued ten bound catalogs, the first in 1845 and the last in 1889, and two broadsides, one in the early 1800s and the other sometime later. Simon T. Atherton was in charge and his first catalog listed 197 medicinal herbs, with eight sweet herbs in canisters, and 13 extracts. He used the common names and botanical names taken from Eaton's last edition; the price per pound and the properties of each herb were given. This was a practice followed in all but the two broadsides and the last catalog under Atherton's direction, which carried the name of his successor in 1889, John Whiteley. These exceptions listed the common name and price only.

The 1849 edition was much the same as its predecessor's but the 1851 issue listed 198 herbs, four sweet herbs in canisters, 13 extracts, and a variety of fruit trees, grape vines, ornamental shrubs, buckthorn hedge plants and seeds, and garden seeds of all kinds, furnished to order.

The catalog for 1853 followed the same pattern. It listed 200 herbs.

In 1853, Simon Atherton had received a great honor from the Massachusetts College of Pharmacy; and he used it as a testimonial in the 1854 catalog:

Boston, Sept. 13, 1853

Mr. Simon T. Atherton, So. Groton, Mass:

Sir:

I have the pleasure to enclose to you a copy of a Resolution passed by the Board of Trustees of the Massachusetts College of Pharmacy in reference to some beautifully cured specimens of Herbs. Their honest quality speaks for itself; and a cursory examination only, will satisfy a judge of such commodities, that they were not mowed down with weeds that had usurped their glory and withdrawn their strength, but that they had been watched and nurtured to a state of perfection rarely equalled and never surpassed.

Very truly yours,

(Signed) Wm. A. Brewer, Rec. Sec.

Boston, September 1, 1835

Massachusetts College of Pharmacy.

Resolved: That the thanks of this College be presented to Simon T. Atherton, for superior specimens of Shaker Herbs, presented this College for their Cabinet, and for the exhibition at the meeting of The American Pharmaceutical Association.

A true copy from the records

Attest:

(Signed) Henry W. Lincoln, Rec. Sec.

On the next page of the catalog Atherton wrote:

Medicinal Herbs prepared in bottles require more labor in preparing and extra care and attention in drying, so as to retain all their valuable properties, which necessarily brings them higher [in cost] by the pound than pressed herbs.

Customers deserving the very best articles prepared in this manner, will have to forward their orders as early in the summer as June, so as to give time for collection in their best condition, and they may rely upon having a superior article, neatly labelled, for $6.00 per doz. quart bottles, or $10.00 per doz. two quart bottles by addressing S. T. Atherton.

The catalog of 1857 offered 213 herbs, for which Atherton gave 167 synonyms stating:

Difficulties having sometimes arisen from the use of the common name being applied to different plants, in different localities, and also from the fact that druggists are frequently called upon for some article which they have, by another name distinct from that by which it is sold under, which they are not aware of, we have appended a list of synonyms, which the seller will please refer to before turning a customer away.

The catalogs of 1860 and 1868 were the same; both listed 212 herbs. In 1873 Atherton offered 213 herbs, but otherwise the catalog did not vary. He issued two broadsides in the eighties as well, listing 226 herbs including sweet marjoram, sage, summer savory, and thyme in cans.

When Simon Atherton died in 1888 at the age of 85 he was succeeded briefly by John Whiteley, as editor of the catalogs and business manager, then the business passed to Elisha Myrick.

The original herb house at Harvard had been a small building, and when the Shakers decided they needed more space, foundations were laid for a new one in 1848. Elisha Myrick wrote a great diary which he started in January 1850.[5] In a preface to round up the business of 1849 he wrote:

This year we cut the timber saw it out at the mill and frame the Herb house ourselves, (the foundation being laid in 1848) get the building so far completed as to be able to occupy the part designed for the herb business Nov. 15th just one year from the day we commenced cutting the timber for the frame. Hire help to cover it [roof it over] and lay two floors and ½ and finish 5 rooms at a cost of about $1800.00 money out.

It also housed a big woodshed where 300 cords of wood were stored for drying herbs.

Arthur T. West who lived with the Shakers at Harvard as a boy from 1884 to 1889 says: "The stone dry-house was where roots were dried by artificial heat. The herb shop was used for stripping, drying by air, and pressing and wrapping the great variety of herbs raised on the broad acres of their estate. There was also the still—no, not what you think, but where rose water was distilled. A very enchanting perfume was made from the real roses."[6]

The daily business of the herb department had been the main occupation of Elisha Myrick who had worked gathering, preparing, and packaging material since he was 11 years old. He was 63 years old when Simon Atherton died. In the first broadside printed as successor to Atherton he wrote:[7]

> Medicinal Herbs, Roots and Compounds were first prepared for the market by the United Society, (called Shakers) in Harvard, Mass. From a small beginning prior to 1820, it has grown to an industry of large commercial importance. These natural remedies have supplanted and retired from use the debilitating nostrums and mineral drugs, and instead of aiding the human assassin, moves directly on the enemies' works, and have become the welcome friends in every household. Much of the success in this business is due to the intelligence and strict integrity of the late Simon T. Atherton, who for more than fifty years has maintained the justly deserved reputation of the genuine *Shaker Herbs*. His motto was "A good name is better than riches." Prime new hops in pound and half pound packages specialty. Call for Shaker Herbs. Also, Rose Water by the Gallon, distilled from Roses. For sale by Wholesale Druggists in Boston and by the Society.

> > E. Myrick, Trustee
> >
> > Successor to the late Simon T. Atherton
> >
> > P.O. address, Ayer, Mass.

Elisha Myrick also wrote in his preface, concerning 1849, that:

> The business this year is carried on by Elisha Myrick, aged 25, and George B. Whitney, aged 22, with the assistance of Isaac Myrick to gather herbs out from home and two sisters to pick over the herbs . . . We do our pressing and keep our stock of pressed herbs at the Ministry's barn and pick our herbs and do other work at the yellow house. We distilled 165 gallons of peach water and made 134 pounds of ointment, 49 gallons of buckthorn syrup and pressed between February 14, 1849 and February 14, 1850, 10,152 pounds of herbs, roots, etc.
>
> The sales for 1849 including all the herbs, and delivered to agents amount to $4,042.31 net. We raise, gather and prepare this year 5,788 pounds of herbs, barks, roots, etc. which is 800 pounds more than was ever collected before.

The last entry, for 1852, notes that "amounts of herbs sold and delivered to agents the past year at 45% off leaving net, $8300." This was double the amount he recorded for 1849.

Excerpts for the years 1850, 1851, and 1852, in the daybook, describe the organization of the business, the herbs handled, the agents dealt with, and the territory covered.

> Jan. 3–9. Elisha works at work bench in the Herb House, packing herbs to go to Boston. . . . Sent some dock root to the mill to be cracked. . . . Commence posting accounts for the agents in Boston. . . . Elisha brings Bills from the Cost Keeper and Office Granary to the Herb House. . . . The Stoves came down from Fitchburg and were brought from the depot. . . . Elisha puts up the Stoves and a lot of herbs for S. W. Fowle and does some writing. After meeting we make 3 herb boxes and Elisha works all night packing and makng out bills.
>
> Jan. 14–31. Elisha up at 3 o'clock in the writing and putting up his herbs. . . . Simon brought 2 bushels of Sage from the Depot and Abel 3 bushels of dock root from the Grist mill. . . . Elisha finishes drawing off last year's accounts. Commences in the new books.

. . . Elijah brought two tubs of horehound from the depot, and a lot of empty boxes. . . . Elisha puts some dampers in the stove pipes in the press and counting rooms, puts up an order to go to Worcester and picks over some Buck Bean. . . . Elisha is up at 4 o'clock putting up herbs to go to Boston. After breakfast goes over to the Grist to carry roots to town. . . . Three sisters pick over dry sage in the evening. . . . Elisha chopping dry herbs. Abel brot 4 bushes of Wormwood and 4 Dock Root from the Depot. . . . Elisha at the herb house all day put up 5 bushels sage to be ground. Sent 1 bushel leaf sage to T. Corbett. Sent 4 bushels of Dock to the Grist mill. Had it cracked. Sent 1 bushel of dock to Providence and put up prepared herbs for the agents in Boston, Salem, and Providence. Simon brot 4 bushels of sage in leaf from the Depot. . . . Elisha goes to the North family and gets 104 pounds of Green Horseradish Root cuts it up and puts it into the Oven to dry for E. S. C. Boston. . . . Elisha papers pressed sage in the A.M. A. Blaisdell of Boston here to make a contract for herbs. . . . Elisha papers Spearmint and packs 5 large boxes of herbs for A. Blaisdell & Co. Boston.

The months of February and March were extremely active filling and labeling cans (63 in one afternoon), sending off orders to Boston and Worcester, and one particular shipment to Charles Dyer in Providence of two barrels of dock root and one of dandelion, all valued at $107.73 net. On February 20 Elisha went to Boston to see about a press and was home the next day and putting up orders. On the 27th he finished putting up 669 boxes of horseradish, which had been dried and ground, also three barrels of dandelion root. One day "after meeting in the evening we got some help and put up 18 dozen large cans of thyme till 12 o'clock."

In March orders were received from William Underwood of Boston, among others, one gross large cans of sage repeated several times during the month. On the 6th "Elijah brot 1,073 pounds of green Horse Radish Root from the depot and dry and ground. . . . March 11th. Put up 4 bushels, 111 pounds of Motherwort and 12 pounds of Bayberry leaves for Chauncey Miller, Watervliet. Put up herbs the remainder of the day to go to Boston." The next day he put up 2 gross small cans of thyme for Underwood and "the Irishmen put the Horseradish in cans labelled and prepared it to go; 980 cans." Elecampane and pennyroyal were papered and ground to a fine consistency.

April 1–14. . . . Build fire in kiln to dry horseradish. . . . Make out bills. In P.M. go to the Corporation Paper Mills after paper. . . . Put up 1 gross small cans Summer Savory for Underwood. Paper some horseradish. . . . Sift 100 pounds Dwarf Elder Root. . . . Work on Herb boxes. Send the Radish Root to the mill to be ground and home again. . . . Put up 560 cans of Horse Radish with the help of some small boys. . . . FAST. After meeting do some cleaning up back of Herb House. . . . Get some help and put up 48 dozen cans for Underwood, work some in the evening. Wrote a letter to S. W. Bullock. . . . Finished making herb boxes for this year. Made 100. 50 past done, making 150 Total.

April 15. Up at 3 o'clock to put up an order to go to Worcester by express. Put up 12 doz. large cans Marjoram and some small orders to go all over the lots.

April 17. Prepared the hot beds for use.

April 22. We repair the centre part of the double press which was liable to fail. . . . Two Irishmen came here this morning and we set them to washing Radish Root. Wrote a letter to S. W. Bullock, N.Y. City ordered up a press.

April 30. Took up two waggon loads of sage roots and carried them over to John Blanchard to cultivate for us this year. He is to cut it and bring it to us green and after it is dried he is to have seven cts. per lb.

May 4. Plowed the garden with horses.

May 10. Help Mary whitewash the herb house interior.

May 11. Sow Hollyhocks and sweet balm seeds.

May 13. Sow Jerusalem Oak, Poppy seed and Lavender and do some hoeing and cultivating.

May 14. Sow Dock seed, Marshmallow, Pennyroyal seed. Do some plowing, hoeing, etc.

May 15. Sowed Horehound seed. . . . To Groton to engage John Boynton to raise Dock Root for 8 cts. per lb. dry and Dandelion Root for 10 cts. per., dry.

May 16. Put up 30 doz. cans for Underwood.

May 22. Finish the writing desk for use. Put up 150 pounds of Fine Elm in pound papers.

May 24. Peel White Oak Bark in the Ox Pasture woods.

May 30. Cut 500 pounds of Sarsaparilla Root, 200 pounds of Sage.

Work during the month of June was much the same, but there were fewer entries. The entries for the summer months of July, August, and September were short and to the point and were contained in six pages of the daybook. Most of the herbs they gathered were catnip, caraway, feverfew, cicuta roots, tansy, wormwood, sweet balm, hardhack leaves, and sumac.

August 6. Commence packing poppy leaves. Cut thyme 5 sheets full.

August 21. Seven sisters and four brethren go out beyond the depot to pick Wintergreen. Get a small quantity.

August 22. Cut the pennyroyal and the thyme.

August 24. Cultivate all the gardens. Spread 30 loads of manure.

August 31. Cut the savory. Put up some orders [a very large one for Underwood]. Set up the still.

Sept. 2. Put up three kettles of peach leaves. Cut the lavender.

Sept. 11. A company of brethren and sisters go to Chelmsford to pick Wintergreen.

Sept. 26. Pound Savin for Ointment. Cut up a lot of Savory.

Sept. 27. Make Savin Ointment at the North House. Put up a barrel of Thyme in cans.

Sept. 28. Finish the Ointment. 155 lbs.

Sept. 30. Pick the Buckthorn Berries, 1½ bushels. Prepare the juice and put up 16 doz. cans to go to New Bedford.

Oct. 1. Make the buckthorn syrup and put up two hundred cans of herbs.

Oct. 3. Go to Leominster in pursuit of herbs.

Oct. 5. Put up 730 ounces of peach water and rose water to go to New York. A great number of herbs, etc. sent to Underwood.

Oct. 21. Go after chestnuts, put up two gross one half cans of sage for Underwood and prepare a lot of herbs, etc.

Nov. 2. Press yellow dock root all day—311 pounds prepared and 48 more in the press, making 359 in all.

Nov. 5. Put up three barrels of dock root to go to Rhode Island.

Nov. 29. Weigh off a lot of herbs bought by a man by the name Vormund Hoyt, of Canada.

10,767 pounds pressed in 1850	
Sold herbs amount to	$3768.18
Delivered to agents	2305.06
Total amount of sales in 1850	$6073.24 net.

Feb. 16, 1851. Elisha takes up the horseradish root in the dryhouse and carries it to the grist mill and gets it ground, also three barrels of dandelion root.

Feb. 26. We work till eleven o'clock in the evening putting up cans of horseradish to go to California.

March 25. Up at two o'clock putting up orders to go to Boston.

May 30. Cut 500 pounds sarsaparilla root and 200 pounds sage.

July 8. Cut horehound and catnip and motherwort.

July 18. Cut the canary seed.

July 31. Hoe the burdock and henbane for the first time in the west garden; slough the carrot field for dandelions.

April 8, 1852. The sisters help cut up some herbs to go to New London.

April 30. Set out wormwood, marshmallow, and thyme roots.

May 2. Transplant hyssop and feverfew to the west garden. Transplant horehound and sage.

Sept. 13. Commence making ketchup in the new furnaces. Cut the marshmallow and sweet marjoram and rue seed. Isaac got a load of life everlasting.

Oct. 24. Put up pumpkin in cans.

Nov. 7. Put up cans of thyme.

Nov. 10. Fill 1,000 cans of summer savory.

Nov. 28. Put up 200 cans of flour of pumpkin. Pack a lot of orders to go to New York.

Christmas Day. After the solemnities of the day are past I paper a lot of herbs.

Dec. 31. This day of the year 1851 closes forever. We have had some hot weather, some cold, some wet, some dry—we have had some joys, some sorrows, some prosperity, and some adversity.

Sold in Worcester and Providence	$ 514.09
Sold to sundry customers	2565.61
Delivered to agents	2573.74
	$5653.44

Elisha Myrick began a new daybook in 1852:

Feb. 16, 1852. Put up ten pounds fine lily root and one hundred pounds ground sage in pound papers. Pack $200. worth of pressed herbs to go to Wilson, Fairbanks & Co. for the California order. Send some herbs to the agents.

Feb. 18. Pack four large boxes of prepared herbs to fit out Weeks & Potter, Boston, who have taken the agency.

In one week 1596 pounds of herbs are pressed. In the year brought in $8300.14.

March 13. 1853. Pack $7500 worth cans of ground herbs for Underwood.

March 14. Pack $7500 worth cans for Davis, Boston.

March 16. Pack $200. worth of prepared herbs to go to Wilson, Fairbanks & Co. for the California order.

March 23. Finish the hops and commence pressing for an order to go to London, England.

March 24. Press 250 pounds and pack 79 different varieties of two pounds each to go to London.

Aug. 11. Take up the poppy capsules and work the dandelion root and cut some thorn apple leaves for ointment.

Aug. 16. We go with a number of sisters to the intervale to collect a load of hardhack. Gather boneset in the swamp. Isaac gets a load of queen-of-the-meadow.

Sept. 20. Make buckthorn syrup.

An honor came to Elisha in 1857 from England.[8] It was a scroll with the handsome royal seal, lions rampant supporting *Dieu et Mon Droit,* at the top of the parchment and it read in print and stylish hand lettering:

ROYAL GARDENS KEW
THE DIRECTOR BEGS TO CONVEY TO
ELISHA MYRICK, ESQUIRE

The best acknowledgements of the Commissioners of her Majesty's Woods and for the undermentioned contribution; Viz:

An interesting set of Extracts of vegetable Pharmaceutical subject,—which together with a large collection of the prepared Herbs in cakes, and deposited in the Museum of Economic Botany.

W. J. Hooker
Director

Royal Gardens, Kew
August 26, 1857

The Shakers of Harvard and other communities had made large shipments of botanical material to England.

Enfield, Connecticut, "shipped out 16 boxes of a variety of herbs for England. . . . paid freight in Springfield."

An account book detailing the work of the "Herb Branch of the Medical Dept" from January 1847 to December 1853 shows that the business had grown sufficiently to warrant the purchase of a new and larger herb press in 1848.[9] This was the press mentioned by a sister from South Union, Kentucky, who visited Harvard in 1869: "They carry on the herb business to a considerable extent; have a remarkably good press, built under the superintendance of an ingenious young man who resided here, but is now a celebrated draughtsman in the city of Washington. This herb business is one of their principal resources, but is now meeting with considerable competition."[10]

Year by year the Shakers of Harvard covered more territory. Selling was brisk each fall on Cape Cod, and in Providence and South Providence, Rhode Island. The Worcester route was greatly enlarged and more hotels were listed for orders. The Adams House and the Quincy House in Boston were steady customers sending in large orders for a variety of culinary herbs, especially for sage.

The account book lists herbs sold to chemists, doctors, "Thomas Corbett and other Societies" and "July 1, 1850 herbs sold to Indian Doctor. $2.90." The total for seven years as recorded in this one book was $33,706.70. (This figure was the gross income.) There are many entries for herbs bought from other societies for home use or for resale. Those communities that were mentioned selling herbs to Harvard were Watervliet ("bought from Chauncey Miller: burdock root, rue and lovage root") and Shirley, New Lebanon, and Tyringham. Yellow dock was purchased in large quantities from the Enfield, New Hampshire, society. Thomas Corbett of Canterbury sold herbs to Harvard and also bought considerable amounts from them: "settled with T. Corbett for short weight on dandelion root."

A Journal of Domestic Work of Sisters, Kept by the Deaconesses, from February 1867 to April 1876, describes what the Sisters' duties were in the department:

> May 29. Cleaning at the Herb house. Some halibut comes tonight.
>
> June 7. Cut some celandine today, pick it over, the first herb this year. Elen, the Irish woman came and helped. We have some fresh halibut and mackerel. Elder Grove and Brother John get some butternut bark this afternoon.
>
> July 4. Independence. Have green pease for dinner.
>
> July 5. The Sisters are picking herbs and poppys.

All during the month of July there are daily entries "picking herbs . . . a great deal of picking to do, herbs, pease, beans and currants. We are going our common rounds." The August records are about the same: "herbs, herbs, herbs, picking over herbs." And finally, "Sept. 30. Finished picking over herbs for this season."

Records for the next years are predictably the same and kept with meticulous care; not always in the same hand or with equal enthusiasm.

> May 22. Clean out the herb house. . . .
>
> July 14. Very warm, begin to pick the peppermint.
>
> July 18. Pick spearmint.
>
> July 21. Picking over wormwood and rue. Herbs, herbs, herbs.
>
> Sept. 1. Picking over Queen-of-the-Meadow.
>
> Sept. 25. We cut coriander seed this week.
>
> Jan. 2. 1869. Papering herbs this week.
>
> Jan. 13. Work in Herb house.
>
> May 7. Clean Herb House.
>
> June 28, 1871. Herbs, herbs, herbs, a plenty of them for all hands.
>
> July 6. Begin to pick over sage.
>
> August 12, 1875. Catnip, catnip, nothing but catnip.
>
> August 13. Very muggy and warm, catnip.
>
> August 21. Catnip. Elder John brought an editer and his wife here. Catnip.
>
> August 30. Horehound.
>
> Sept. 2. Sage, sage, the Eldress came.
>
> Sept. 3. Work on sage. The Ministry Sisters come.
>
> Sept. 8. All hands work on horehound.

Sept. 9. Work on horehound. Elder Henry Blinn from Canterbury come. We see Elder Henry some, he goes at noon. Horehound and rue.

Sept. 23. Finish horehound and rue. Have fresh fish for dinner.

Orders from many big companies in Boston and in the Providence and Worcester areas are listed in account books from January 1879 through the year 1888.[12] Deliveries were made in March soon after the devastating blizzard of 1888. S. S. Pierce of Boston placed monthly orders for sage, thyme, marjoram, sweet savory, five dozen cans at a time, and gallons of rosewater. Park and Tilford of New York City bought about the same amount of sage and thyme and placed orders for 106 pounds of hops at a time as well as rosewater by the hundreds of gallons. A typical order they placed with the Shakers included 27 to 35 cans of thyme, sage, marjoram, savory, peppermint, and horehound pulverized or ground fine.

The Shakers at Harvard had a very good account with the Deerfoot Farm Co., makers of sausage. Their buyer, W. W. Rogers, had orders filled in November and December 1885, as an example, for 289 pounds of kiln dried sage, "in stem, fine and powdered." In 1886 Mr. Rogers bought 295 pounds; in 1887, 220 pounds; and on January 10, 1888, Mr. Rogers purchased for Deerfoot Farms 668 pounds of sage, in stem and ground.

Other companies doing business with the Harvard Shakers over a long period of years were the F. W. Hensman and Co. of Augusta, Maine, which ordered quantities of lobelia in bulk and pressed; Cheney and Myrick, Boston; Howe and French, and Peek and Velson, New York. In all, 266 accounts were active from 1879 to 1888 and a prodigious amount of material was shipped out.

However, the herb business began to decline in the eighteen-nineties. It is mentioned in "Home Notes from Harvard" in a Manifesto for February 1892 as being "ably managed," but account books concentrate more on the sale of brooms, and Shakers recorded fewer companies and doctors sending in orders for herbs. Henry S. Norse writing the history of Harvard, Massachusetts, in 1893 says of the Shakers:[13]

> Financially the Society is very prosperous and has invested savings. Its resources and support have been largely derived from horticulture farming and the sale of standing wood and timber. Brooms are manufactured to the value of six or seven hundred dollars, yearly and herbs are pressed and packed for the retailers, the sale of which amounts to seven or eight thousand dollars per annum. Eight or ten laborers are permanently employed, besides the members of the community. The chief farm product from which an income is arrived is milk. This is sent to the Boston Market, though the sisters make all the butter used. The variety of herbs, barks, leaves, roots and flowers used for culinary or medicinal purposes, here dried and ground or pressed, packed and labeled, is very large. Many are cultivated or gathered upon the premises, others are bought by the bale. A boiler of ample capacity and a small engine furnish heat and power for the herb-packing department, laundry and dairy, all of which are provided with the most recent scientific and labor saving machinery and economic devices. A very large business was done in the raising and packing of garden seeds; the making of cider, applesauce and the drying and preserving of fruit; in the braiding of palm leaf and straw; the knitting of hosiery.

Writing in the last years of the Shakers at Harvard Clara Endicott Sears asked one of the Believers: "Eldress where has the fervor gone and all the ardor and enthusiasm, and all the spiritual fire that swayed these men and women? The wind or the Spirit has swept through this place and borne the soul of it away on its wings. Only the outer shell of what was here remains to designate the spot through which it passed."

And she answered: "But nothing that has gone before is lost. The Spirit has its periods of moving beneath the surface, and after generations pass, it sweeps through the world again and burns the chaff and stubble."[14]

NOTES

1. Clara Endicott Sears, *Gleanings From Old Shaker Journals* (Boston: Houghton Mifflin Co., 1916), p. 235.

2. Physician's journal, January 1, 1834–November 8, 1842, Cleveland, Shaker Collection, Western Reserve Historical Society.

3. Journal kept by the Sisters of the Church family, Harvard, Mass. (1824), Library of Fruitlands Museum, Harvard, Mass.

4. Daybook kept by Joseph Hammond, May 1, 1820–July 15, 1822, Harvard Society, Harvard, Mass., Library of Fruitlands Museum, Harvard, Mass.

5. Elisha Myrick, *Day Book kept for the Convenience of the Herb Department*, Harvard Church 1850, Harvard, Mass., Library at Shaker Community, Inc., Hancock, Mass.

6. Arthur T. West, "Reminiscences of Life in a Shaker Village," *The New England Quarterly* (June 1938), p. 347.

7. Broadside, Elder Simon T. Atherton's picture on cover, Library of Fruitlands Museum, Harvard, Mass.

8. Scroll from Kew Gardens acknowledging contribution of herbs from Elisha Myrick, 1857, Library of Fruitlands Museum, Harvard, Mass.

9. Account Book, herb branch of medical department, January 1947–December 1853, Harvard, Mass. Andrews Collection, Library of Henry Francis du Pont Museum, Winterthur, Del.

10. Travel journal, Ministry of South Union, Ken., May 1, 1869–September 1869, Shaker Collection, Library of Congress, Washington, D.C.

11. A Journal of Domestic Work of Sisters, Kept by the Deaconesses, February 1867–April 1876, Library of Fruitlands Museum, Harvard, Mass.

12. Account Book, January 1879–1888, Harvard, Mass., Church family, Library of Fruitlands Museum, Harvard, Mass.

13. *History of the Town of Harvard, Massachusetts*, printed for Warren Hapgood, 1894, Library of Fruitlands Museum, Harvard, Mass., p. 257.

14. Clara Endicott Sears, *Gleanings From Old Shaker Journals* (Boston: Houghton Mifflin Co., 1916), p. XII.

7. SHIRLEY, MASSACHUSETTS

The first step to greatness is to be honest.

Manifesto, January 1887

There was a saying common in that part of
the country that when you bought Shaker
garden seeds you were sure what you were
paying for.

Clara Endicott Sears

Garden seeds were one of the several prosperous industries the Shakers conducted at Shirley, which supported "Harvard's twin sister" during its 116-year existence. Over the years the society acquired some 2,000 acres of farmland including several outlying farms; one 40 miles away in lower New Hampshire was used to graze stock during the summer. The raising and selling of cattle produced a steady income for many years, but the largest income was from garden seeds.

Two years after the community was organized, the Reverend William Bentley of Salem, Massachusetts, in July 1795 visited the "Pleasant Garden," its spiritual name. He[1] reported that, although the soil was not good, the cultivation was the best; that there were two fields of 30 acres each planted to rye, a large field of corn, and that "their flax was in admirable order."

The Shakers enlarged their garden-seed business, and they converted fields they had previously mowed for hay to cultivate and plant the seed plants. The production of seeds was first mentioned in a record book kept by Asa Brocklebank, dated August 5, 1805. His first entry states: "We begin to make seed bags."[2] The seeds raised for sale then included 14 for vegetables and six for herbs, those being caraway, parsley, sage, saffron, lavender, and summer savory. By December 24, 1815, Asa records that balm, fennel, and burnet also were being sold.

Another gardener's daybook of 1806 lists 65 firms and individuals the Shirley brethren were doing business with for a total income of $1835.18, "before discount."[3]

Asa Brocklebank's journal presents a picture of ceaseless activity and substantial accomplishments.

Nov. 29, 1805. We stamp bags. 21 vegetables, lavendar, sage, parsley.

Dec. 31. The amount of garden seed sold this year we find to be $1062.

January 1806. Brothers selling in Bolton, Lynn, Groton, Lancaster and Boston.

Feb. 26. Oliver Burt and Joshua go to Boston and stay three days. [This was unusual as the trips were seldom more than one day.]

May the first. Asa goes to Harvard in the morning to inform Elder Eleaser [Rand] that Deacon Daniel Goodrich has come from Hancock.

May 4–7. Spent raking and hoeing in the new garden and Herb garden.

May 16. Oliver goes to Lancester with the widow Burt [his mother] Plough Vine Ground [vineyards] and sow peppergrass, sage and parsley.

May 24. Oliver does what he has a mind to.

June 4. Mother Lucy [Wright] arrives here at half past 2 o'clock. [This remarkable woman had been appointed "to lead in the female line" succeeding Mother Ann and served for 25 years at Mt. Lebanon.] Oliver kills worms in the garden. Sister Ruth gathers two quarts of worms, but will not kill them and so she scolds them to death.

Herbs were gathered and raised to be made into medicines for the family's use at Shirley and were carefully collected and processed, but the Shakers' herb business did not comprise an industry as extensive as their garden seed business. A broadside dated in ink 1810 is probably the earliest catalog to be issued by the Shakers in Shirley.[4] It lists 28 garden seeds of which six are herbs. Other broadsides were issued in 1826, 1830, and 1855, offering 43 seeds.

A handwritten book of formulas is dated Shirley Village, July 12, 1866, and was prepared for the use of the "Nurse-Sisters at The Infirmary."[5] It contains seven "Medical prescriptions given by an Indian Spirit Doctor named Pohatton, through James Parker of Shirley Village to G. B. Blanchard." There are remedies for gallstones; for the blood, stomach, and liver; and for a bad back. The ingredients include onion juice, angelica root, bark of the root of prickly ash, bitterwort, seneca, bloodroot, cayenne pepper, brandy, lobelia pods and seeds, burdock leaves, and good pure water.

Shirley supplied planed board for herb boxes for Harvard, according to Elisha Myrick's journal, and could be counted on to supply "green herbs." Thus, 200 pounds of hops were delivered to Harvard in February 1851. The "twin sister" was supportive to Harvard rather than competitive.

NOTES

1. Diary of Rev. William Bentley, D.D., Gloucester, Mass., 1962, vol. 2, pp. 149–51, Peter Smith Collection, Yale University Library, New Haven, Conn.

2. Record book, Asa Brocklebank, 1805, Library of Fruitlands Museum, Harvard, Mass.

3. Record book, 1806, Library of Fruitlands Museum, Harvard, Mass.

4. Broadside, garden seeds, 1810, signed by Oliver Burt, Shirley Society, Williams College Library, Williamstown, Mass.

5. "Medical Formulae Prepared for the Use of the Nurse-Sisters at The Infirmary, Shirley Village, July 12, 1866," Library of Fruitlands Museum, Harvard, Mass.

8. CANTERBURY, NEW HAMPSHIRE

Henry Clay Blinn described his beloved home as being located on gently rising ground, overlooking most of the surrounding country, "high up on the Canterbury hills, twelve miles northwest of the beautiful City of Elms— Concord, the capital of the state." Love for his Shaker home grew from the first sight of it when he went there as a boy of 14 against protests of his friends in Providence, Rhode Island. They thought "the wild scheme of going among the mountains of New Hampshire" and with such strange people was not only folly, but also extremely dangerous.

His first impression of the village never left his mind and as a talented Shaker teacher, botanist, bee-keeper, journalist, printer, and dentist this dedicated elder returning from the many journeys which were a part of the ministry's life always thrilled with pride and expectation as he had on that youthful trip in 1838.

Writing about the occasion later he said: "On reaching this last elevated spot, the whole of the Church Family was presented to view and the presentation was a beautiful picture on the mind. At that date, the white and yellow houses with bright red roofs, heightened the beauty of the village very much and to my mind, after a long and tedious journey, it seemed to be the prettiest place I had ever seen."

Isaac Hill, writing in his paper *The Farmer's Monthly Visitor*,[1] gave a full account of the Shakers' botanical medicine industry:

> The Botanic garden and Herbiary at the Shakers' first family contains probably a greater variety of the useful medicinal plants than any other establishment of the kind in New England. This garden was commenced by Thomas Corbett, one of the family and a self taught botanist and physician, twenty-four years old; it has been enlarged by the introduction of new species and new varieties until it covers a full acre and a half. We have before us a catalogue of Medicinal Plants and Vegetable Medicines prepared in the United Society of Canterbury, N.H. "printed at Shaker Village" (for they print here as well as perform almost every other mechanical business) consisting of about two hundred varieties. When this business was first commenced by Dr. Corbett the editor of the Visitor well remembers the aid he gave him in the way of his vegetable preparations in connexion with the celebrated Rocking Truss invented by the same self-taught disciple of Aesculapius. The trusses have since become extensively used, and are one of the very best articles of the kind that were ever invented to alleviate the pains of humanity. The vegetable preparations have grown annually into an establishment probably more extensive than any other in the United States. The vegetables were introduced in the shape of dried leaves pressed into a solid cake

weighing a specific quantity, in shape like a brick. When these articles of different kinds, such as chamomile, coltsfoot, elecampane, goldthread, horehound, johnswort, rose flowers, saffron, sage, summer savory, and the like were first introduced and left at the apothecary stores in Boston, they were the food of merriment to some of the regular physicians. Gradually, however, Dr. Corbett has succeeded in their introduction until the prejudice of the doctors has been so far conquered that many of the faculty are constantly applying for them. The medical establishment at the Shakers is not confined to articles raised by themselves— they purchase all the varieties of vegetable articles of extensive use in the materia medica. As a single item of purchase at one time was mentioned six tons of the *ulmus fulva* or bark of slippery elm, which was procured from the northern part of Vermont and Canada. This article, like many other barks and roots, is pulverized into fine flour and pressed into pound cakes; it is a most valuable medicine to be used in inflammation of the mucus membrane, in catarrhs, influenza, pleurisy, dysentery, strangury, and inflammation of the stomach and bowels.

   Not only as medicine, but as articles of extensive family use in cooking, are the preparations of vegetables invented by the Shakers, two of which are of great value to the inhabitants of cities; they are *sage* and *summer savory*, two articles of vegetable growth which impart the finest flavor to various items of cookery. They are preserved and pressed into that compact form that they may be carried anywhere and used with as much convenience as a compressed hand or roll of manufactured tobacco. In all these productions and preparations, as in almost every other enterprise they undertake, the Shakers find their account to be a constant gain. If others undertake to imitate their inventions and improvements, by the time their articles are finished, they will find the United Brethren in advance of them in some other improvement which always makes theirs to be preferred.

   Mr. Hill also wrote about some of the other brethren who were responsible in the matters concerning farming:

   William Tripure the Botanist who has the personal charge of the Botanic Garden, and who at the same time practices physic in the Shaker families, the individuals of which seldom need medicine of any kind, was taken by the Shakers when very young, a poor boy from Elliot in the State of Maine. Probably there is not the second individual in the United States of his age who had so extensive a practical knowledge of botany as this young man. There is not a plant in the herbiary that he cannot give both its common and its botannical name with a description of its peculiar qualities. This young man takes upon himself a large share of the personal labor of the Botanic garden; he excused himself for the few weeds that had recently got under way in it by saying, that as they were short-handed on the farm he had been at work haying a greater part of the time for four weeks. The Botanist is making the experiment on his garden of the efficacy of the oil manure. He had planted side by side, three hills of medicinal beans. One hill he manured with peat and a solution of potash—another with vault manure—and the third with oil; the second hill was larger and more vigorous than that manured with peat; and the hill manured with oil was three times as large as either of the others.

   The first medicine herb catalog prepared in the Canterbury society was printed in 1835.[2] This catalog offered 180 herbs, with common botanical names and the price per pound, and 12 extracts: butternut, cicuta, clover head, cow parsnip, dandelion, garget or poke, henbane, garden lettuce, nightshade, poppy, thorn apple, and thoroughwort. Any other kinds not mentioned could be made to order. Oils made from cedar, fir, goldenrod, snakeroot, wormwood, and wormseed were listed.

   Three compound syrups were offered: Syrup of Liverwort, "a safe and valuable medicine for coughs, spitting of blood and consumption," Syrup of Black Cohosh, "one of the most powerful deobstruents, and alternatives in the vegetable kingdom; and as such has proved an effectual remedy in rheumatism, gout, chronic lameness; and in scrofulous, glandular and eruptive diseases," and Syrup of Sarsaparilla, "taken in doses of an ounce, four or five times a day, will fulfill every indication that the boasted panaceas and catholicons can perform; is free from the mercurial poison such nostrums contain; and is much more safe and efficient as a medicine for cleansing and purifying the blood."

Other medicines listed in this 1835 catalog are similar to those in the early catalogs issued by the Watervliet and New Lebanon societies.

"We recognize Vegetable Antidyseptic Restorative Wine Bitters, a superior tonic guaranteed "to restore the appetite, tone up the stomach, dispel torpid feelings and headache and warm the system." Vegetable Bilious Pills, Digestive or Stomach Pills, and Vegetable Rheumatic Pills were listed with familiar ingredients, much the same as those offered by other societies. The Rheumatic pills were endorsed by six doctors, who stated: "This may certify that the subscribers have examined by request the formula for the Vegetable Rheumatic Pills made by Doctor Thomas Corbett of the United Society of Shakers at Canterbury, New Hampshire, and having compared it with that for the celebrated Dean's Rheumatic Pills, are of opinion, that the substitution of 'Extracts' in the former, for the vegetables in substance in the latter, with some alterations, gives to his formula a decided preference as a mild and efficient cathartic over that of Dean's."

Other medicines listed were:

Cephalic Pills; Vegetable Cough Pills; Bitter Root, highly valued by the Southern Indians; Compound Emetic of Lobelia; Flour of Slipper Elm; A Chemical Liniment for bruises, sprains, rheumatism, pain in the neck, chilblains, etc.; Nitrous Salts, a new and valuable medicine for physic in fevers, influenzas and colds and also in St. Anthony's fire and most kinds of eruptive diseases. In cases where the food lays hard on the stomach, it is an infallible remedy; and Beth Root [trillium] one of the mildest but most efficient remedies in Haemoptysis as well as all kinds of hemorrhage.

A broadside printed a few years later listed 200 herbs with common and botanical names, but the next bound catalog was not issued until 1847. The back cover listed the Reimproved Rocking Trusses, "Single, Double, and Umbilical adapted to all ages and sexes, for the relief and permanent cure of Hernia, or Rupture; invented, manufactured, applied and sold in the United Society of Shakers, in Canterbury, N.H. All orders to be addressed to Thomas Corbett." The ointments offered were bone or Kittredge, savin and thorn apple. Sweet marjoram, sage, summer savory, and thyme were sold in canisters, small and large. Without giving specific ingredients five syrup compounds by the gallon bottle were listed. They were called black cohosh, liverwort, poppy, sarsaparilla, and wild cherry pectoral.

The Shakers published their catalog in 1848, which was similar to their last one, but it also carried a detailed description of Corbett's Compound Concentrated Syrup of Sarsaparilla, and four pages of signed testimonials from physicians and agents. David Parker, trustee for the community, claimed that Corbett's syrup of sarsaparilla was composed entirely of vegetables and herbs. One ounce of pure iodide of potassium was added to every twelve bottles "to insure a pure article." The society stated that the formula was a combination of the roots of sarsaparilla, dandelion, yellow dock, mandrake, black cohosh, garget, Indian hemp, and the berries of juniper and cubeb. He further stated that "this medicine had proved to be most valuable in the following diseases: chronic inflammation of the digestive organs, dyspepsia of indigestion, jaundice, weakness and sourness of the stomach, rheumatism, salt rheum, secondary syphilis, functional disorders of the liver, chronic eruptions of the skin, and all scrofulous diseases. Also it is found to be an invaluable remedy for the erysipelas, and the distressing disorder of asthma. It has proved highly beneficial in some cases of dropsy, dysentery, and diarrhea."

Thomas Corbett was not a doctor, but took up the study of medicine in 1813 when he was 33 years old at the request of the leaders in his community. Brother Thomas became known as a good physician outside the Shaker boundaries, and built up a large and profitable business in pressed herbs, pills, and syrups. Corbett's Shaker Vegetable Family Pills, "that medicine which goes slowly and without irritation along the intestinal canal," was endorsed by the celebrated Professor of Surgery of Dartmouth College, Dr. Dixi Crosby, who helped Corbett work out the sarsaparilla formula.

Corbett's Wild Cherry Pectoral Syrup was also endorsed by several distinguished doctors and was said to have been given their highest commendations.

The following account from the *Granite Monthly*, for September 1885, gives the best of many descriptions of the origin and ingredients of this medicine:[3]

> Some fifty years ago Dr. Dixi Crosby, the celebrated physician of Hanover (New Hampshire), gave his counsel and advice to the Shakers, Dr. Thomas Corbett and David Parker, to aid them in the preparation of a curative compound of herbs and roots, which should meet the wants of the medical fraternity. The learned doctor wanted his prescription honestly and conscientiously mixed; and, reposing confidence in the fidelity of the Shaker community, he and his friend Dr. Valentine Mott gave the new medicine the benefit of their approval, and widely advertised its merits. . . . From the most euphonious of its constituent parts, it was called "sarsaparilla," and became so famed for its curative properties, that great fortunes have been made in manufacturing imitation or bogus articles of the same name. The medicine was designed for impurities of the blood, general and nervous debility, and wasting diseases; and, for the half century during which it has been prepared for the public, it has been an inestimable boon to the sick and suffering.
>
> To fully appreciate the care given to the preparation of this remedy, one should visit the Shaker community in Canterbury, the home of Dr. Thomas Corbett and David Parker,—both long since gone to their final reward,—and see their successors in the field and in the laboratory, working to compound the sarsaparilla. A little north of the kitchen garden of the First Family, and east of the great barn, near where the saintly Elder Henry [Blinn] caresses his pet bees, and jovial Friend George attends to the grape, the pear, and the apple, the brothers of the family cultivate the curative herbs in a garden especially tilled by them. At the proper season the plants are gathered into storehouses, the roots and berries subjected to chemical changes by skillful hands, dirt and impurities are absolutely banished, and in time Shaker *Sarsaparilla* is ready for the market.

The records of the amount of sarsaparilla sold from Canterbury is impressive:[4]

1849	551 bottles sold.
1850	668 dozen bottles and 10 jugs sold.
1853	Eleven barrels sold.
1857	303 dozen bottles sold.
1859	154 dozen bottles and 6½ dozen jugs sold.
1861	400 dozen bottles and 20 gallons in jugs.
1879	154 dozen bottles and 6½ gallons in jugs.
1894	100 dozen bottles sold.

In 1853, David Parker circulated a handbill soliciting the gathering of herbs by people outside the community.[5]

WANTED

The following Roots and Herbs are wanted, delivered at Shaker Village, Merrimac Co. N.H. for which a fair compensation will be given, if the following directions are observed.

All herbs must be well cured by being dried in the shade that they may retain a bright appearance, and must be freed from all other articles, as dirt, grass, etc. and those having large stalks must be stripped therefrom. They should be gathered in time of blossoming or soon after.

Roots must be cleansed from dirt, and if large, split and well dried. None will be received unless the above directions are strictly regarded.

Roots should be gathered in the fall or very early in the spring.

June is the best time for peeling barks.

                                                          1853.   David Parker.

Avans Root
Alder Bark, Black
Bittersweet
Blackberries
Blue Flag Root
Bugle, Sweet
Burdock Leaves
   Root
   Seed
Catmint
Coltsfoot
Dragon Root

Dragon's Claw
   Crawley root
Dwarf Elder Root
Harvest Lice
Horsemint
Horseradish Leaves
Lobelia, Herb and Seed
Marigold Flowers
Motherwort
Peppermint
Rose Flowers, red and
   white (Separate)

Scabish
Spearmint
Snakehead
Stonebrake (Purple
   Thoroughwort)
Sumach Leaves
Sweet Flag Root
Thoroughwort
Vervain
Witch Hazel Leaves
Yarrow

David Parker, in his day, was doubtless one of the most widely known of all the Canterbury Shakers. He was remarkable for his industry, thrift, and shrewdness, but combined with absolute honesty, which stamped him with the reputation of being perfectly reliable in every business transaction. He was admitted to the society at Canterbury when he was ten years old in 1817.

Parker was 17 years older than Henry Blinn and had been at the Canterbury community 21 years before young Henry was admitted. In spite of the difference in years the men were congenial and Brother Henry was under the watchful eye of the experienced trustee. It was this early training which was to be so valuable to Henry Blinn.

The Shakers of Canterbury published their last catalog of medicinal plants and vegetable medicines in 1854. Two hundred and two herbs with common and botanical names and prices were offered, and 36 properties were listed. They also offered the same extracts, oils, ointments, syrups, and sundries for sale.

Although not in the category with their catalogs, the Shakers issued a little booklet of 34 pages, called *Mary Whitcher's Shaker House-Keeper*, to sell Shaker medicines. Originally published in Boston in 1882 this is the earliest cookbook in Shaker culinary literature. Sister Mary had been a member of the Canterbury community since early childhood; she was a kitchen deaconess and a trustee. In her introduction she says: "The Shakers recognized the fact that good food, properly cooked and well digested, is the basis of sound health." The novelty of her book was that it introduced, she said, for the first time, "bills of fare for the dinner of each day of the week."

Corbett's Shakers' Sarsaparilla was described as "The Most Economical Medicine," the best for "Mothers When Worn Out," a restorative for "Good Appetite and Rich Blood," and was endorsed by doctors, druggists, and chemists. Menus and recipes in one column were side by side on each page with testimonials and "kind words" as to what Corbett's would do. In a column beside "Brown Bread No. 3 and Graham Gems" was a note of gratitude: "Mary Whitcher whose portrait adorns this book, has been a conspicuous figure in Shaker history, for more than a half a century, and has done more to adapt the Sarsaparilla to the wants of mothers and children, than any other person."

But, in spite of all the advertising and testimonials, the last of Corbett's sarsaparilla was made in the syrup house at Canterbury in 1895. Competition with commercial firms had become increasingly stiff, and, as the trustees were counseled not to sell inferior articles, it was impossible to maintain their high standards and realize a profit.

NOTES

1. *The Farmer's Monthly Visitor*, Concord, N.H., August 31, 1840, pp. 113, 118, Vol. 2, No. 8. Dartmouth College Library, Hanover, N.H.

2. *Catalogue of Medicinal Plants and Vegetable Medicines,* 1835, Emma B. King Library, Shaker Museum at Old Chatham, N.Y.

3. *The Granite Monthly—A New Hampshire Magazine* (September–October 1885), 8:310–11.

4. Record of 1841, Canterbury, N.H., Shaker Society, in Phyllis Shimki, *Sarsaparilla Bottle Encyclopedia* (Aurora, Ore.: 1969), p. 54.

5. Handbill circulated by Trustee David Parker of the Canterbury Society, 1853, Emma B. King Library, Shaker Museum at Old Chatham, N.Y.

9. ENFIELD, NEW HAMPSHIRE

Enfield is situated near the western border of New Hampshire, 13 miles southeast of Hanover, home of Dartmouth College. Although not as close geographically as the "twin villages" Harvard and Shirley, these two, Enfield and Canterbury, on opposite sides of their state, were close in spirit.

"Shaker Hill," the rich farmland on the west shore of Mascoma Lake, belonged to James Jewett, and eventually became the site of the society when it was formed in 1793. As more farmers joined and gave their land to the society it increased to about 3,000 acres, productive uplands of the Connecticut River further enriched by acres of alluvial mowing grounds. There was also a never-failing water supply from a lake far up on a mountain 1,500 feet above the village.

Here again we have a contemporary account of a Shaker village and again we see that it has been located in an ideal spot, the land is rich, the farming productive, and the water supply abundant. Isaac Hill reporting in the September 20, 1839, issue of *The Farmer's Monthly Visitor* on his trip to the Enfield Shakers wrote that the garden of the Center family covered five acres of ground on the margin of the Mascomy pond. He said:

> Of the garden one half an acre was sage, a portion of which had been forced in early hot beds. The Shakers also raise large quantities of summer savory. The preparation of sage and summer savory is by drying and pressing into a solid mass. The profits of these and other botanical preparations are best understood by those who are well acquainted with the best methods of raising and preparing them.
>
> Five hands, two men and three boys, are sufficient for the labor of these five acres of garden, which yields annually in cash its thousand, if not its thousands of dollars.

The Enfield Shakers manufactured a list of medicines "composed of native vegetables" as stated on the labels.[1] They prepared a Family Cough Syrup; and a big seller called Arnikate of Tannin which was a specific for all choleric diseases. This was "first recommended to a Company going to California, in 1849, by whom its virtues have been fully tested and is now put up by their advice expressly for that numerous portion of our countrymen who are going to the infected region for gold."

They claimed that their Vegetable Pills were an almost sure preventive of epidemic complaints, such as cholera morbus, bilious colic, and bilious and typhous fever. They were also "a safe and powerful cathartic," the label read. An Alterative Syrup, "A Compound Concentrated Decoction of Rumex highly recommended as a natural efficient and safe alterative to the system affected with scrofulous, cancerous and other accidental or hereditary diseases," was in general demand.

Extract of Dandelion was made in large quantities at Enfield, as it was in the medical departments of other Shaker communities, to act upon "the derangement of hepatic apparatus, Liver and Gall and of the digestive organs generally. In Congestion and Chronic Inflammation of the Liver and Spleen; in cases of suspended or deficient biliary secretion, etc., if employed with due regard to the degree of excitement, our own experience is decidedly in its favor. Nothing further need be said, its use is so common and generally understood."

Among other preparations manufactured at Enfield were a gargle for the throat and tongue; pure Jamaica ginger which was highly recommended for dyspepsia and indigestion, a tonic for debilitated systems, "which if taken in season" would cure colds and coughs and was the best known remedy for summer complaint, toothache, earache, cramp, and cholera; Mother Seigel's Curative Syrup for Dyspepsia and Brown's Extract of English Valerian.[2] *Valeriana officinalis* was the botanical name of the principal ingredient of this extract which the Shaker catalog said "is the best remedy yet discovered for the cure of Nervousness, Lowness of Spirits, Debility, Hypochondria, Neuralgia, Hysteria, Restlessness, Tic Douloureux, Sick Headache, and every other disease arising from mental affection and nervous exhaustion. One trial will prove its great superiority over all other remedies now in use. It is also an invaluable remedy for outward application, in all cases of Cuts, Bruises, Sores, Sprains, Scalds, Burns, Lameness, Skin Diseases, and every affection requiring external treatment."

The Enfield Shakers printed advertising circulars and broadsides and two pamphlets of several pages each containing facts about Brown's Extract in 1879 and 1880.[3]

The medical department of this community also published a seven-page catalog of medicinal plants and vegetable medicines, with their most prominent medical properties. Although it was not dated, it was probably an earlier issue than the pamphlets published in 1879 and 1880 because it listed valerian as an available root for medicinal purposes but did not list the manufactured product, presumably because it predated the medicine.

In selling the extract in their printed material the Shakers gave this information about valerian:

> This highly valuable article is a preparation manufactured by the United Society of Shakers, at Enfield, N.H. It is simply an extract from the pure green roots of the Valerian plant; and owing to their favorable position for obtaining the fresh, green roots of the Valerian plants at the proper season for digging when they are strongest, they claim greater efficacy for their preparation than is secured by that made in the usual way from dry roots of uncertain age and strength.

For years the Enfield Shakers enjoyed a well-earned prosperity, their farm and garden operation accounting for a large part of it. In 1874 they were doing a business of $30,000 in the sale of seeds and $4,000 in distilled valerian. Boston was their best marketplace.

Sister Frances Carr, today a member of the Sabbathday Lake society in Maine writing in *The Shaker Quarterly* for the summer of 1963, said: "Brown's Fluid Extract of English Valerian compounded at Enfield, New Hampshire, by Br. Samuel Brown of that Society, remained in demand as late as 1897, though he died in 1856. From his youth and for many years, he worked closely with Br. Ezekiel Evans, who was charged with raising and preparing herbs for the market. Their work contributed considerably to the advance of the herb industry at Enfield."

After 125 years this community, which at one time counted 330 members, closed its doors in 1918, and the remaining seven Shakers of "The City of Union" moved to Canterbury.

NOTES

1. Labels on medicine bottles, Canterbury Shaker Society, Canterbury, N.H.

2. Advertising circular for Brown's Shaker Extract English Valerian, 1879, Cleveland, Western Reserve Historical Society.

3. Ibid.

10. THE MAINE SOCIETIES

ALFRED

Alfred is about 30 miles southwest of Portland and the Alfred Shakers' 1,200 acres were situated between sizable hills and included a large pond which provided them with important waterpower. Charles Nordhoff reported in 1875 that the land was not very fertile or easily cultivated and when an outlying tract of timberland was sold for $28,000 the Shakers "were glad to be rid of it."

Sister R. Mildred Barker, now of the Sabbathday Lake society, formerly a member of the Alfred community, writes in *The Shaker Quarterly:*[1]

> The herb and medicine business does not seem to have gained the prominence in Alfred that it did in most Societies, though their use within the family itself was prevalent. During the latter half of the [19th] century, Elder John Vance, who had studied medicine to some degree, provided the family with a most capable physician during most illnesses. There were, however, some herbs gathered and sold to Harvard and some of the other Societies where the herb industry prevailed to a larger extent.

The raising of garden seeds was a much larger business; the Shakers started growing them in Alfred as early as 1835. A broadside dated 1850 lists 47 seeds including ten herbs: summer savory, sage, lemon balm, sweet balm, rue, parsley, saffron, English sorrel, marigold, and hyssop.[2]

The herb business became sufficiently successful for the trustees to issue a broadside listing 82 medicinal herbs, including rose flowers, belladonna, poppy flowers, raspberry leaves, Roman wormwood, and sumac berries. However, this business did not compare in size with that at Sabbathday where almost twice as many herbs were offered for sale, but it was a good source of income.

Editor Hill once again furnishes an account of a Shaker village. In *The Farmer's Monthly Visitor* for July 31, 1840, he says of Alfred:

> Their garden for the production of vegetables and seeds was what we always expect to see when we visit a Shaker family in the summer season; they had recently erected an extensive seed house, in the lower story of which were preparation rooms for labelling and packing seeds, and in the two upper stories ample space was given for drying, curing, thrashing and cleaning the seeds as they are collected from the field.
>
> The perservering attention which the several Societies of Shakers have paid to the produc-

86

tion of Garden Seeds for many years, commends them to the public patronage. They have steadily pursued this business for more than half a century; and they are not a people to relax in any laudable effort which is likely to be crowned with success. Others following their example have gone extensively into the production of garden seeds; but the growth of the country still affords the consumption which induces the Shakers to continue this as a profitable business. Of them useful lessons may always be taken in every thing connected with domestic economy and in the productions of the earth. If they raise garden seeds, they know how to preserve the pure varieties of onions, beets, carrots, cabbages, melons, squashes, etc., not suffering them to intermix by growing in the near contact; and they are in advance of most other horticulturists in a more sure and better method of curing and preserving seeds.

SABBATHDAY LAKE

In 1794 this Maine community, the last of the eastern societies to be organized, was formally covenanted. It was first called New Gloucester, then West Gloucester; it was given the present name of Sabbathday Lake after 1890. The society owned 2,000 acres of land when Nordhoff wrote about it in 1875 and according to him its income was derived from the raising and selling of garden seeds, the making of brooms, and quantities of woodenware and old-fashioned spinning wheels. He said: "Its most profitable industry is the manufacture of oak staves for molasses hogsheads, which are exported to the West Indies. . . . They made last year also a thousand dollars worth of pickles; and the women make fancy articles in their spare time."

Eldress Betsy Smith from Pleasant Hill visiting the eastern societies writes in her journal in July 1869:[3]

> First Order, New Gloucester, their dwellings have the neatness of a flower bed. . . . There are about 60 persons in this Society composed of two families, the Church and the gathering order, Poland Hill, and they are a little band of very clever, social good folk. They have a very nice terraced garden on the hillside just west of the road and buildings that looked lively and thrifty where they raise herbs and vegetables for sale. . . . They have a tolerably good farm, fine for meadows and tolerably good for grain potatoes, good barns and stables. They have a grist mill including a machine shop with circular saws planing mill. This is the mill that brought them into trouble by the Trustees speculating in wheat and flour clandestinely and one Charles Vining absconding full handed and leaving them hopelessly involved. But there is a little band there struggling to survive it all and are making it a success.

The Shakers grew and processed medicinal herbs at Sabbathday in the beginning, as those in other Shaker communities did, only for the benefit of their own families. When they grew a surplus, they sent the excess to market. The Shakers did manage to produce a surplus of herbs and accordingly issued "A Catalogue of Medicinal Plants Prepared in the United Society of Shakers, New Gloucester, Cumberland County Maine" with prices per paper in 1840. In broadside form 83 herbs were offered.[4]

James Holmes (1771–1856) was a deacon in the society and also the author of three little books which he printed in the Garden Seed House.[5] The first one of 81 pages printed in 1850 gives instructions for the treatment of hydrophobia; recommends camphor to destroy lice on cattle; gives a cure for piles; and recommends human urine in a bucket of water as a simple cure for "Cough in Horses," and heather root for treatment of whooping cough in children.

In 1853 *The Farmers' Second Book,* a collection of useful hints for farmers and many valuable recipes, collected and compiled by James Holmes, appeared with this preface: "The compiler of this little work in his leisure moments, has collected the following recipes, maxims and useful hints in farming and other matters of economy, considering them worth preserving and believing they might be useful and of great benefit to those who may wish to avail themselves of every improvement, and the best methods of performing business." This volume was 152 pages in length.

The third little book with much the same kind of information was of 44 pages and Deacon Holmes's preface read: "The publisher an Octogenarian who has neither press nor fixtures for printing, the types excepted, but those of his own invention begs leave to say that, if the reader detects errors, either in typography or in the mechanical execution, he hopes the above assertion may be received as sufficient apology for any lack of propriety which may be discovered in the rules of printing." The garden seed house, where these little books were produced, was razed around 1920 and all the contents destroyed.

The Shakers increased the garden-seed business both from Alfred and Sabbathday Lake (which did not find favor with their brethren in New Hampshire). The following three letters concerned with encroaching upon the areas of selling are given here as they reflect so precisely the business attitudes between the societies.[6]

> Canterbury. October 18, 1828. Much respected Deacons. The object of our writing at this time is to form a more correct understanding between us concerning the distribution of our Garden Seeds. We have formerly understood the line between the States of New Hampshire and Maine divides the districts for distributing Garden Seeds although there are some few towns in the upper part of this State which have been inconvenient for us to supply and we have therefore given them to the Societies in the East say Conway, Milton, and the Three Ponds, but the towns of Portsmouth, Dover, Sommersworth (or Great Falls) we have invariably considered as belonging to our districts and cannot feel right in giving up any part of them as our route is very small comparatively speaking, so small as to hardly make it an object for us to raise seeds.
>
> Several of the merchants in these towns particularly at Great Falls are often calling on us to supply them but knowing the Eastern Brethren brought seeds there we would not interfere. We wish to come to some proper agreement concerning the above for this good reason to promote the cause of union and leave no place for the World to say we are not united. If the Brethren from other societies continue to crowd upon us much longer we shall soon be obliged to give up our own establishment at home.
>
> With these few lines be so kind as to accept our Best Love and well wishes from the Deacons at Canterbury. N. B. Be so kind as to write an answer to this, the first opportunity Direct to Israel Sanborn, Canterbury, Shaker Village Post Office, New Hampshire.

> From Trustees at Canterbury to Nathan Freeman at Alfred, November 24, 1828:

> Beloved Deacons,

> We received your letter of the 3rd, Inst. concerning the distribution of Garden Seeds. We should be sorry to have any strife between us on that subject or any other *For We Are Brethren.* We think that you have three or four times the scope that we have for Seeds. Ours is so small it is hardly worth attention. But we intend to make some improvements about seeds and try it yet longer. Were it necessary we would give you the names of all the Towns we supply. Suffice it to say that the Society at Harvard supply the best part of our State viz almost all of the Counties of Cheshire and Hillsboro.
>
> The Deacon says that he agreed that you should have Milton and Three Ponds and Wakefield, and we now say we are willing you should have them, and Ossipie, Effingham, Eaton, and Conway, (except one box which Dr. Chadbourne will take here and return here for he *will* have our seeds). But he (the Deacon) says *we* were to have Rochester and that there was *no* agreement made about it as he recollects as Sommersworth years past had been of no importance for seeds and Dover not very good. But since the Factorys have started at Dover and Great Falls in connexion and so many

people have gone there who used to sell our seeds and yet *claim* them and *will* have them and as we trade largely there in other things and they are also in our State we should be thankful to have your union for us to supply them. And we wish that the line between the States from *Norraway Plains* to the sea shore would divide the Districts as we think it would be the most proper and not unreasonable.

We have very much omitted sending our wheels, etc. to Norraway Plains for years past because you wished that Privilege as it was nearer to you and we were willing to accommodate you and we think we ever ought to have that feeling.

With these few lines we send you our Best Love.

However, the issue cannot have been settled for it was still of concern ten years later.

Canterbury, November 1838.

Much Beloved Deacon Nathan.

We wish to state to you in short our views concerning the Garden Seed Route of which something has heretofore been said. Without doubt you will at once say, with us that it is not only convenient but absolutely necessary in the world to have *Elbow Room* this admitted, we will endeavor to show to you that we have not this desirable and necessary requisite in our seed route. In the first place on the South we have Harvard and Shirley, who come within 33 miles of us; and not only due South of us they have an east route which extends to the sea at Cape Ann. Next we have Enfield on the West and North of us who border down close *very close* and last though not least our good Brethren at Alfred venture over the State line by including Chatham, Conway, Eaton, Effingham, Wakefield and Milton which are all in New Hampshire.

Now Beloved Deacon do you not think that we stand in rather a squeezed situation? Without any means of enlarging our routes, hedged on all sides by bounds which we consider sacred and inviolable until removed by mutual agreement. We are unlike our brethren at Alfred who have a great unbounded territory North and East of which no one holds a right or privilege and a means of extending the same especially since the grant from Gloucester. Just compare the extent of your district with ours and upon mature deliberation we think you will readily concede that we are asking no more of you than you would ask of us were you placed in our circumstances. All we ask is the privilege of our State by having the towns above named included in our district and have the State line a boundary. Just place a map of New Hampshire before you and a glance of the same will convince you of the truth of the above. You will also see that it makes a crooked notch over the line of New Hampshire which if the State line be made the division (which we think of right and ought to be) it makes all straight and gives us desired *Elbow Room* of which we so much need and which we confidently believe you can spare to us without materially discomoding yourselves and for which we would in duty bound feel ever grateful.

With this please receive our best and warmest love and extend the same to the Ministry and as far as you feel.

Israel Sanborn

William Willard

P.S. Do you wish to purchase any of the following seeds as we have them to spare. Early cucumber, common cucumber, red and blood beed, carrot, savory cabbage. Please answer this by return of the Bearers.

W. W.

Although it seemed to be difficult to settle on a division of territory between the Maine and the New Hampshire brethren, the two Maine societies had agreed on this subject in 1837, a year before the November letter to Brother Nathan.[7]

Memorandum of Agreement made and entered into this sixteenth day of October A.D. 1837 by and between the Deacons or Trustees for and in behalf of the United Society in Alfred, County of York and State of Maine on one part, and the Deacons or Trustees for and in behalf of the United Society in New Gloucester, County of Cumberland and State aforesaid on the other part to establish a line of division for the distribution of Garden Seeds in said State for each Society.

It is hereby agreed by the parties aforesaid that the Society in Alfred is to supply with Garden Seeds all the towns in the County of York in said State, viz. Hiram, Porter, Brownfield, Denmark, Freyburg, Lovell, Sweden, Waterford, Stowe, Albany and Batchelder; and in the County of Cumberland, the towns of Scarboro, Standish, Gorham, Baldwin, Sebago, Bridgton, Harrison, Naples, Raymond and Windham, (Portland is free for either Society) and in the County of Lincoln (It being expressly understood that the town of Bath belongs to the Society in New Gloucester); in the County of Waldo, the towns of Camden, Lincolnville and Northport and all east and south of these three towns in said County; in the County of Penobscot, the towns of Ovington, Brewer, Eddington, Javis, Gore, Milford and Greenbush, and also the whole of the County of Hancock, and the whole of the County of Washington in said State.

It is further agreed by the parties aforesaid that all the rest, residue and remainder of said State of Maine are to be supplied with Garden Seed by the Society in New Gloucester and Poland.

It is further agreed by the parties aforesaid and they hereby obligate themselves and their successors in trust, that they will not directly or indirectly consign any Garden Seed whatever to any person or agent to supply any person or persons with seeds residing out of their own route as described aforesaid, but each Society are to supply their own route as before described unmolested.

In Witness thereof the Parties aforesaid have hereunto set their names this 16th day of October A.D. 1837.

Nathan Freeman

Alfred

Edward Goodrich

James Holmes

New Gloucester

Levi Holmes

Sage was the culinary herb grown in the largest commercial quantities, and from all accounts it was a large crop. There are several entries in Elder Otis Sawyer's journal bearing on this:[8]

March 6, 1873 Brother William Dumont went to the depot in the afternoon with four barrels of Sage for Thompson and Leighton of Portland.

The next year:

March 25, 1874. Brother William Dumont ground and put up a barrel of Dockroot for Brother Samuel.

March 31, 1874. Brother William Dumont went to the depot with 5 barrels of herbs. Brought back 10 bushels of corn.

January 14, 1878. Brother William Dumont took garden seed to the depot to be sent to Portland. Three barrels of Carrot Seed. Two barrels of Beet Seed.

January 16, 1878. Herbert West took five barrels of sage to the depot to be shipped to Portland.

January 18, 1878. Herbert West took another five barrels of sage to the depot to be shipped to Portland.

The society issued only one bound herb catalog, in 1864. It listed 155 herbs, barks, roots, and powdered articles. Herbs were ground and pulverized and sweet marjoram, sage, summer savory, and thyme were sold in canisters, in two sizes, for $2.00 per dozen for the large and $1.00 per dozen for the small. Also offered for sale were grape vines, plants, garden seeds, horseradish in jars, apple sauce by the gallon or barrel, peach water and rosewater by the gallon or bottle, and sieves and brooms.

(Whatever Charles Vining's shortcomings as a businessman were, the catalog is one of the nicest looking of all those put out by the Shakers and happily it was reproduced in 1972 by the society in its "Hands to Work Series" of publications.)

Many Shaker communities specialized in producing one product in the medicinal herb department which provided a source of income larger than all of the other medicines they also made. At Mt. Lebanon, Seven Barks and Veratrum Viride were in this category. At Canterbury it was Corbett's Sarsaparilla, and at Enfield, New Hampshire, it was Brown's Pure Extract of English Valerian. At Sabbathday Lake it was The Shaker Tamar Laxative, a fruit compound. How this came to be manufactured by the community is told in the *Church Record:*[9]

October 5, 1881. Brother Benjamin came to offer the Church a chance to prepare and put up a new medicine compounded and invented by A. J. White of New York who gives preparations to the amount of twelve hundred dollars and New Lebanon gives two hundred [both Mt. Lebanon and New Lebanon are used in this entry]. The Church gladly and gratefully accept the offer.

Brother Benjamin went around to the Laundry, the Herb House and other places to see where the business could be carried on and decided that the large Herb room in the chamber of Middle Wood House was a very appropriate place. The medicine is to be made in the shape of Lozenge and to be called "The Shaker Tamar Laxative." A meeting of the principal part of the family was called and decided in favor of prosecuting the business.

October 8, Saturday. Brother Hewett went to New York to meet Brother Benjamin Gates to learn more about the preparation of medicine.

October 24. Monday. Brother Hewett is making preparation for the manufacture of the Shaker Tamar Laxative. He has purchased a kneader to work the stuff through.

October 28. Friday. Brother Hewitt went to Lewiston. He is having a machine made to cut out the Losenges [sic].

November 24. . . . *The New Medicine* started this afternoon. Brother Hewitt and Sisters mixed one batch of *The Shaker Tamar Laxative* and cut a few tablets. That it may prove a profitable business is the prayer of every person in the Church.

December 29. Elder William and Sisters are making the Tamar Tablets with a hope to make sales and render the medicine Popular.

January 16, 1882. Monday. The first order for Shaker Tamar Lozenges came Thursday, January 12, from Dr. Russell of Minot; 4 boxes. Tall oaks from little acorns grow.

March 22. A large lot of Tamar now packed for parties in Boston, New York City, Philadelphia, Chicago and Troy, New York.

And so a medicine was manufactured which from the very first and for 30 years was an outstanding success. The last batch was made in 1911. A four-page leaflet of testimonials, directions for its use, and the admonition "The West Gloucester Society are the only Shakers who make the Shaker Tamar Laxative, and all others bearing the name of Shaker are not genuine" was distributed under Brother William Dumont's name who was the trustee in charge of its manufacture.

Sister Frances Carr, a member of the Sabbathday Lake society, gives the formula:

> Take Cassia Fistula, crushed, 400 lbs; Tamarinds 135 lbs; Prunes, 100 lbs; Digest each in warm water and strain through sieve or fine cloth. Then mix the strained liquid and evaporate in vacuo to a thick extract. Then take of this compound, Fruit extract, 579 oz; Fruit of Cassia Obovata, 192 oz, Glycerine, 24 oz; Sugar, 80 oz; Powdered Hyoscyamin, 1½ oz. Mix thoroughly and make into Tablets of 53 grains each which are then to be covered with Gelatin.[10]

Sister Frances explains that after the compound was cut into lozenges, each one was put on specially prepared drying boards which were studded with wire pins. On these the lozenges were placed by hand and remained there until the coating was thoroughly dried and they could be packed. Each box, when ready for sale, had both the compound's formula and the directions for its use printed on the bottom. (The above formula does not include wintergreen, but a church journal with a March 13, 1884, entry states: "Laxative rolled into sheets today. Two pounds of glycerine and two ounces oil of wintergreen put into full batch.")

NOTES

1. *The Shaker Quarterly*, vol. 3, no. 4 (Winter 1963), pp. 114, 115, 116, Shaker Society, Library at Sabbathday Lake, Me.

2. Broadside listing forty-seven vegetable and herb seeds, 1850, Cleveland, Western Reserve Historical Society.

3. Diary of Eldress Betsy Smith, July 1869, Pleasant Hill, Shaker Collection, Library of Congress, Washington, D.C.

4. Broadside listing eighty-three herbs, 1840, Shaker Society, Library at Sabbathday Lake, Me.

5. *The Farmers' Books*, 1771–1856, vol. 1 (1850), 81 pp.; vol. 2 (1853), 152 pp.; vol. 3 (1856), 44 pp., Shaker Society, Library at Sabbathday Lake, Me.

6. Three letters, 1828–1838, Sabbathday Lake Library.

7. *The Shaker Quarterly*, vol. 3, no. 4 (Winter 1963), p. 115, Shaker Society, Library at Sabbathday Lake, Me.

8. Journal of Elder Otis Sawyer for 1873, Shaker Society, Library at Sabbathday Lake, Me.

9. *Church Record*, vol. 2 (1881), Shaker Society, p. 57, Library at Sabbathday Lake, Me.

10. *The Shaker Quarterly*, vol. 2, no. 1 (Spring 1962), p. 40, Shaker Society, Library at Sabbathday Lake, Me.

11. THE WESTERN SOCIETIES IN OHIO, KENTUCKY, AND INDIANA, AND THE SOUTHERN SOCIETIES

Three members from the Mt. Lebanon society, John Meacham, Benjamin S. Youngs, and Issachar Bates, set out for the west traveling mostly on foot to see for themselves the religious fervor which was sweeping over the southwestern part of Kentucky. This journey of more than a thousand miles was begun on the first day of January 1805, and the missionaries arrived in Kentucky about the first of March, weary, but exalted, having experienced great hardship and many indignities. They carried the "true Gospel" to the land of the great awakening and in the spirit of renewal and revival they survived. Their hymn, from the Kentucky Revival, by Richard McNemar, was:

> Shout Christians, Shout! The Lord is come!
> Prepare, prepare to make Him room.
> On earth He reigns; we feel Him near;
> The signs of Glory now appear.

As many a cause carried its disciples onward so did theirs and the arduous journey resulted in the eventual founding of six Shaker societies in the west between 1811 and 1826, two in Kentucky, and four in Ohio. (A community at Busro, Indiana, was organized in 1810, but lasted a few years only; its members moved to Union Village, Ohio, in 1812.) Union Village, Ohio, and Watervliet (Dayton), Ohio, were founded in 1812 and 1813; Pleasant Hill, Kentucky, in 1814; Busro, Indiana, in 1810; South Union, Kentucky, 1811; North Union (Cleveland), Ohio, 1826; and Whitewater, Ohio, in 1824.

The Shakers followed the same pattern for organizing the western villages as others had in the 11 eastern societies. Each community bought land, continuously, amassing from one to six thousand acres to pasture their fine herds of cattle and sheep, graze horses, and to grow their diverse crops. At first, the settlers had to build dwelling houses, huge barns, large sheds for many different uses, and mills and shops. Then they established industries to manufacture goods to provide first for the needs of the members of the families and then to sell materials in the general markets to produce necessary cash income.

All the western societies raised herbs for the use of their families as was the custom of the day on the frontier. And in most of these societies the Shakers sold the surplus of herbs or medicines to the outside world. In some cases this practice became a good business. In others it was more of a thrifty procedure to avoid waste.

93

Actually, all seventeenth- and eighteenth-century families in the United States relied on herbs for homemade medicines, and it was just as essential for the Shakers to include herb gardens, with drying houses, in each community, although herbs were first gathered in their natural habitat. Eventually the Shakers cultivated herbs in short supply in the outside markets and those in greatest demand by themselves. To do so, they accumulated and relied upon Indian lore.

Thus Peter Boyd, one of the Shakers of Union Village, notes on February 26, 1845, that the Indians had brought gifts of herbs and roots.[1] He also tells about I. Bates and R. McNemar visiting the Shawnee Indians. At Union Village, as was the case at Mt. Lebanon, the Shakers used herbal material provided by Indians.

UNION VILLAGE, OHIO

Union Village, situated between Cincinnati and Dayton, three miles west of Lebanon, had as its spiritual name, "Wisdom's Paradise." It was the largest in size and population of the western communities and for a short while it was as large as Mt. Lebanon. Six families lived there comprising 600 members when it was at its height. It prospered for 98 years, until, after a period of decline, it was sold in 1910.

O. H. Hampton, who joined the community in 1822, frequently audited diaries and in 1849 compiled a summary, not always in chronological order, from several covering the life of the society from March 1805 to 1819.[2]

> We were at this time [1849] still running many of our former branches of business such as the tanyard, seed selling, preparing of herbs, roots, extracts and oils. The woolen factory operated in 1819 as did a fine garden of sage and sassafras. In 1834 among the other methods of making a living at this time and for many years previous was the distilling of oils and fragrant waters which paid as well as almost any other resort, considering the small expense of procuring raw material. And sometimes in the distilling, we would occasionally double distill a barrel of Whiskey for the sake of the Alcohol for medical purposes. In 1854 the Church family agreed on February 7, to send to England for a lot of fine blooded Durham stock.

Brother Oliver continues:

> In 1857 seed business carried on by West Families was transferred to the First Order of the Church and the Church proper in consideration of this transfer paid to the West Families, $7,000. Transfer made about the 14th of January. . . . March 28, 1859. A new arrangement was made this season in regard to the seed garden. Taking the Medical and Seed gardens both into consideration, the grounds were equally divided between the First and Second Orders. . . . *1866* by the 22nd. of September we had made 125 gallons of good Catawby wine which was used for medical purposes and was far more reliable than anything in that line we could get from outside, besides being cheaper.

It is also from Brother Oliver's diary we learn of a fire on March 4, 1865, which destroyed the Old North House and its contents containing the tin shop, broom shop, carpenter shop, and sarsaparilla laboratory.

An anonymous auditor has added: "In 1897 still cultivated gardens and orchards, only 32 members" [the number in the entire village].[3]

Another journal titled "A Register of Work performed by Second Family Sisters, Together with the Most Important passing Events, Recorded by Amy Slaters" is full of minutiae, all of it forming the picture of a busy family. From January 10, 1848, with few dates given until May, the entries cover many industries and household chores.

Jan. 10th. Had boiled eggs for breakfast. I took the number [counted] of 240. The 28th, had eggs again. Picked geese, hackled flax, made soap, spooled yarn, dyed yarn, cut rags for carpets, made candles, wove carpets. Aseneth Edie came here to see the sick. Whitewashed rooms, tagged the sheep, gave the sisters pins, picked cotton for fine light gowns. April 10th. Two letters from East, one from Canterbury, the other from Hancock bringing information in relation to spinning machine. . . . Blue vat finished and brought to coloring house. A mother takes her children away. . . . A step father brings his little girl for us to keep if willing, her name is Harriet McCurdy. . . .

May 13th. Picked the geese. The silk worms came out [hatched].

May 26th. Had strawberry short cake for supper. Put butternut bark to soap for coloring, begin to spin wool, put the wool in the butternut dye. Four of the sisters stained the floors in the new house.

June 1st. The nurses now in the new house [infirmary]. Had short cake and strawberrys. Colored blue wool. Commenced spinning worsted and wool.

June 26th. Made green apple pie. Gathered blackberries.

August 10th. Commenced drying apples.

October 22nd. Commenced painting chairs.

November 3rd. Received 4 lbs. coffee for the strangers' kitchen. Weaving tape, dyeing cloth madden red.

December 21st. Changed the time of rising in the morning, from ½ past four to five o'clock. Also change our evening meeting from ½ past seven to eight.

December 25th. Christmas went to the Meetinghouse and had a very comfortable meeting. Divided pins to the sisters.

Sister Amy continues her "Register":

July 5th. Had two hired hands to cook for.

July 22nd. Rained again today, picked the saffron. [She also picked saffron on the 24th and 26th.]

July 27th. Rhoda Evens here today to pick the saffron. [Also picked saffron the 31st].

August 2nd. Amelia went with her brother [left the community], picked the saffron.

August 5th. The brethren gathered boneset, the sisters commenced stripping it off the stems.

August 6th. Continued stripping boneset, picked the saffron.

August 25th. Stripped boneset.

September 1st. Gathered elder berries to make wine.

September 2nd. Brother Abner come here to show about the wine.

September 3rd. Gather more elder berries. Visitors from Shaker Villages, and from Lebanon, Cincinnati, and Kentucky. Watervliet brethren tarried overnight.

October [no date]. Stewed and dried pumpkins. Gathered husks for mattresses.

The entries for 1848 and 1849 are concerned with the dates when strawberries, new potatoes, green apples, and eggs for breakfast were offered the family. There are also two other references to winemaking which was of sufficient volume to sell to the world and to print an illustrated 11-page booklet on the subject.[4]

Shaker Community Wines. A treatise on Pure Wines and its Beneficial Uses. Shaker Community Wine Growers, William G. Ayer, Assistant Trustee, Union Village, Ohio. Vineyards on the Shore of Lake Erie. Established 1805.

Shaker wines are medicinal wines. They are for medicinal purposes. . . . Above all things they are not incentives to drunkenness.

The Shakers had started and had been expanding an herb business for several years. By the time Sister Amy recorded the wagonload of boneset in 1847, the Shakers had been able to issue a four-page catalog listing 170 medicinal herbs and 18 extracts.

In 1847 they offered 156 herbs, 25 extracts, 9 essential oils, and 4 culinary herbs: pulverized sage, summer savory, sweet marjoram, and thyme. Seven fragrant waters were also listed in this eight-page catalog. Thirty-four properties with abbreviations were explained and there was a lengthy testimonial from R. D. Mussey, Professor of Surgery at the Medical College in Cincinnati:

> I have the pleasure in saying that I have used the extracts of Sarsaparilla, Hybrid Colocynth, and the Belladonna prepared at Union Village by A. Babbit & Co. and that I have never found better articles of the kind. From the fidelity with which these articles are prepared, I can have no doubt that other medicines prepared and vended by them are of prime quality, and may be fully relied on.

Dr. Mussey had written half a page discussing a hybrid plant developed at Union Village. It was a cross between the colocynth and a watermelon and had been success-fully cultivated by the Shakers. It yielded a bitter fruit which had the medical virtues of colocynth and was an important addition to the medical plants grown at the village.

Six preparations were advertised on the back cover of the catalog: "Fluid Extract of Sarsaparilla and these simples which for their important therapeutic qualities deserve to be more extensively known and used, Bugle, Button Snake Root, Golden Seal, Indian Hemp, and Pleurisy Root." The diseases for which these preparations were recom-mended were the same as those set forth by the eastern Shakers as were the doses and properties.

A three-page catalog was printed the next year listing 206 herbs, 18 extracts, 7 essential oils, and 26 powdered herbs, roots, and barks. (As was the case in all Union Village catalogs, the botanical names were taken from *Eaton's Manual of Botany*, *Griffith's Medical Botany*, and *Raffinesque's Medical Flora*. Common names were such as were in use in the cities of Cincinnati, St. Louis, Louisville, and New Orleans.) Prices were given per pound and a 25 percent discount was allowed regular retail customers.

In 1850 a 12-page "Annual Wholesale Catalogue"[5] was offered by Peter Boyd. Seven classes of drug plants and drug plant products were listed:

252 drug plants; leaves, roots, seeds, bark, flowers, and berries.
 46 extracts
  8 inspissated juices
 15 essential oils
  4 pulverized sweet herbs; sage, summer savory, sweet marjoram, and thyme.

Extracts and essential oils produced from herbs raised at Union Village were given and are listed here in full for the purpose of comparing them with similar products offered in the eastern Shaker catalogs:

EXTRACTS

Belladonna	Dock, yellow	Poppy
Bittersweet	Foxglove	Snakehead or Balmony
Boneset	Garget or Poke	Thornapple
Butternut	Henbane	Tomato
Cicuta	Horehound	White ash bark
Cow parsnep	Lettuce, garden and wild	Wood sorrel
Colocynth, simple and	Mayapple	Wormwood
compound	Nightshade, garden	
Dandelion	Popular bark	

The essential oils offered were fennel, fleabane, pennyroyal, peppermint, spearmint, summer savory, tansy, wormseed, and wormwood. The catalog also included seven double-distilled and fragrant waters: rose, wild cherry, peppermint, elderflowers, peach, sassafras, and spearmint, and 31 roots, herbs, and barks "in a powdered state." The price per pound was given for all of the items, as well as both the common and botanical names. Thirty-four properties with abbreviations were explained.

The catalog also stated that other kinds of extracts would be made to order and said: "Of the above, though placed under the general head of EXTRACTS, the following are always INSPISSATED JUICES: Belladonna, Cicuta, Poke, Henbane, Lettuce, Thornapple and Tomato. As mere Extracts of the Narcotic plants are nonofficinal preparations, we never make them; but follow carefully, the directions of the United States Dispensatory. The prices however of these articles, are set down at the common rate of extracts, though it is customary to charge double for Inspissated Juices. Hence it will be seen that our articles of this class are very low." The prices for one-pound amounts ranged from $1.00 to $2.50, except for foxglove which was $3.00.

A note explained colocynth:

> Both the Simple and Compound Extracts of Colocynth, are prepared from the Hybrid Colocynth, which was originated at Union Village, Ohio, in 1842. This Hybrid was produced by planting seeds of the genuine colocynth, and at the proper time the flowers of the colocynth plant were fecundated with pollen from those of the watermelon. Hence we have given the plant thus derived, the Botanical name of *Cucumis colocynthis hybridum*. But we propose to call it the American Colocynth, and give it the Botanical name *Colocynthis Americana*. The following reasons for this are respectfully submitted. It is now reduced to a certainty that the Colocynth does not belong to the genus Cucumis where botanists have placed it. It has no resemblance to the cucumber; but both the plant and its fruit have a striking similarity to the Watermelon; and the fact that it freely mixes with the latter plant demonstrates that it belongs to the same genus. It ought therefore to be put in the genus *Cucurbitas*.
>
> In all the editions of the *United States Dispensatory* previous to that of 1845 (sixth edition) the Colocynth is called the "bitter cucumber," and said to bear considerable resemblance to the cucumber of our gardens. This mistake was pointed out by the writer to the learned and much respected author of the *Dispensatory* previous to issuing the sixth edition. Consequently the description was altered and the plant described as resembling the watermelon and the following note appended by the author:
>
> In a letter from R. W. Pelham, of the Shakers' Village near Lebanon Ohio, the author was informed that a hybrid plant between the colocynth and the watermelon had been successfully cultivated in that place, and yielded a bitter fruit having the medical virtues of Colocynth. With the letter I received some seeds of the plant, and a portion of the extract prepared from the pulp of the fruit. This was found upon trial to be actively cathartic. The seeds planted in the garden of the author, produced vigorous plants, which perfected their fruit. The plant appeared intermediate between the colocynth and the watermelon. The fruit was globular, about four inches in diameter, green like the watermelon externally, having the same odor when cut, but of an extremely bitter taste.

The author of this "Note" was R. D. Mussey, Professor of Surgery, Medical College of Ohio at Cincinnati, which he wrote in 1846.

The Union Village catalogs not only listed botanical products and medicines, but as in the case of the 1850 publication, the Shakers made the statement in the front:

TO OUR PATRONS

The articles contained in the following catalogue are prepared and put up with the greatest care and fidelity. The various Herbs, Roots and Barks, are gathered in the

season proper to each; the stalky and coarser part being rejected; they are then uni-
formly dried under shelter, after which they are neatly prepared and papered in
assorted packages for the convenience of the purchasers.

Our Extracts are prepared by experienced persons; they are vaporized by steam,
and great care is used that they are not burned, or otherwise injured. Our Inspissated
Juices are of superior quality and excellence.

We pledge ourselves that our preparations shall be inferior to none offered in market, and that they shall be such as will meet the approbation of dealers and practition-
ers generally, to whom we confidently recommend them.

Orders for such Native Plants as are not in the Catalogue will receive due attention.

They advertised another business as well:

Druggists, Merchants and others who desire Garden Seeds, will be allowed a commission of
33 per cent. We can supply them at the proper season of the year, with an excellent assort-
ment, for esculent vegetables, *fresh* and *genuine*: and which for quality, are unsurpassed in
any section of the Union.

It would be well to send orders as early as the middle of November, in order to secure a
full and complete variety.

The back cover was devoted to Compound Fluid Extract of Sarsaparilla and testimonials by Dr. Mussey, Dr. Andrew Campbell of Middletown, Ohio, and a resolution
from the Lebanon, Ohio, Medical Society:

That this Society have entire confidence in the purity of the Pharmaceutical preparations of
the Shakers at Union Village, Ohio, and that we heartily recommend these preparations to
the profession; especially the extracts of the Narcotic Plants and of Sarsaparilla.

Joshus Stevens, M.D. President

W. D. Charters, M.D. Secretary

The final paragraph states:

We wish the public to understand that, as we never on any occasion obtain any patents for
our medicines, or sell any receipts, or sell any medicine of which the materials are secret;
any publication purporting to have obtain receipts of us, is a fraudulent attempt to obtain
money on our credit.

A catalog similar to that published in 1850 was issued in 1856; in the meantime,
several broadsides were printed during the years between the two larger publications.
One was for Shaker Cough Syrup and another was for The Extract of Sarsaparilla. The
basis of the Cough Syrup was fresh wild cherry bark, squills, and seneca snakeroot, to
which was added rhubarb and in very small proportions, morphine and antimony. A
paragraph states:

Notwithstanding the prejudices of ignorance, physicians know the value of opium and
antimony in pectoral affections. The one allays irritation, the other acts as a sedative, expectorant and febrifuge; in combination they meet many indications in diseases of the respiratory organs, better than almost any other medicament; and when united with the other
ingredients of this preparation, they complete, as we verily believe, the best Cough
Medicine ever offered to the Afflicted.

The broadside advertising sarsaparilla claimed the medicine could be successful in
cases of chronic rheumatism, scrofulous affections, obstinate skin diseases, derangement of the liver, internal organs, and nervous system:

It is a fact well known, that the general character of the Extract of Sarsaparilla, now in market, is deficient in quality. The truth is, a perfect article costs more than can be afforded for the price at which it is generally sold; therefore, we would say to the public, and will appeal to the medical profession for the truth of the statement, that wherever a quart bottle of "said to be" Sarsaparilla Extract is offered for One Dollar, it is utterly deficient in quality, and can not be a true and legitimate article.

Peter Boyd wrote journals, diaries, and letters from 1833, the year the medicine garden came into importance in the late 1850s when he was in his eighties. These records give a good idea of the meticulous care he took building up and maintaining the industry. Writing in 1833 he says:[6]

January. Have had a frame built, a cold frame, a hot house frame. It is well ventilated and elevated, banked with sod and leaves to the waist height. Seed will begin to do well when planted here in February and March. It being well protected.

In June of the next year he says: "I will build and frame a hot house to enter and work within."

Some material in Peter Boyd's diaries is cut out, but enough remains to follow his numerous activities.[7]

January 16, 1844. David Parkhurst and Peter Boyd start to Cincinnati and sell a two horse waggon loaded with sage and brooms. . . . January 25th. Peter Boyd starts to Cincinnati with brooms, sage and other herbs. . . . February 19, 1844. Peter Boyd went to Dayton after flax, bought 419 pounds.

Later, Peter Boyd wrote:

April 10th, 1844 David Parkhurst and Peter Boyd start to Kentucky after squaw root, weather is warm. April 13th. Got home, planted corn. April 14th. The apple trees are in full bloom at this time. 15th. Ministry start to the East on their visit. April 29th. We begin to plant the peppermint south east of the apple orchard. I seed [sic] red clover in bloom last Saturday in the dooryard. The grass and trees are very forward. April 30th. We finish planting the peppermint. May 1st. Richard Pelham and Peter Boyd start to Watervliet, or in the neighborhood of Dayton after roots with two colts and the light waggon.

On May 4 they returned with a load of roots and on the eighth Peter was off again to sell herbs and brooms and to buy a casting "for grinding herbs."

February 6, 1845, Peter sold brooms, herbs, and extracts in Cincinnati in weather very warm for the season and a few days later "he was notified by Elder John [Rankin] of his intended removal to the Meetinghouse to take part in the Ministry." He [Rankin] also informed Richard W. Pelham that he must move into the office to take Peter Boyd's place there. The diary notes that on April 9 the thermometer dropped to 16 degrees above and "the peach trees which were in full bloom and arrayed in all their glory at the commencement of this cold spell, are now dressed in sadness. The land mourns and nature wears a general gloom." On the eleventh they finished the hotbed and put the sweet potatoes in it.

In 1850 the Shakers issued a four-page illustrated leaflet advertising Extract of Sarsaparilla, signed S. D. Howe and Co., Cincinnati. It shows a Shaker brother on the back cover, holding a sarsaparilla bottle. A testimonial signed D. M. Bennett states that this is the same recipe as that used by the Shakers in New York and New Hampshire. Bennett, formerly a physician to the New Lebanon Shakers, seceded in 1846, and it can be assumed that he furnished Dr. Howe with the formula for Howe's Shaker Sarsaparilla.

The Shakers issued another publication the same year, *The Influence of the Shaker Doctor*,[8] a ten-page illustrated advertising circular for medicines made at the Shaker Village. It showed a Shaker residence; the medical laboratory, exterior and interior; the office building and pictures of Peter Boyd, Dr. J. R. Singerland, and Dr. Louis Turner. And it said of the latter:

> Dr. Louis Turner a regular graduate of medicine, of high repute, number of years ago, engaged in the manufacture and sale of medicines, made from the formulas he used in his extensive practice, and found to be specifics for those troubles, he recommended them for.
>
> The merit of those remedies, having received for them a most extensive sale, it became necessary for the doctor to increase his facilities, owing to the difficulty he experienced, in supplying the demand, and at the same time attend to his other duties. The chief source of embarrassment which presented itself at this time, was the trouble of obtaining a sufficient quantity of crude material, such as Roots, Barks, Buds, Berries, Blossoms and Seeds, which had been gathered at the proper time, to secure their best medical effect.
>
> It was under these perplexing circumstances that the Doctor concluded to arrange with the Shakers, his old friends, as being the best prepared to help him out of the difficulty. . . .
>
> From his knowledge of the Shakers, the Doctor concluded to select the Community at Union Village, Warren County, Ohio, as being the best suited for his purpose. This society is the parent community of the west, being the most important west of the Allegheny Mountains and dates from 1805, they own 4,500 acres of land in one tract, which for fertility, and other qualities, is perhaps unexcelled by any body of land of equal size on the continent. The special reason Dr. Turner expected to find here exactly what he needed, was that he knew here was founded in 1833, a special Botanical Garden for raising medicinal plants, under the care of the scientific members of the Shakers, prominent among which may be mentioned Dr. Abiathar Babbitt, and Dr. Andrew Houston, who at the same time acted as physicians to the community and neighborhood. The following endorsement will serve to show the great advance they have also made in skillfully preparing their "nature's remedies" into medical products.

The story as told by the Shakers continues:

> After signifying his intention Dr. Turner paid a visit to this community and was met at Lebanon the nearest R.R. station by the oldest member of the society, and on the way was impressed by this venerable man that here was evidence, of not only a knowledge of the laws of health, but a keen insight into scientific, and experienced medication, and how life may be prolonged in its full vigor. Dr. Turner was first shown through the Botanical Garden which had been established for so many years, and which he saw was in the best possible condition. Such plants as are improved by the care of man were here seen to almost give out their medical qualities without any manipulation, while those which flourish best under the retiring influence of shade and moisture remained undisturbed.
>
> Men and women were busy collecting portions of the plants, which had reached the proper state, under the direction of the Shaker Doctor J. R. Singerland, who was introduced to Dr. Turner, and informed of the object of his visit.
>
> They together paid a visit to the Laboratory, where the plants were being carried and where they were to be made into powerful and palatable medicines.
>
> This is done by those intricate and interesting chemical manipulations which cannot be described in a phamplet [sic] of this size, but caused Dr. Turner to be more than pleased when he saw how everything seemed to be made especially to meet his requirements.
>
> Dr. Turner, under the guidance of the Shaker Doctor went over the Farm, carefully noting all the surroundings, which he afterward had reproduced to illustrations, so that a fair conception could be had by those knowing and using his remedies.
>
> Nothing could be more complete than the arrangement of vats, receivers, etc., which he saw in the interior of the medical laboratory.
>
> The Shaker Doctor before referred to [Singerland], asked to examine the formulas for his medicines which Dr. Turner had brought with him, and he was not long in discovering that

the advice and influence of the Shaker Doctor would be worth considering. A discussion arose as to some worthy changes, and after a full and free exchange of ideas, which had the combined experience and learning of these two men, resulted in producing a line of medicines; which have accomplished wonderful results for good, and which is alike gratifying to patient and doctor.

Right here Dr. Turner wants it understood by all, that these remedies are made by the Shakers, and they will vouch for their purity and curative action.

If anyone doubts this statement write Dr. J. R. Singerland, Union Village, Warren Co., Ohio, who will cheerfully give an endorsement wished.

The community is also provided with a large and convenient office building, to which the Doctor after having been assured by his companion that the community was able in every particular to meet all requirements, was invited, where the serious consideration of his business was to take place.

The remaining pages of the booklet are devoted to Dr. Turner's Wonder Herbs, "the great Shaker Blood Cure, for all altered, changed and poisoned conditions of the blood," and Turner's Wonder of Shaker Pain Cure. These two medicines were prescribed for rheumatism; neuralgia; sick, nervous, or bilious headache; burns and scalds; diarrhea, cramps, colic, cholera morbus, and cholera; corns; earache; sprains, bruises, and cuts; sore throat and diphtheria; catarrh; inflammation of the kidneys; piles; pains in the side, breast, back, or any part of the system; asthma and phthisic; dyspepsia; contracted cords or muscles; deafness; chilblains or frosted feet; toothache; fever and ague; nervous prostration and general debility; and skin diseases. A final paragraph was directed

> To the Ladies—who suffer Periodical Pains in the Back, burning sensation at the top of the head, dragging down pains below the waist, palpitation of the heart, smothering sensations and general lassitude of the system, take from ten to thirty drops in a little sweetened water from one to three times a day, at the same time using the Wonder as directed for Rheumatism, also use Slingerland's Shaker Granules.

The granules referred to were made like all the rest of Shaker medicines, the advertisement said, and, for the ladies "to whom life has become a wearisome burden and whose power and nerve force seems gone," this botanic drug was guaranteed to be "nature's proper restorer."

Dr. Turner also advertised a Consumption Cure or Shaker Cough Remedy. He said that there were more than 200,000 deaths from consumption each year in the United States, and in more than two thirds of the cases there was no trace of hereditary consumption. Most cases, he claimed, started with a slight cold which could have been cured easily by a single bottle of his consumption cure.

With the medicine business increasing each year it was quite natural that Deacon Peter Boyd's duties as business manager increased more and more.[9] His account books and letters for 1851 and 1852 tell the story:

> To G. H. Reynolds, Cincinnati. We should be thankful to obtain your check and will be pleased to supply you with more items on our most libral terms. We have made considerable additions to our gardens and other conveniences for pulverizing, by which our assortment is improved and we prefer selling low. For the cash we make a liberal discount according to the amount ordered.

> To Means and Wilder: We have an excellent assortment of Medicines on hand and will sell low for cash, lowering from our catalogue price according to the amount ordered. Thank you also for the Information concerning J. H. Reynolds, Your friend Peter Boyd.

> William Glowny: Respected Friend. We have to state that we sell our Sarsaparilla syrup for $8.00 per gallon, always cash. If you wish a supply we can send it to the City almost any

week by our own market waggon which stands at 5th Street Market on Fridays in each
week. The name of the person with whom you can make the payments is Moses Miller. You
can furnish him with a vessel of suitable size to contain what you wish free of charge to us
and it will be sent down the next week. Your Friend, etc. P.S. Send for but little at this time
as we are scarce of the article.

Peter Boyd was very strict in allowing commissions:

We are not in the habit of distributing our medicines on commission. We sell low for cash as
you will perceive by our catalogue which we have sent you. Your order accompanied by a
remittance will be personally attended to. The Garden Seed one [catalog] kept by C. Hallo-
way and I think he has distributed all he expects to send out this season.

Deacon Boyd had some difficulty in filling orders on his own however.

Union Village July 21, 1851. W. W. Brown: Estimed Friend; Your order of the 15th. Inst. is to
hand and we have all the articles ordered ready, except the s. marjoram which will be ready
to send in about two weeks, but some of them we cannot sell at your prices as we have to
pay for some of them considerable higher in New York City for instance. Barberry bark you
price at 20 cents, we pay about 10 cents higher in this instance besides the freight from New
York. Poppy flowers we cannot sell at less than our catalogue price which is 75 cents. But our
uniform way of doing business is where the customer purchases from $150.00 to $200.00 per
year we allow a discount of 20 percent off less than that amount, 10% off and above that
amount 25% off. We will delay sending your order for the present and wait your reply.
Hoping to hear from you soon, I remain your friend, Peter Boyd. By W. H.

A letter regarding tansy oil indicates that the deacon was having some help with
the correspondence.

None at present due to failure of crop. Cause miserable drought—but one house in our
village can supply 18 to 20 bottles which they will furnish for $1.00 cash per.

In a letter to Edward Fowler, dated September 12, 1850, Peter Boyd asks him to
supply at the lowest price the following herbs and roots: aconite root, black elder,
borage, balmony leaves, cancer root, centaury (*Centaurea cyanus*), lavender seed growth
of 1851, cow-parsnip root, frostwort, hardhack leaves, laurel leaves, lady's slipper root,
fevertwig [bittersweet] root.
To Chauncey Copley of Watervliet he wrote:

Dear Brother; Will you please be so kind as to affix your lowest prices to the following
articles and oblidge your friend, Peter Boyd.
    Prices in bulk and in paper pressed: 40 lbs. aconite leaves, 40 angelica root, 30 lbs.
evans root, 40 lbs. Black elder, 10 lbs. borage, 50 lbs. Balmony leaves, 10 lbs. cancer
root, 40 lbs. centaury (sabatia angularis) 40 lbs. centaury (s. paniculata), 20 lbs. coriander seed herb, growth of 1851, 20 lbs. cowparsnip root, 10 lbs. frostwort, 5 lbs. hardhack, 20 lbs. laurel leaves, 30 lbs. lady slipper roots, 40 lbs. male fern roots, 400 lbs.
pipsisaway, 20 lbs. wild indigo, 20 lbs. extract of aconite.

He wrote a letter dated December 12, 1851, to:

Beloved Brother David Parker: We shall be glad to have your order for a large amount of oils
of peppermint and wormseed. Perhaps it might answer you to make an arrangement with
Jonathan Wood, New Lebanon. We are indebted there and should like our oil to pay the
same. Anything that you can do that would be mutually benefical we should be glad and
thankful for. Your friend. P. B.

It is easy to understand the indignation of Deacon Peter when bills were not paid. To Dr. H. Snizer:

> You should have a better thinking about doing business with our concern. You have our medicine, we do not have your money. The information you give in your letter is untrue and we expect a speedy correspondence with remittance to correct the situation.

He also had trouble in this respect with one H. P. Turner in Kentucky and there ensued several very brisk letters regarding some large orders without remittance.

> Sir: How do you suppose we should think of them [the material] being seized on the way by your creditors when you had not paid the insurance. Henry, we shall hold you in honor bound to pay the debt to us by any bank in Cincinnati.

Again H. P. Turner gave him trouble. "Respected Friend: I would be glad to accommodate you with the drugs if I could do so and see myself safe for the payment. You owe $75. plus $23. since 12 months past." And finally Boyd sought outside help in collecting:

> March 25, 1852, Postmaster, Hopkinsville, Kentucky. Respected Friend: My object of addressing you at this time is to get you to do me the favor of giving me the name of some suitable person to collect a claim I have on a man in your place by the name of P. Turner. I think he is in the drug business, perhaps he practices medicine. My claim is a note of hand given last March for $75. and $23. Any information on this subject will be thankfully received. Peter Boyd.

In 1875 the society at Union Village was free of debt and, according to Noyes, "one of the families had a fund at interest." And still, this lovely village, this "pattern of neatness," this affluent community, suffered from unfortunate business management and deceitful members who plunged the society into bankruptcy, making it necessary to sell the land and eventually to liquidate the community.

NORTH UNION, OHIO

The Parent Ministry of the United Society of Believers organized the society at New Lebanon (later named Mt. Lebanon) in 1787. It presided over all 18 communities of the sect for 160 years and was particularly concerned with the eastern brethren. It was assisted but not exceeded in its authority by the ministry at Union Village, Ohio, whose responsibility was the western societies. This ministry, while subordinate to that at Mt. Lebanon, ruled or had a general responsibility over the societies in Ohio and Kentucky.

These two societies were concerned with the founding in 1826 of North Union. Sixty-three years later the community which, once founded, proved to be successful and also important in the development of that portion of the Western Reserve, nonetheless closed its doors.

From account books, journals, and letters of visiting Shaker brethren we have a complete picture of the life at North Union and the products raised by the families. The seed and herb gardens were enormous. They and the orchards took up one-third of all the premises of the East family. The garden house at the East family was mentioned as being spacious and used as a dryhouse also. The garden nursery and the orchards at the Center family farm were large, and there was also a fine toolhouse, notable for its size.

A map of the lands of the Center family in 1880 shows large gardens and orchards and a sage hedge covering an area as big as the pear orchard on the map. In all Shaker settlements sage was a major crop. It is the one herb which is mentioned in Prescott's manuscript when he writes that the seed garden was fenced off in 1835.

Later, Elder James S. Prescott writes:

> Brother Samuel being a successful gardner wished the society to have an extensive garden in order to enter the seed business. To this end we had fenced off six acres on the east side of the road opposite the Center house and it extended as far as the old cabin grounds. Christian Slade came to us direct from Germany. He too is a gardner and will assist.

At North Union, the Shakers, like other pioneers, raised herbs and medicinal plants for their own use. Caroline Piercy in *The Valley of God's Pleasure* tells us about the cultivation of herbs at North Union:

> In the fine gardens were rows of tansy, horehound, feverfew, thyme, marjoram, marigold, foxglove, dandelion, boneset, numerous mints, roses and lavendar. . . . The sisters went gathering in the wild berry-tea, penny royal and catnip for teas; poke berries for ink and sundry roots and herbs for poultices and steeps. The neatly kept rows of red roses with no thought of their beauty and fragrance, were raised to be converted into delicate rosewater with which the sisters bathed the feverish brow or flavored the crisp apple pies or the enormous silver cakes—especially produced for Christmas and Mother Ann's birthday. Nor was the making of wild-cherry bitters, various tonics or medicinal wines ever neglected.

In a recent history of Shaker Heights (now a suburb of Cleveland) the North Union community is discussed and the industries of the Shakers are described. In the order of their productivity and chief source of income they were the manufacture of woolen goods, and the dairy business, which supplied quantities of milk, butter, cheese, and eggs to the Cleveland market. "The seed business was carried on very extensively, as well as the sale of medicinal herbs which they gathered and prepared for the market. Large amounts of fruit were prepared and canned, not only for their own consumption but for the sale to the outside world in which they found a ready market. People soon learned that there was a better flavor to the Shakers canned goods. . . ."

If the Shakers at North Union had circulated seed or herb catalogs or handbills to sell produce, it seems likely that careful researchers would have found them. Dr. Harry D. Piercy, for example, presented a paper on Shaker medicines to the Ohio Academy of Medical History, May 1, 1954, at Columbus, Ohio. Dr. Piercy's paper refers to the Shaker herb industry in some detail at Mt. Lebanon, Harvard, Canterbury, Union Village, and South Union, but he does not mention North Union at all. A few years later in August 1959, Charles O. Lee, Professor of Pharmacy at Ohio Northern University, presented a paper at the annual convention of the American Pharmaceutical Association in Cincinnati, "The Shakers as Pioneers in the American Herb and Drug Industry." He does not mention North Union either as being involved in the herb industry. It seems safe to assume that the herb business at this community was not a source of income or a business; it only served to provide medicines for its members.

Several Shaker societies in their early days followed the Thomsonian practice of herbal medicine. This was logical because of their thinking that herbs could cure all ailments, as herbs were the first medicine used by man. (Samuel Thomson was born in Alstead, New Hampshire, in 1769. One of six children, he was often taken into the woods to help a botanic practitioner gather herbs and plants. When very young he experimented with the herb lobelia, which he discovered to be an emetic. He cut his leg badly when he was 19 years old and against advice to have it amputated he applied a poultice of comfrey root and saved his leg. Having proved the emetic qualities of lobelia he advocated the necessity of eliminating waste materials from the body to restore it to the natural condition of health. He also stressed steaming the body outwardly and using herb stimulants to produce inward heat. These were the rudiments of Thomsonian medical practices.)

In his *History of North Union*, James S. Prescott writes:[10]

> *Doctoring.* Their former mode of practice for curing physical disease was Thomsonian more than any other, but of late years (1880) since they have paid more attention to ventilating

their sleeping apartments and dwelling rooms and have become better informed with regard to the laws of life and health, sickness is almost unknown among them, consequently they have but little use for lobelia, drugs or doctors of any kind, not withstanding.

Deaths. No pestilential diseases have ever been known among them—in time of cholera, no case has ever been known, this may be attributed in great measure to their regular habits and clanliness [sic].

PLEASANT HILL, KENTUCKY

Elisha Thomas's 140-acre farm, located on the Shawnee Run, high above the Kentucky River, was the nucleus of the Shaker society founded and organized at Pleasant Hill in 1814. Situated between Harrodsburg and Lexington in the midst of the famous blue-grass region of the state, the beautiful rolling meadows of this farm on a level limestone plateau eventually totaled over 4,300 acres.

A writer has given an account in *The Cultivator* for September 1856 of Pleasant Hill.[11] This farm journal notes that the Shaker farm at Pleasant Hill includes about 5,000 acres of land and that the buildings "are excellent and commodious and several of them remarkably well proportioned, if not absolutely tasteful, their principles being opposed to extraneous show and ornament." The article praised the Shakers for being careful and systematic farmers being "among the first in giving attention to improved stock," and commented upon their self-sufficiency:

> With the exception of cotton and sugar only, we believe they are the producers of nearly all their own foods and clothing and necessities, bringing into requisition quite a wide range of raw material and giving occasion for many labor saving contrivances, which last, like the best economists everywhere they think it the wisest policy to invent or make use of whenever possible.
>
> The main sales of the community are of garden seeds in which they do a large business in the south, and west, and of preserved fruits. Of the last they dispose of jars and cans to the amount of twelve to fourteen hundred dollars worth last year. They are preserved of course with the utmost neatness, and put up so that they will keep for any length of time.

Travelers have said little about the herb industry of Pleasant Hill. It was not conducted on a scale such as that of the Shakers of the eastern societies or of Union Village, Ohio. Nevertheless journals and diaries written from 1843 to 1888 record considerable activity in the raising and selling of herbs.

Dr. Benjamin Dunlavy's diary for January 1843 notes: "Today we ploughed up a piece of meadow on the west side of the south shed for the purpose of removing the medical garden to that place. Same day ploughed up a piece of meadow, on the west side of the south street, twice as large, as we need more space. Medical garden by John Shain, length 28 feet by 11 feet."[12]

A family journal kept by Order of the Deaconesses of the East House between 1843 and 1871 is concerned with many events and activities:[13]

June 1st [1843]	We make a general turn out to gather herbs for sale.
June 2nd.	We gather herbs again.
June 3rd.	We gather first meal of strawberrys.
June 29th.	The sisters went to the Mill to gather elder flowers for sale.
July 13th.	The sisters began to gather cherrys to dry.
Aug. 19th.	The sisters went to the Shawney [sic] Springs after boneset. A medical herb.
Sept. 1st.	Sisters gathered medical herbs.

May 3rd [1844]	Some of the sisters from each family went with John Shain and James Cooney to Harrison after hoarhound [sic] for sale.
May 7th.	Went after hoarhound.
May 29th.	The first herb was cut in John's garden.
Aug. 21st.	The sisters began to dry apples. Same day went for loblia [sic].

Produce in 1845 for sale . . . 1175 pounds of herbs.

May 5, 1846	The sisters began to gather herbs.
May 12th.	Five hands began to gather herbs.
May 23rd.	All hands turned out to gather herbs.
June 6th.	All hands engaged in gathering cherries and herbs.
June 17th.	Gathered herbs again.
July 15th.	These times are chiefly occupied in gathering herbs.
July 25th.	Still going on with fruits and herbs.
Aug. 20th.	Another trip was taken after herbs.

Produce for sale 1846, 550 pounds of herbs.

May 6, 1847	Gathered some herbs.
June 2nd.	. . . Gathered herbs.
Aug. 26th.	Gathered lobelia in the rye field.
Sept. 30th.	Gathered hops and apples.
Oct. 1st.	The sisters went after hoarhound.
Oct. 16th.	Dug and roasted meadow roots, also went after herbs.

Produce for sale, 1847. 761¾ pounds of herbs.

The journal continues:

June 24, 1848	Went after elder flowers.
July 23rd.	Went after wild plants.
Sept. 7th.	Went to the cliff pastured after life everlasting, found lobelia there very unexpectedly. Gathered it.
Sept. 8th.	Gathered life everlasting and lobelia.
Oct. 24th.	Began to put up herbs again.

Produce for sale, 1848, 529 pounds of herbs.

June 1, 1849	Gathered hoarhound and finished gathering herbs in the garden.
June 5–22.	Gathered hoarhound, catnep and elderblow.
June 26th.	William and the sisters went after mint and elderblows with the waggons.

Several entries follow as to picking elder blows and blackberries to make into cordials.

| Sept. 28th. | The brethren commenced pressing herbs. |

Produce for sale, 1849, 504 pounds of herbs.

May 1, 1850	The Center and West sisters trimmed off the thyme and tanzy in John's garden.
May 3rd.	Gathered hoarhound in the hen lot.
May 4th.	Cleaned the garden house and press house.

John Shain not only managed the medical garden, but also took to the road to peddle garden seeds, herbs, and brooms. It was on these excursions that he kept an eye open for children orphaned by the cholera epidemics of 1833 and 1849, bringing them home to be cared for by the Shakers, perhaps to remain at Pleasant Hill for many years.

A financial journal kept by one family, but not identified, lists the pounds of herbs they produced: In 1850, 417; 1851, 600; 1852, 271; 1853, 107; 1854, 160; and 1855, 282.[14]

A journal kept by Kitty Jane Ryan commencing January 1, 1839, records an herb industry in the Center family.[15]

July 25, 1949	Gathered sage and other herbs in the garden. The largest cutting ever known. Gathered blackberries at the Cove spring.
Sept. 29th.	Gathered hops, grapes and walnut roots for dye. Went after herb roots with Joel and three sisters and all the boys, but got none.
May 1, 1850	Trimmed off the thyme and tanzy in John's garden.
May 1–4th.	Cut herbs in the garden, burned caterpillars, gathered hoarhound, tanzy, bugleweed in the hen lot, cleaned herb house and press house.
June 16–19th.	Gathered and shipped off catnep, gathered sage, thyme and other garden herbs.
June 31st.	Gathered blackberries and mint.
Aug. 6th.	The whole society of sisters went out after supper and cut sage. William went to Harrodsburg after roots.
Aug. 24th.	The young sisters set up the night previous and cut peaches and apples to fill dry house and press herbs. The sisters generally took a walk to the Cliffs with the North Union [Cleveland] Visitors.

The Kentucky River was a great channel of transportation that the Shakers used to ship products from their farms and shops southward. One of the marketable medicines which traveled this route was the Shaker Aromatic Elixir of Malt. A broadside advertising it claimed: "Manufactured exclusively by the Shakers at Pleasant Hill, Mercer Co., Ky., under the supervision of R. B. Rupe, M. D. Pharmacist. Orders to be addressed to E. S. Sutton, General Agent, Louisville."[16] But the manufacture of the elixir, from 1880 to 1883, was a short-lived enterprise, for the lack of profits caused the Shakers to abandon the undertaking. The label on the bottle showed a Shaker brother and stated:

This elegant elixir may be used in all cases where the extract is indicated and it will prove far superior, for it is Carmative, Nutrient and Tonic. It may be administered in Consumption, Debility, the Loss of Flesh and Strength, Variable Appetite, Dispepsia, Headache, Flatulence, Diarrhoea, etc., etc.

This preparation of malt is grateful to the most delicate Stomach, and can be prescribed in many cases, where the common extract of Malt can not be taken.

It is also a good vehicle for the administration of Quinine, Iron, Cod Liver Oil, etc., etc. . . . R/x Aromatic Elixir seven parts; Pure Extract of Malt (our own make) eight parts. Dose for adults one tablespoon three times a day after meals. Children less in proportion to age. Retail per bottle, $1.00. Six bottles for $5.00.

Dunlavy and Scott, Trustees.

Another advertisement, dated 1877, informs the public:[17]

Pure and Reliable Medicines: Manufactured and for Sale by the Shakers, Pleasant Hill. We append to our Catalogue of Preparations our Remedies, with the methods of the U.S.P. (Pharmacopaea) 1877 so that all parties concerned may compare the results of each and in this way may draw their own conclusions as to which method is the best to Secure Pure and Reliable Medicines of *full strength* in acts of principle and menstrums. N. B. Spurious and fraudulent imitations may be sold for much less than the Real and Pure, but are vastly more costly in the end.

Orders again were directed to Dunlavy and Scott.

One might feel that some of the testimonies concerning material produced by the Shakers are boastful, but in reality the claims were true. So much attention and care were devoted to making a perfect article the Brethren felt justified in selling it with praise.

SOUTH UNION, KENTUCKY

Sixty-two years after its founding in 1811, the society at South Union was prosperous and appeared to have recovered from the disastrous years of the Civil War. While all of the communities in Ohio, and to a much lesser degree the eastern families, suffered from the war and its aftereffects, nothing could compare to the harassment, destruction, and desolation experienced at South Union and Pleasant Hill. But the beautiful rich farmlands at South Union were producing bumper cash crops in 1873. Other sources of income were the preserved fruit business, leasing of farmland, and the raising of garden seeds, an extensive operation.

During the three decades prior to the Civil War the society had been almost entirely self-sufficient, and the members provided nearly all of the food and clothing they needed. They had planted large orchards of peach, cherry, and apple trees and acres of gardens to produce vegetable seeds for the market. They grew medicinal herbs for their own use and sold the surplus along with the garden seeds.

In South Union seeds were first marketed in 1821; ten years later the business had expanded so that the Shakers could record that on one day in March, 5,525 paper seed bags were pasted with labels printed on the village's own press. In October 1831 the sisters had prepared 33,290 packets of seed for sale down the Mississippi to New Orleans by flatboat.

The large seed boxes, divided into compartments to hold the seed packages, had a printed label on the inside cover which read:[18]

> If you want a splendid Garden buy the Shakers' [South Union, Kentucky] GARDEN SEEDS. They are more reliable and better adapted to the climate of the South than seeds grown in a colder region.

The label on the Shakers' Winter Turnep seeds said: "Winter Turnep makes the best and earliest greens in the Spring of any vegetable. Sow at the end of Summer or early in the Fall, in light rich soil, and in drills 18 in. apart. Hoe when the leaves are two or three inches long, and when the plants are somewhat larger hoe again, and thin them to 9 in. apart. When sown broadcast in the field they are excellent for sheep."

The earliest "Catalogue of Shaker Garden Seeds" grown at South Union was an 1843 broadside. It lists 34 varieties. From 1850 on, 17 were distributed selling seeds from the garden crops of 1853, 1856, 1857, 1858; 1861, 1866, 1867, 1868, 1869; 1870, 1871, 1872, 1873, 1875, 1877. A four-page catalog was issued in 1884.

The Shakers' cholera remedy carried on its label: "This remedy was discovered by Dr. J. P. Holmes, deceased, late member [of the society] from whom we obtained the formula."[19] A statement of the efficacy of this medicine in the London epidemics is signed by Dr. Holmes.

The South Union Shakers used herbal remedies in their nursing. There are records that herbs were gathered in the wild state but that the Shakers grew and sold sage themselves. Hervey Eades writes on June 12, 1833: "*Herb Press*. Samuel McClelland finished and put up a new herb press for pressing herbs for sale."

A Shaker record from 1804 to 1836, later transcribed by Hervey Eades in 1870, and also one of Eades's own journals contain many interesting details of the lives of the Believers and the medical procedures and herbs they used:[20]

Nov. 6th. Spider Bite! Andrew Barnett while rising was bitten by a spider and soon life despaired of. A great many things done, given Black snake root. Plantain, sweet oil clysters, warm baths, drafts of raw onions, spirits of Harts Horn. Did not get about until the next 3rd day and not entirely well for over two weeks. Note: [from H. L. Eades] The Spirits of Hart Horn perhaps was the only thing that did any good. In a precisely similar case, I gave the patient nearly a half gill of *Hartshorn and Brandy* mixed and though previously screaming with pain, was relieved in 5 hours and well as common next day.

In their river trade the Shakers refer to peddling garden seeds, herbs, brooms, straw hats, socks, and jeans down the Red, the Ohio, and the Mississippi rivers to New Orleans. Material was traded for needed commodities, and other necessities were purchased. A journal of such a trip was kept from October 6, 1831, to February 2, 1832, by Thomas Jefferson Shannon.[21]

Brother Jefferson, or "T.J.," as he is referred to in his diaries, lists the sale of "Garden Seeds by the Box, $1,773.41," ten times the amount of any other single item sold. In the final accounting the sale of herbs is not itemized, but there are 15 references to selling herbs in the lengthy journal. Sage was sold most frequently, "A pound of sage. . . . Sage $10.00. . . . Sold some herbs worth $9.00. . . . Sold 52 ozs. essential oils at 25 cents per oz., $13.00. . . . Sold some sage. . . . Sage to John W. Swains' Drug Store and exchanged it for some medicines."

The records kept by Hervey L. Eades from October 1836 to April 1868 reveal the day-to-day activities of a busy family. He noted that the garden seed business continued to grow with increasing acreage put under cultivation for this industry. "Sept. 9th. Finished boxing garden seed . . . whole amount 170,000 papers."

He continues:

1847   June 30th. White walnut bark. Brothers George Rankin and Deacon Reubin Wise get it at Frazers. . . . Whole amount of wheat this year 829½ bushels.
        July 23rd. Lobelia gathering. Elder Brother S. Shannon, Olive and Lucy Shannon and Denise Barker go to Stokes' oil field for this purpose.
        July 27th. Eli and Sisters gather lobelia again at Stokes.
1848   October 3rd. Gardners finished putting up seed. 103,143 papers.
        October 6th. Gather chestnuts. . . .
1850   October 7th. Finished papering 110,000 papers of seed. . . .
1854   July 12th. Blackberries. Teams and hands, Sisters especially, into the country to gather blackberries to make wine and cordial. . . .
1857   January 23rd. T. J. Shannon and L. Pearce Field returned. This seed trip brought $4310. [A February seed trip brought $2,425.]

The next four years covered in Eades's diary are still concerned with the events in the families (but he is mostly concerned with the Civil War). Hervey Eades, now an elder, continues his record, in 1864, by stating "the money wealth of the Society, $45,000 in bonds and cash." There were also "210 souls, 1st, 2nd, and Junior Orders."

1864   February 25th. Seed trip south down the Mississippi River, the first since the War got under way. Elder H. L. Eades and Brother Jackson McGown start by Railroad to Louisville thence down Ohio and Mississippi Rivers with 150 Boxes, 30,000 papers and garden seeds. Late for a southern trip.
        March 22nd. Return of Elder Hervey. Successful as could be expected. $1450. Expenses were enormous, $400.

The outbreak of the Civil War placed the Believers of Kentucky in a difficult position. They had never owned slaves, and did not approve the institution which permitted it, and on that account were regarded with distrust and suspicion by the pro-slavery element of the neighborhood, while their principles of pacifism, which forbade them to take up arms in the defense of the Union, brought them into conflict with the authorities at Washington. Much tact was required on the part of the leaders to steer safely through those troubled times. Their settlements were often occupied by northern and southern forces, and the bands of irresponsible guerrillas were a constant source of anxiety, but their greatest loss came from the almost total cessation of business. Nevertheless Eades could write:

> The garden seed [business] has become good. Sales better than for many years. A large business is done in the seed line . . . and also in the Chh [Church family] in pressed and prepared herbs and roots, besides many tons in bulk . . . considerably many tons of powdered herbs and roots . . . and many tons of Extracts, both solids and fluids. The War makes great demand for all these articles. They sell in large quantities. We cannot prepare enough to meet the demand.

> 1865   January 30th. Ex. Elder Soloman Rankin and James Richardson started south west and west with a small load of seeds. This trip is extra hazardous having to pass through guerilla country. I do not look for them to return with their horses as one looks well and is about sure to be taken, if the guerillas come across them, we hope they may return with their lives.
>
> February 2nd. Brother Joseph Averett started south with small load of seeds. Springlike weather.
>
> February 7th. Elder William Ware started from the Junior Order with a horse load of seeds, 1400 papers. He goes via Gallatin out to middle and east Tennessee. We cannot but have unpleasant forbodings for him. . . .
>
> February 12th. Ex-Elder Soloman Rankin and James Richardson returned this evening. Succeeded tolerably well in sales. Brought home with them $390. Were not molested by guerilas. . . .
>
> November 29th. Elder Asa Ware and John Perryman returned. Profit of trip $857.
>
> December 11th. *Seed Trip*. H. L. Eades and C. Blakey took the cars this morning for Louisville via Memphis and Mississippi Central Railroad to dispose of garden seeds. They have 27,000 papers.
>
> 1866   October 28th. *Seed soliciting trip*. Brother T. J. Shannon returned home today in good health. He succeeded well in getting orders for seeds. He sent and brought home orders for about 150,000 papers to be delivered at 5 cents per paper.
>
> October 31st. Nutting and pleasure excursion. Two Brothers, two Sisters, Jane Cowan, school teacher, and thirty-three girls took jaunt to forest today.

When peace was restored after the Civil War, Elder Hervey Eades, a Shaker for all 55 years of his life, applied himself with great energy to building up and maintaining the size of his community, by intense recruiting and receiving orphans. Keeping the members in good health was a constant burden and worry. Eades also had to repair the financial damage his community had suffered. He was successful at that, but as the years went on he was pained to see the steady decline in the number of members. Julia Neal in commenting about the society after the war says:[22]

> Practicing their economic precepts in the reconstruction years as they had in the beginning period of the society, the trustees took advantage of every possible source of income, offering for sale such nonrelated items as 181 pounds of Jamestown weed or "Strammon"; 1,121 pounds of honey "the most ever got in one season"; and tanyard leather, the 1867 sale of which brought $1,296.57.

The reference to "Jamestown weed," or *Datura stramonium*, is the only one this author has encountered in records of the western societies. It was an energetic narcotic poison and, although handled by some of the eastern Shakers in their medical department, was eventually dropped as being too dangerous.

The vigorous and well administered Society at South Union which Elder Henry Blinn praised during his visit in 1873 diminished gradually in numbers and in prosperity. Over a long period of years, at most fifty, the members under good leadership for the most part worked with characteristic energy to maintain their industries and trade.

After the thirteenth amendment was ratified in December 1865, the Shakers were pleased to be able to hire men who had been slaves, and it was lawful to pay them directly. This came at a time when because of their reduced membership extra hands were needed to increase the output of the community. Even so, when Elder Henry died in 1892, there were less than 200 souls under his ministry and thirty years later, only ten.

The society closed and the property was sold in 1922. This brave band of Believers had withstood the invasions of both the Union and the Confederate armies, raging epidemics and national financial panics, but changes in the outer world, in material, industrial, and social conditions, were not favorable toward enticing even the most sympathetic into their restrictive society. Against this trend, the Shakers were helpless.

WATERVLIET AND WHITEWATER, OHIO, AND BUSRO, INDIANA

Third in size to Union Village and North Union in Ohio was Watervliet, founded in 1813, a year after Union Village. It was a prosperous community until it closed in 1900. During its 87 years its membership rose to 100 and then declined, until it was necessary to merge with Union Village.

Elder Henry Blinn wrote in his journal in 1873 that the society owned 5,000 acres of excellent land and that the garden covered five acres. He said, "They cultivate this for the market & have a stall in the city which is kept by one of the Brethren." However, there is no mention of the growing of herbs, nor are there examples of printed matter, either broadsides or catalogs, connected with the medicine business. It must be surmised that, although the society may have raised herbs for home consumption, they never grew a sufficient surplus to sell.

This is the same conclusion we must draw concerning four other Shaker societies not mentioned before. They are Whitewater, Ohio, 32 miles from Union Village, and West Union or Busro, Indiana.

WHITE OAK, GEORGIA, AND NARCOOSSEE, FLORIDA

The last two societies the Shakers organized were at White Oak, Georgia, started in 1896 but soon abandoned, and Narcoossee, Florida, organized in 1894 and dissolved several years later. These two efforts to extend the range of the society into the South, at a time when the northern communities were waning, are hard to understand in view of the realistic attitude of the Shakers in most matters. It seemed hardly to matter that their numbers were diminishing. The determination to survive and grow was as apparent as in the early days of the struggle of Mother Ann.

NOTES

1. Journal of Peter Boyd, Union Village, Ohio, March 1, 1805–December 15, 1850, Library of Congress, Washington, D.C.

2. Journal compiled from other journals made between March 1805 and 1894 by O. H. Hampton, added to in 1856 and 1857 by anonymous editor. Shaker Manuscript Collection, Library of Congress, Washington, D.C.

3. "A Register of Work performed by Second Family Sisters," recorded (1846–1849) by Sister Amy Slaters.

4. *Shaker Community Wines. A treatise on Pure Wines*, Assistant Trustee William G. Ayer (Union Village, Ohio, n.d.), 11 pp., p. 4. Library of Congress, Washington, D.C.

5. Botanical catalogs (Union Village: Press of Richard McNemar, 1847, 1850), Library of Congress, Washington, D.C.

6. Manuscript journal, Peter Boyd, January 1833–September 1837, Library of Congress, Washington, D.C.

7. Manuscript journal, Peter Boyd, 1844, Library of Congress, Washington, D.C.

8. *The Influence of the Shaker Doctor*, issued by Union Village Society, 1850, Cleveland, Western Reserve Historical Society.

9. Account book of Peter Boyd with copies of letters, 1851–1852. Library of Congress, Washington, D.C.

10. James S. Prescott, *History of North Union*, 2nd ed. (Printed by North Union Society, 1880), Cleveland, Western Reserve Historical Society.

11. The Albany [N.Y.] *Cultivator*, September 1856, Library of Congress, Washington, D.C.

12. Diary of Dr. Benjamin Dunlavy, 1843–1868, Library at Shakertown, Pleasant Hill, Ky.

13. Family journal kept by Order of the Deaconesses of the East House, 1843–1871, Library of the Filson Club, Inc., Louisville, Ky.

14. Financial journal of Pleasant Hill, Library of the University of Southern Kentucky, Bowling Green, Ky.

15. Center family journal, Pleasant Hill, 1843–1869, Library at Shakertown, Pleasant Hill, Ky.

16. Calendar, 1974, Library at Shakertown, Pleasant Hill, Ky.

17. Calendar, 1972, Library at Shakertown, Pleasant Hill, Ky.

18. Individual herb labels, Shaker Collection at Shakertown, South Union, Ky.

19. Ibid.

20. *History of South Union Colony 1804–36*, vol. 1-A (1804–21), transcribed 1870 by Hervey L. Eades from original journals and diaries pertaining to South Union, Western Kentucky State College, Bowling Green, Ky.

21. Journal of Thomas Jefferson Shannon, October 6, 1831–February 2, 1832, Library, University of Kentucky, Bowling Green, Ky.

22. Julia Neal, *By Their Fruits* (Chapel Hill, N.C.: University of North Carolina Press, 1947), p. 221.

12. SUMMARY AND CONCLUSION

Since the beginning of time man has depended upon herbaceous plants to cure his ailments and diseases. It is known how many plants the ancients used for medicinal purposes, how they made their choices among them, and what the effects were, for good or bad. Hippocrates, the Greek physician living in the fourth century B.C. (460-377), became an herbal practitioner in his attempt to disassociate medicine from the supernatural. In his writings he names about 400 simples for their medical value. This was a significant contribution, for up to his time the records of the great nations of antiquity, such as the Sumerians, Egyptians, Assyrians, Persians, Indians, and Chinese, prove that these people believed that it was the gods who first possessed the knowledge of plants and their healing properties.

The herbal written in the first century A.D. by the Greek Dioscorides, said to have been Antony and Cleopatra's private physician, includes as many as 600 medicinal plants and was accepted as an almost infallible authority throughout the Middle Ages. For more than 16 centuries this was regarded as one of the authoritative works on medical botany and formed the main source of the herbals written after his time. Scores of Latin editions of Dioscorides' work were printed during the period of the Renaissance, and they were translated into many European languages. Yet, strangely enough, there was no modern edition in English until 1934.

From the time of the ancients onward, in each century, in every country, each generation has produced its herbalists and their herbals. The English writer Mrs. C. F. Leyel says that "the eighteenth century in England was a period of rationalistic theorizing and systematizing, in which the art of herbalism, while steadily continuing to be practised throughout the country, was nevertheless ignored by English scientists preoccupied by other matters." Herbal remedies were much used and enjoyed great popularity among all classes. There was a remedy for gout which went by the name of the Duke of Portland's Powder. The Duke had been cured by this mixture and had the formula printed and distributed for the benefit of other sufferers. It was composed of gentian root, the leaves of germander, birthwort, and centaury. All of these were herbs used by the Shakers in their remedies.

In England until the nineteenth century illness and wounds were treated at home, usually by the mother of the family, or some woman specially skilled in the making and application of plasters, ointments, and medicines. In early America it also was the housewife's business to prescribe for her household and to provide the necessary reme-

113

dies, most of which were herbal. We are familiar with the stillroom in colonial houses. It usually was located in nearly every dwelling as close to the kitchen as possible. Here the mistress distilled her medicines and fragrant cosmetics and concocted healing salves and syrups.

The Shakers were no different from their fellow countrymen and neighbors in their dependence upon herbal remedies. Like the earlier colonists they brought their herbal lore and craft with them and were, as they had been in England, self-sufficient in maintaining good health by the use of herbs. Their health was of paramount importance to the early Shakers, for their numbers were few, and every soul counted. Thus they organized a form of medical treatment with herbs from the earliest days they had arrived in this country, and from this rather insignificant start we have traced the growth of a prosperous industry.

Healing in the eighteenth century was a ready field for the sharper, the quack, and the flamboyant purveyor of nostrums and cure-alls. But the Shakers, who many regarded as "religious quacks," brought herbal medicine to a plane of probity and respectability and, of course, their business in pure herbs accordingly became the source of enormous profit to the order. Relying on the account books and journals kept by those in authority in the medicine departments of the larger Shaker societies, we can make some calculation of the profitability of this business. During the 75 years when it was at its height, the business at Watervliet and Mt. Lebanon, New York; Harvard, Massachusetts; Canterbury, New Hampshire; and Union Village, Ohio, was averaging an aggregate gross of at least $150,000 annually. And this figure does not include the income of some of the smaller societies.

Even after the height of the herb business had passed, the members at Enfield, New Hampshire, could send a note to *The Manifesto* dated December 1889, stating that:

> The Brethren have finished the drying of the Dock root and have shipped some forty-four thousand pounds to the firm of J.C. Ayer and Co., Lowell, Mass. Of this quantity the Second Family raised 27,856 lbs., the First Family 11,139 lbs. and the North Family 5,031 lbs.

Dock root was selling around 50 cents per pound at this time.

The annual gross output under Jefferson Whyte's direction at Enfeld, Connecticut, was in excess of $30,000 and a good part of this was from the sale of herbs and herb seeds. It seems conservative to estimate that the industry in the smaller societies was producing an annual gross of at least $50,000 for a total yield of over $200,000, a business that today would be reckoned upwards of $2,000,000.

Modern science has long been contemptuous of herbal folk remedies. But in his book, *Plant Drugs That Changed the World*, Norman Taylor lists some botanicals, that will be found in the herbal section of this book, which formed a good part of the Shaker herb and drug industry. Mr. Taylor says:

> But in spite of much fumbling, science has given us priceless remedies, many of them derived from the plant lore of people quite innocent of science.[1]

In a way this epitomizes the Shaker excursion into the drug business. There was the need, and they supplied the herbs and helped to determine their proper use. So, if along the way some of the brethren fell ill of the "Mandrake malady," having ill-advisedly chewed on the root while gathering it, a brother could supply a remedy. If he were "baffled beyond art or skill," a physician was called to administer with more sophisticated skills and pathology, but many times he, too, used only herbal remedies.

Twentieth-century biologists all over the world continue to analyze plants which have been in the materia medica for centuries, and they are discovering properties which have been overlooked before. It is possible that researchers will come up with astonishing cures using plants which were relied upon by the Shakers and those who bought from them.

Elder Joseph Holden of Hancock, writing to a beloved brother on February 15, 1900, said: "The Gospel of Mother Ann is just as good today as it ever was and will bring the same peace to poor humanity, if they will only come to its requirements."

Are we not fortunate to have inherited so many aspects of her gospel. The faith to "live each day as if you had a thousand years to live, but as though you were to die to-morrow" and the hopeful exhortation of a strong but immensely gentle leader who said:

> It is now the spring of the year, and you have all had the privilege of being taught the way of God; and now you may all go home and be faithful with your hands. Every faithful man will go forth and put up his fences in season, and put his crops into the ground in season, and such a man may with confidence look for a blessing.

NOTES

1. Norman Taylor, *Plant Drugs That Changed the World* (New York: Dodd, Mead and Co., 1965), p. 2.

The Herbal Compendium

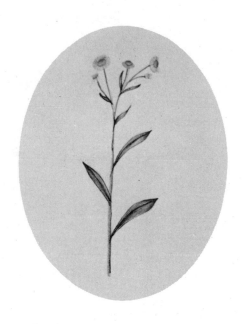

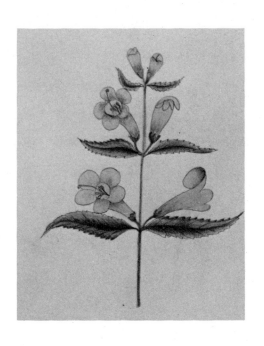

INTRODUCTION

Every herb employed for a medicinal purpose, whether in its natural state or after processing, belongs to the herbal materia medica. This section of the book lists those herbs that the Shakers collected, grew, or purchased for use in their own societies or for resale, together with the names of the communities participating and the years they did so.

Three hundred and two plants, shrubs, and trees with their roots, barks, flowers, and berries have been compiled, many of which were included in the Shaker pharmacopoeia of most of the Shaker societies at some period in their history.

The botanical names and the properties ascribed to the plants were taken from Shaker catalogs which covered a 64-year period from 1830 to 1894. The major source for this herbal compendium was the *Druggist's Hand-Book of Pure Botanic Preparations, &c. sold by Society of Shakers, Mount Lebanon, Columbia County, New York,* published in 1873. That catalog listed 304 herbs with their Latin names, the medical properties ascribed by the Shakers, and a synopsis of the various diseases in which they were used. There were two indexes, one of the botanical names and the other of 860 common names which included 557 synonyms. It eliminated many of the early herbal remedies and continued to offer for sale only those herbs which were most constantly in demand and relied upon by the medical profession.

The reader is urged to regard this list of medicinal plants and their uses as an addendum to the history of the Shaker herb industry. The botanical information given here is not intended to foster use of herbs by the amateur in cases of illness nor to replace the services of a physician. While every herb given here was classified at some time or other as medicinal in some degree, however slight, we are quoting the evaluation given them by the Shaker herbalists of the eighteenth and nineteenth centuries and not by present-day botanists.

Not every Shaker medicinal herb catalog carried every plant, of course, but all of the material the Shakers in five eastern states and three midwestern states prepared and sold has been listed.

The reader may also note minor omissions of information and discrepancies within the entries for individual herbs, and these are simply repetitions of the gaps or discrepancies in the original catalogs.

The herbs were sold in various quantities and forms, i.e., leaves, roots, bark, flowers, buds, berries, whole herbs, and in ground, fluid, pulverized, or solid form.

To make this herbal a more practical guide for today's student of botany, we have, in many cases, updated the nomenclature and corrected the Shakers' early spelling, having in mind that fixed or rigid botanical nomenclature in Latin or the vernacular is unattainable. The sources which were referred to in order to help resolve these inconsistencies were: *A Field Guide to Wildflowers* by Roger Tory Peterson and Margaret McKenney, *A Field Guide to the Ferns and Their Related Families* by Boughton Cobb, *A Field Guide to Trees and Shrubs* by George A. Petrides, *The Herbalist* by Joseph E. Meyer, *A Modern Herbal* by M. Grieve and Mrs. C. F. Leyel, *Hortus Second,* compiled by Liberty Hyde Bailey and Ethel Zoe Bailey, and *Manual of Botany,* 8th edition, by Asa Gray.

Opposite each herbal entry are listed several abbreviations. These indicate the major healing principles according to the old Shaker catalogs, listed in the order of priority given in those catalogs. The abbreviations are defined in the key that precedes the herbal entries. In addition, there is a glossary of medical and other terms that may be unfamiliar to readers, appearing at the back of this compendium.

To help identify the plants listed in this section we have arranged them alphabetically under their most familiar names. We have adopted this method used by two English herbal authorities, Mrs. Maud Grieve, compiler of *A Modern Herbal,* and Mrs. C. F. Leyel, who edited Mrs. Grieve's monumental work. The listing in the compendium differs from some other methods. We expect that interest in Shaker herbs will be largely a historical one for the amateur botanist. We hope the professional botanist will understand that the arrangement has been made to conform to that used by the Shakers in their catalogs. Should the reader be looking for a name such as Sweet Balsam, for example, not finding it under S he should check under B, where he will find it. In other cases, double names will be treated as a unit and will be alphabetized under the first letter of the first name. For example, Lady's Slipper will be found under L.

Common names listed in Shaker catalogs differed from place to place among the three major areas, Northeast, Midwest, and South, and these listings have been retained. Different parts of plants were used and different uses made of the herbs in the various communities and the Shaker catalogs also reflected this.

ABOUT THE ILLUSTRATIONS

During 1886 and 1887, Cora Helena Sarle, a sister at the Canterbury society, drew and painted these delicate but realistic herbs, finishing the work in her twentieth year. She had been in the society five years at that time and lived at Canterbury until her death in 1956 when she was 89 years old.

She did the drawings under the direction of Elder Henry Clay Blinn, a Canterbury Shaker from 1824 to his death in 1905, who wrote the description of each plant. Elder Henry was greatly interested in botany and in teaching it to the children in the society.

It is characteristic of the Shakers that these colorful drawings served also as a teaching device. Like the "Sacred Sheets" which were beautiful and articulate symbols of their religion, these drawings, annotated in Elder Henry's fine hand, were used to familiarize the Shaker schoolchildren with their native plants.

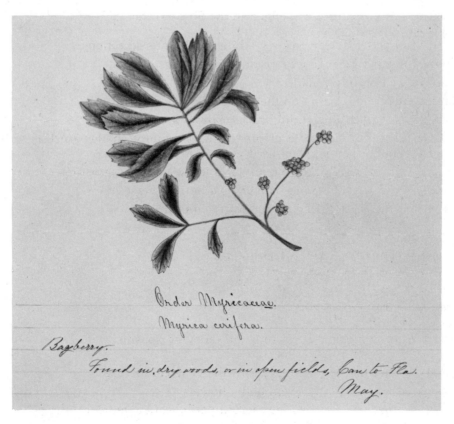

The illustration above is a sample of Cora Helena Sarle's art and Elder Henry Clay Blinn's description. Wherever such illustrations appear in the following herbal entries, the handwriting of Elder Blinn has not been included, but quotations from his descriptions appear near each drawing, preceded by the initials CHS.

KEY

Abbreviations of properties, as defined in the Shaker catalogs:*

A-BIL. ANTIBILIOUS Correcting the bile and bilious secretions.

ABO. ABORTIVE Capable of producing abortion.

ACR. ACRID, biting caustic.

ADEN. ADENAGIC Acting on the glandular system.

A-LITH. ANTILITHIC Preventing the formation of calculous matter.

ALT. ALTERATIVE Capable of producing a salutary change in disease through catalytic action when used with another substance.

ANAPH. ANAPHRODISIA Capable of blunting the venereal appetite.

ANO. ANODYNE Relieving pain or causing it to cease.

ANTHEL. ANTHELMINTIC Destroying or expelling worms.

ANTI-SCOR.,
A-SCOR.,
A-SCORB. ANTISCORBUTIC Opposed to scurvy.

ANTI-SEP.,
A-SEP.,
A-SEPT. ANTISEPTIC Opposed to putrefaction.

ANTI-SPAS.,
A-SPAS. ANTISPASMODIC Correcting and relieving spasms.

ANTI-SYPH.,
A-SYPH. ANTISYPHILITIC Acting against the venereal disease.

APE. APERIENT Gently opening the bowels.

A-PER. ANTIPERIODIC Arresting morbid periodical movement.

A-PHL. ANTIPHLOGISTIC Opposed to inflammation.

* In the individual herbal entries, abbreviated properties are listed in order of precedence, as they were in the original catalogs.

ARO.   AROMATIC   Agreeable, spicy.

AST.   ASTRINGENT   Contracting the organic textures.

BAL.   BALSAMIC   Mild, healing, and soothing.

CAR.,
CARM.   CARMINITIVE   Allaying pain by expelling the flatus.

CATH.   CATHARTIC   Increasing the number or the alvine evacuations.

CEPH.   CEPHALIC   Relating to the head.

CHOL.   CHOLAGOGUE   Causing the flow of bile.

COR.   CORROBORANT   Strengthening and giving tone.

DEM.   DEMULCENT   Correcting acrid conditions in the humors.

DEO.   DEOBSTRUENT   Removing obstructions.

DET.   DETERGENT   Cleansing parts of wounds.

DIA.,
DIAP.,
DIAPH.   DIAPHORETIC   Promoting moderate perspiration.

DIS.   DISCUTIENT   Repelling or resolving tumors.

DIU.   DIURETIC   Increasing the secretion of the urine.

DRAS.   DRASTIC   Operating powerfully on the bowels.

EME.   EMETIC   Capable of producing vomiting.

EMM.   EMMENAGOGUE   Favoring the discharge of the menses.

EMO.,
EMOL.   EMOLLIENT   Relaxing and softening inflamed parts.

EXC.   EXCITANT   Stimulant.

EXP.,
EXPEC.   EXPECTORANT   Facilitating or provoking expectorations.

FEB.   FEBRIFUGE   Abating or driving away fevers.

HER.,
HERP.   HERPATIC   Attacking cutaneous diseases.

HYDR.   HYDRAGOGUE   Capable of expelling serum.

HYP.   HYPNOTIC   Promoting sleep, somniferous.

LAX.   LAXATIVE   Gently cathartic.

MUC.   MUCILAGINOUS   Resembling gum in its character.

NAR.   NARCOTIC   Having the property of stupefying.

NAU.   NAUSEANT   Exciting nausea.

NEPH.   NEPHRITIC   Relating to the kidney.

NER.   NERVINE   Acting in the nervous system.

NUT.   NUTRITIVE   Relating to nutrition.

PART.   PARTURIENT   Inducing or promoting labor.

PEC.   PECTORAL   Relating to the breast.

PHRE.   PHRENIC   Relating to the diaphragm.

PURG.   PURGATIVE   Operating on the bowels more powerfully than a laxative.

REF., REFRIG.	REFRIGERANT	Depressing the morbid temperature of the body.
RUB.	RUBEFACIENT	Causing redness of the skin.
SEC.	SECERNANT	Affecting the secretions.
SED.	SEDATIVE	Directly depressing the vital forces.
SIAL.	SIALOGOGUE	Provoking the secretion of saliva.
STI., STIM.	STIMULANT	Exciting the organic action of the system.
STO., STOM.	STOMACHIC	Giving tone to the stomach.
STY.	STYPTIC	Arresting hemorrhage.
SUD.	SUDORIFIC	Provoking sweat.
TON.	TONIC	Exciting slowly the different systems of the economy.
VER., VERM.	VERMIFUGE	Capable of expelling worms.
VUL.	VULNERARY	Favoring the consolidation of wounds.

THE HERBS

ABSCESS   ROOT   Alt. Dia. Ast.

Polemonium reptans

Greek Valerian. Blue Bells. Jacob's
   Ladder.

Serviceable in pleurisy, fevers, and inflammatory diseases.

New Lebanon   1851, 1860
Mt. Lebanon   1873, 1874

ACONITE   LEAVES   Nar. Sed. A-phl. Dia.

Aconitum napellus   ROOT   Nar. Sed. A-phl. Dia.

Monkshood. Wolfsbane.

Used in scarlatina, inflammatory fever, acute rheumatism, neuralgia, etc. Must be used cautiously. Although monkshood in the hands of the intelligent physician is of great service, it should not be used in domestic practice. As a sedative and anodyne it is capable of many beneficial uses in the hands of a skilled person.

Watervliet   1850, 1860, 1861, 1863
New Lebanon   1849, 1851, 1860
Mt. Lebanon   1872, 1873, 1874
Harvard   1857, 1860, 1873, 1880
Union Village, Ohio   1850
New Gloucester   1864

AGRIMONY   HERB   Ton. Alt. Ast. Dia.
Agrimonia eupatoria
Cockleburr. Stickwort.

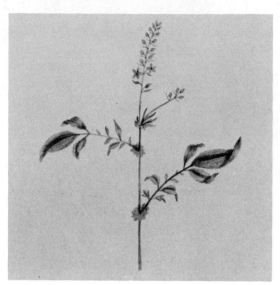

Highly recommended in bowel complaints,
gravel, asthma, coughs, and gonorrhea.
Used as a tea sometimes infused with licorice root. Also used as a gargle for throat and
mouth irritations.

CHS: "Found by the roadsides and borders
of fields, Can. and U.S. common, July."

Watervliet   1847, 1850, 1860, 1863
New Lebanon   1851, 1860
Mt. Lebanon   1872, 1873, 1874
Harvard   1853
Union Village, Ohio   1847, 1850

ALDER, BLACK   BARK   Ton. Alt. Ver. Ast.
Prinos verticillatus   BERRIES   Cath. Ver.
Striped Alder. Winterberry. Fake Alder.

Used with good effect in jaundice, diarrhea, gangrene, dyspepsia; the berries used for worms in
children. Used by dyers, tanners, and leather dressers; the bark powdered and used as a basis for
blacks.

Watervliet   1830, 1833, 1837, 1843, 1845, 1847, 1850, 1860, 1862, 1863
New Lebanon   1836, 1837, 1841, 1849, 1851, 1860
Mt. Lebanon   1872, 1873, 1874
Harvard   1849, 1851, 1853, 1854, 1857, 1860, 1873, 1880
Canterbury   1835, 1847, 1848, 1854
New Gloucester   1864

ALDER, RED OR TAG   BARK   Alt. Emm. Ast. Ton. Deo.
Alnus serrulata   TAGS   Alt. Emm. Ast.
Tag Alder. Smooth Alder. Brook Alder.

Valuable in scrofula, syphilis, and diseases of the skin. Bark, leaves, and berries used. Used also
in bitters and as an astringent.

Bark of black and red alder used by dyers, tanners, and leather dressers, also by fishermen for their nets. The young shoots dye yellow and when cut in March will dye a cinnamon color. The catkins dye green.

Watervliet   1850, 1860

New Lebanon   1850, 1851, 1860

Mt. Lebanon   1872, 1873, 1874

Harvard   1848, 1849, 1851, 1853, 1854, 1857, 1860, 1873, 1880, 1890

Canterbury   1835, 1847

New Gloucester   1864

Union Village, Ohio   1850

ALUM ROOT   ROOT   Ast. A-sep. Det.

Heuchera pubescens

Cranesbill. Splitrock.

Wild alum root is powerfully astringent without bitterness or an unpleasant taste and is useful in diarrhea. Boiled in water and mixed with sugar and milk, it is easily administered to children. Also used as a gargle for throat irritation.

New Lebanon   1849, 1851, 1860

Mt. Lebanon   1872, 1874

ANGELICA   LEAVES   Car. Sto. Ton. Bal.

Angelica atropurpurea   ROOT   Bal. Aro. Stim. Carm. Diu. Sto.

Purple Angelica. Masterwort. High   Emm.

   Angelica. Archangel.   SEED   Car. Acr. Aro. Sti.

Used in flatulent colic, heartburn, and debility. The seeds used in syrup for pain in the stomach and side. Serviceable in promoting elimination through the urine and skin.

Watervliet   1829, 1830, 1833, 1837, 1843, 1845, 1847, 1850, 1860

New Lebanon   1830, 1833, 1836, 1837, 1841, 1849, 1851, 1860

Mt. Lebanon   1872, 1873, 1874

Harvard   1849, 1851, 1853, 1854, 1857, 1860, 1873, 1880

Canterbury   1835, 1847, 1848, 1854

New Gloucester   1864

Groveland, N.Y.   1842

Union Village, Ohio   1850

ANGOSTURA   BARK   Eme. Cath. Ton. Feb.
Galipea officinalis

Used in bilious diarrheas and dysentery, intermittent fevers and dropsy.

Mt. Lebanon   1873, 1874

ANISE   SEED   Stim. Carm. Aro. Pec.
Pimpinella anisum

Valuable to remove flatulent colic of infants, allay nausea, and as a corrigent of griping or unpleasant medicines.

New Lebanon   1851, 1853, 1860
Mt. Lebanon   1872, 1873, 1874, 1888

APPLETREE   BARK   Ton. Feb. Ast.
Pyrus malus

For intermittent, remittent, and bilious fevers; also for gravel.

Watervliet   1850, 1860   Mt. Lebanon   1872, 1873, 1874
New Lebanon   1850, 1851, 1860   Union Village, Ohio   1850

ARNICA   FLOWERS   Sti. Dia. Vul.
Arnica montana   ROOT   Sti. Dia. Vul.
Leopardsbane. Mountain Tobacco.

Used in gout, dropsy, and rheumatism; the tincture of arnica used for bruises, wounds, irritation of nasal passages and chapped lips, sprains, and the bites of insects. This flower should be used externally only as it may produce a serious reaction if taken internally.

NOTE: A salve, used for the same purposes, is made by heating one ounce of the flowers with one ounce of lard for a few hours. For another external use, take two heaping teaspoons of the flowers to a cup of boiling water. Apply cold to sores or wounds.

New Lebanon   1850, 1851, 1860
Mt. Lebanon   1872, 1873, 1874

ASH, MOUNTAIN   BARK   Ast. Ton. Det.
Pyrus americana   BERRIES   Verm. A-scor. Ast.
Roundwood.

The bark is used in bilious diseases to cleanse the blood; the berries for scurvy, and as a vermifuge.

Watervliet   1860

New Lebanon   1850, 1851, 1860

Mt. Lebanon   1872, 1873, 1874

Harvard   1849, 1851, 1853, 1854, 1857, 1860, 1873, 1880, 1885

Canterbury   1835, 1847

New Gloucester   1864

ASH, PRICKLY   BARK   Stim. Ton. Alt. Sial. Aro. Dia.

Zanthoxylum americanum   BERRIES   Stim. Carm. A-spas.

Toothache Bush. Yellow Wood. Suter
    Berry.

A valuable tonic in low typhoid fevers; used in colic, rheumatism, scrofula, etc. The berries are a most valuable agent in Asiatic cholera. They contain a volatile oil and are aromatic. The bark is used for flatulence and diarrhea.

Watervliet   1830, 1833, 1834, 1837, 1843, 1845, 1847, 1850, 1860, 1862, 1863

New Lebanon   1836, 1837, 1841, 1849, 1851, 1860

Mt. Lebanon   1872, 1873, 1874

Harvard   1851, 1853, 1854, 1857, 1860, 1873, 1880, 1885

Canterbury   1835, 1847, 1848, 1854

Union Village, Ohio   1847, 1850

New Gloucester   1864

Groveland, N.Y.   1842

ASH, WHITE   BARK   Ton. Cath. Ast.

Fraxinus americana

Beneficial in constipation, dropsy, ague cake, etc. The seeds are said to prevent obesity.

Watervliet   1860   Mt. Lebanon   1872, 1873, 1874

New Lebanon   1849, 1850, 1851, 1860

ASPARAGUS ROOT   ROOT   Ape.

Asparagus officinalis

Valuable in dropsy and enlargement of the heart.

New Lebanon   1850, 1851, 1860   Hancock   1821

Mt. Lebanon   1872, 1873, 1874   Union Village, Ohio   1847, 1850

Aspen, Quaking   BARK   Feb. A-scor. Ver.
Populus tremuloides
European Poplar

· The active principles of the bark are salicin and populin. Used as a vermifuge by veterinaries.

Union Village, Ohio   1850

Avens, Water   ROOT   Ton. Ast. Sto.
Geum rivale
Chocolate Root. Throat Root. Cure-All.
   Evans Root.

Valuable in hemorrhages, chronic diarrhea and dysentery, leucorrhea, and active ulcers.

Watervliet   1830, 1833, 1837, 1843, 1845, 1847, 1850, 1860, 1863
New Lebanon   1830, 1836, 1837, 1841, 1849, 1851, 1860
Mt. Lebanon   1866, 1872, 1873, 1874
Harvard   1851, 1853, 1857, 1860, 1873, 1880, 1885
Canterbury   1835, 1847, 1848, 1854
Union Village, Ohio   1847, 1850
New Gloucester   1864

Backache Brake   ROOT   Anthel. Ver. Pec. Dem.
Athyrium filix-femina
Female Fern

Used to expel worms.

New Lebanon   1851, 1860
Mt. Lebanon   1866, 1872, 1873, 1874

Balm, of Gilead   BUDS   Pec. Stim. Ton. Diu. A-scor.
Commiphora opobalsamum   Bal. Sto.
                                                     BARK   Ton. Cath.

Tincture of the buds is used in affections of the chest, stomach and kidneys, rheumatism and scurvy. Applied to frost and fresh wounds. The bark is useful in gout and rheumatism.

Watervliet   1829, 1837, 1843, 1845, 1847, 1850, 1860
New Lebanon   1836, 1837, 1841, 1849, 1851, 1860
Mt. Lebanon   1866, 1872, 1873, 1874
Harvard   1849, 1851, 1853, 1857, 1860, 1873, 1880
Canterbury   1835, 1847, 1848, 1854
Union Village, Ohio   1847, 1850
New Gloucester   1864

BALM, LEMON   HERB (LEAVES AND STALK)   Sto. Diap.
Melissa officinalis   A-spas. Sud.
Bee Balm. Blue Balm. Cure-All. Dropsy Plant.

Useful in low fevers, and to assist menstruation. A warm infusion taken freely produces sweating; is made more palatable by adding lemon juice.

Lemon balm tea, a pleasant drink; sometimes a little rosemary or spearmint may be added and a few cloves. Alone, it is agreeable as a summer beverage iced and slightly sweetened.

Watervliet   1830, 1832, 1833, 1834, 1837, 1843, 1845, 1847, 1850, 1860
New Lebanon   1836, 1837, 1841, 1849, 1851, 1860
Mt. Lebanon   1866, 1872, 1873, 1874
Harvard   1851, 1853, 1854, 1857, 1860, 1873, 1880, 1885
Canterbury   1835, 1847, 1848
Union Village, Ohio   1847, 1850
New Gloucester   1864

BALM, MOLDAVIAN   LEAVES   Aro. Sto. Dia.
Dracocephalum moldavica
Sweet Balm. Tea Balm. Dragonhead.

Useful in low fevers, and to assist menstruation.

Watervliet   1830, 1833, 1834, 1837, 1843, 1845, 1847, 1850, 1860
New Lebanon   1836, 1837, 1841, 1851, 1860
Mt. Lebanon   1866, 1872, 1873, 1874, 1888
Harvard   1851, 1853, 1854, 1857, 1860, 1873, 1880, 1885

Canterbury   1835, 1847, 1848, 1854
Union Village, Ohio   1850
New Gloucester   1864

BALMONY   LEAVES   Ton. Cath. Anthel. A-bil. Ver.
Chelone glabra
Snakehead. Turtlebloom. Turtlehead.
Salt Rheum Weed. Fishmouth. Shell
Flower. Bitter Herb.

Especially valuable in jaundice and hepatic diseases, to remove worms and excite the digestive
organs to action, particularly the liver. An ointment made from the fresh leaves is valuable for the
itching and irritation of piles.

Watervliet   1850
New Lebanon   1849
Mt. Lebanon   1873
Union Village, Ohio   1850

BALSAM, SWEET   HERB   Ast. Sto. Dia. Sud. Sed.
Gnaphalium polycephalum
Life Everlasting. White Balsam. Indian
   Posy. Old Field Balsam.

Irritations of the mouth and throat are said to be relieved by chewing the leaves and blossoms; the
leaves applied to bruises and other local irritations are very efficacious.

Watervliet   1833, 1837, 1843, 1845, 1847, 1850, 1860, 1863
New Lebanon   1836, 1837, 1841, 1849, 1851, 1860
Mt. Lebanon   1866, 1872, 1874

BARBERRY   BARK   Ton. Lax. Ref. Ast.
Berberis vulgaris   BERRIES   Ton. Lax. Ref. Ast.
Sowberry

Employed in all cases where tonics are indicated; has proved efficacious in jaundice. The berries
are used as a wash in canker. The berries form an agreeable acidulous drink. The bark of the root
is the most active, a teaspoon of the powdered bark acting as a purgative. A decoction of the bark
or berries will be found of service as a mouthwash or gargle.

New Lebanon   1851, 1860, 1866
Mt. Lebanon   1872, 1873, 1874
Harvard   1851, 1853, 1857, 1860, 1873, 1880, 1885
Canterbury   1835, 1847, 1848, 1854
Union Village, Ohio   1850

BASIL, SWEET   LEAVES   Aro. Sti.
Ocimum basilicum

To allay excessive vomiting. This plant is aromatic with the added advantage of value in cooking
and use as a tea.

Watervliet   1830, 1833, 1834, 1837, 1843, 1845, 1847, 1850, 1860
New Lebanon   1836, 1837, 1841, 1851, 1860, 1866
Mt. Lebanon   1872, 1873, 1874, 1888
Canterbury   1835
Union Village, Ohio   1847, 1850

BASSWOOD   BARK   Emo. Dis. Sto.
Tilia americana   FLOWERS   Emo. Dis. Sto.
Linden. Lime-Tree. Spoonwood.   LEAVES   Aro. Stim. Ast.

Used as a poultice in painful swellings. A
tea of linden flowers and leaves promotes
sweating. An admirable remedy for quieting coughs and relieving hoarseness resulting from colds.

CHS: "A common forest tree in the northern
and middle states. June."

New Lebanon   1851, 1860
Mt. Lebanon   1866, 1872, 1873, 1874

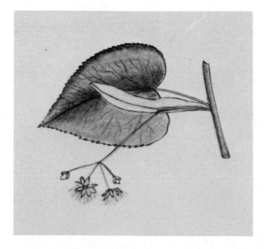

BAYBERRY
Myrica cerifera
Wax Myrtle. Wax Berry. Candle Berry.
  Myrtle.

BARK	Stim. Ast. Eme. Err.
BERRIES	Stim. Ast.
LEAVES	Aro. Stim. Ast.

Valuable in jaundice, diarrhea, dysentery,
canker in the mouth, throat, and bowels,
and as a wash for spongy gums. The leaves
are used to treat scurvy. Powdered, it has
been employed as a snuff with good effect
in nasal congestions or catarrhs. It is sometimes applied in poultice form to cuts,
bruises, scratches, etc., but it is better for
these when combined with bloodroot. The
wax possesses mild astringent properties.

CHS: "Found in dry woods, or in open
fields, Can. to Fla. May."

Watervliet   1830, 1833, 1837, 1843, 1845,
  1847, 1850, 1863
New Lebanon   1836, 1837, 1841, 1851, 1860
Mt. Lebanon   1866, 1872, 1873, 1874
Harvard   1851, 1853, 1854, 1857, 1860, 1873,
  1880, 1885
Canterbury   1835, 1847, 1848, 1854

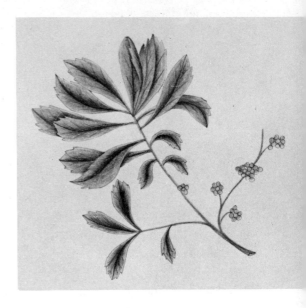

Union Village, Ohio   1850
New Gloucester   1864

BEECH
Fagus ferruginea

BARK	Ast. Ton. A-syph.
LEAVES	Ast. Ton. A-syph. Alt.

Useful in diabetes, cutaneous diseases, ulcers, and dyspepsia.

CHS: "A common forest tree in U.S. and
Can. 50 to 80 ft. high. May."

New Lebanon   1851, 1860
Mt. Lebanon   1866, 1872, 1873, 1874
Union Village, Ohio   1850

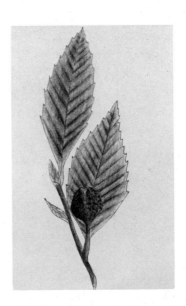

BEECHDROPS   WHOLE PLANT   Dis. Ast.
Epifagus virginiana

An eminent astringent. Applied locally to minor cuts, wounds, and bruises.

Union Village, Ohio   1847

BELLADONNA   LEAVES   Nar. Ano. Dia. Diu.
Atropa belladonna
Deadly Nightshade. Dwale.

Used in convulsions, neuralgia, rheumatism, mania, gout, and painful conditions of the nervous system. Requires caution in its use. In the hands of skilled herbal physicians this botanical has great virtues, but it is too powerful and dangerous for general or home use. The leaves should be gathered while plant is in flower.

Watervliet   1830, 1834, 1837, 1843, 1845, 1847, 1850, 1860, 1863
New Lebanon   1837, 1849, 1851, 1860
Mt. Lebanon   1866, 1872, 1873, 1874
Harvard   1853, 1854, 1857, 1860, 1873, 1880, 1885
Canterbury   1848, 1854
Union Village, Ohio   1847, 1850
New Gloucester   1864

BELLWORT   LEAVES   Ton. Dem. Ner. Her.
Uvularia perfoliata
Mohawkweed.

For sore throat, inflammation, and as poultice in erysipelas and wounds.

CHS: "A handsome plant in the woods. Can. and U.S. May."

Watervliet   1834, 1837, 1843, 1845, 1847, 1850
New Lebanon   1836, 1837, 1841, 1851, 1860, 1866
Mt. Lebanon   1866, 1872, 1873, 1874

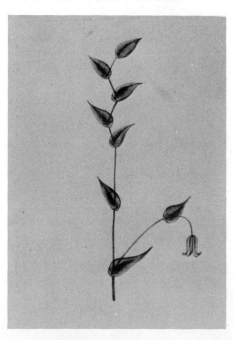

BENNE   LEAVES Dem. Lax. Emo.
Sesamum indicum   SEEDS   Dem. Lax. Emo.
Sesame. Gingili. Tell.

The seeds are used in cookery, cosmetics, etc. The leaves are used as a demulcent and emollient, sheathing or lubricating.

Watervliet   1850, 1860   Mt. Lebanon   1866, 1872, 1874
New Lebanon   1851, 1860   Union Village, Ohio   1847, 1850

BETHROOT   ROOT Ast. Ton. A-sep. Pec. Alt.
Trillium pendulum
Birth Root. Indian Balm. Ground Lily.
  Cough Root. Pariswort. Truelove.
  Wake Robin.

Valuable in coughs, asthma, hectic fever, bloody urine.

Watervliet   1837, 1843, 1845, 1847, 1850, 1860, 1861
New Lebanon   1836, 1837, 1841, 1851, 1860
Mt. Lebanon   1866, 1872, 1873, 1874
Harvard   1851, 1853, 1854, 1857, 1860, 1873, 1880, 1885
Canterbury   1835, 1847, 1848, 1854
Union Village, Ohio   1850
New Gloucester   1864

BETONY, WOOD   HERB Ner. Ton. Dis. Ape.
Betononica officinalis

For headache, hysterics, and nervousness, and used as a cordial.

New Lebanon   1851, 1860   Mt. Lebanon   1866, 1872, 1873, 1874

BIRCH, BLACK   BARK Aro. Ton. Ast. Stim. Diap. Nar.
Betula lenta   Ano. Diu.
Cherry Birch. Sweet Birch. Mahogany
  Birch. Spice Birch.

Used in diarrhea, dysentery, cholera infantum, and to tone the bowels after exhausting discharge.

Watervliet   1850, 1860
New Lebanon   1851, 1860
Mt. Lebanon   1866, 1872, 1873, 1874

Harvard   1851, 1853, 1857, 1860, 1873, 1880, 1885
Union Village, Ohio   1850
Groveland, N.Y.   1873
New Gloucester   1864

BIRD PEPPER   FRUIT   Stim. Cath. Rub.
Capsicum frutescens
Cayenne Pepper. Chillies.

A powerful stimulant used in colds, rheumatism, spasmodic affections, and cholera.

Mt. Lebanon   1866, 1873

BITTER HERB   TOPS AND ROOTS   Aro. Ton. Feb.
Erythraea centaurium
Lesser Centaury. European Centaury.

Aromatic and bitter, used to dispel fever, allaying fever heat.

Mt. Lebanon   1872   Canterbury   1835

BITTERROOT   ROOT   Alt. Sud. Eme. Diu. Ver. Dia.
Apocynum androsaemifolium   Ton. Cath.
Honey Bloom. Milk Ipecac. Dogsbone.
   Wandering Milkweed. Flytrap.
   Dogbane.

Valuable in chronic liver complaints, syphilis, scrofula, intermittent and low stage of typhoid fever. In conjunction with yellow parilla, it is excellent for dyspepsia.

Watervliet   1837, 1843, 1845, 1847, 1850, 1860, 1862
New Lebanon   1836, 1837, 1841, 1851, 1860
Mt. Lebanon   1866, 1872, 1873, 1874, 1851, 1853, 1854, 1857, 1860, 1873, 1880
Harvard   1885
Canterbury   1835, 1847, 1854
Union Village, Ohio   1847, 1850
New Gloucester   1864

BITTERSWEET, FALSE   BARK OF ROOT   A-bil. Dis. Alt. Dia. Diu.
Celastrus scandens   BERRIES   Emo. Dis. Alt. Dia. Diu.
Staff Tree or Staffvine. Waxwork.
   Climbing Orange Root.

Used in scrofula, syphilis, leucorrhea, and obstructed menstruation.

Watervliet   1850, 1860

New Lebanon   1851, 1860

Mt. Lebanon   1873, 1874

Harvard   1851, 1853, 1854, 1857, 1860, 1873,
   1880, 1885

Mt. Lebanon   1866, 1872, 1873

Canterbury   1847, 1848, 1854

Union Village, Ohio   1850

New Gloucester   1864

BITTERSWEET

Solanum dulcamara

Garden Nightshade. Woody Nightshade. Violet Bloom. Fever Twig.
Scarlet Berry.

HERB   Nar. Alt. Diu. Sud. Dis. Her. Deo.

TWIGS AND BARK OF ROOT   Her. Deo. Alt.

Employed in cutaneous diseases, scrofula,
syphilitic diseases, jaundice, obstructed
menstruation, rheumatic afflictions, and for
the relief of skin irritation. It is a purifying
tea and a pectoral tea.

CHS: "A well known climber with blue
flower and red berries. N. Eng. to Ark. The
berries are said to be poisonous. July."

Watervliet   1830, 1833, 1834, 1837, 1843,
   1845, 1847, 1849, 1850, 1860, 1861, 1862

New Lebanon   1836, 1837, 1841, 1851, 1860

Mt. Lebanon   1866, 1873, 1874

Harvard   1851, 1853, 1854, 1857, 1860, 1873,
   1880, 1885

Canterbury   1835, 1847, 1848, 1854

Union Village, Ohio   1847, 1850

Groveland, N.Y.   1842

New Gloucester   1864

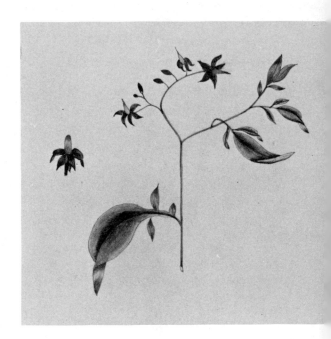

BLACKBERRY

Rubus villosus, Rubus occidentalis

Dewberry. Bramble. Gout Berry. Cloud
Berry.

HERB   Ast. Ton.

ROOT   Ast. Ton.

Excellent in cholera infantum, diarrhea, dysentery, and relaxed condition of intestines of children;
as an injection in gleet, gonorrhea, and prolapsus uteri and ani. Also used by some for offensive
saliva. The fruit was made into wine and brandy and used to treat diarrhea.

CHS: "In damp woods and by the roadside. Can. to Carolinas. Trailing several feet. May and
June."

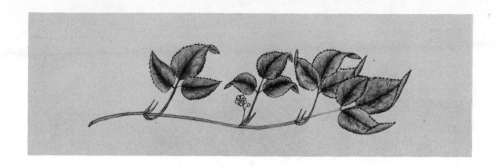

Watervliet   1830, 1833, 1837, 1843, 1845, 1847,
   1850, 1860, 1861
New Lebanon   1836, 1837, 1851, 1860
Mt. Lebanon   1866, 1872, 1873, 1874

Harvard   1880, 1885
Canterbury   1835, 1847, 1848, 1854
Union Village, Ohio   1847, 1850
New Gloucester   1864

BLAZING STAR
Aletris farinosa
Devil's   Bit.   Unicorn.   Stargrass.
   Colic Root. Ague Root.

ROOT   Nar. Ton. Eme. Cath. Sto. Diu.
   Stim.

Used in chronic rheumatism, dropsy, and colic. The decoction was useful as a gargle in throat irritations.

Watervliet   1860
New Lebanon   1851, 1860

Mt. Lebanon   1866, 1872, 1873

BLOODROOT
Sanguinaria canadensis
Indian Paint. Red Puccoon. Tetterwort.

Valuable in typhoid pneumonia, catarrh, scarlatina, jaundice, dyspepsia, ringworm, and in affections of the respiratory organs. In small doses, it stimulates the digestive organs, acting as a stimulant and tonic. It appears to be used chiefly as an expectorant.

CHS: "In woods. Can. and U.S. When bruised the plant exudes an orange red fluid. The juice is emetic and purgative. Apr. May."

Groveland, N.Y. 1842

Watervliet   1830, 1833, 1837, 1843, 1845,
   1847, 1850, 1860, 1862, 1863

ROOT   Eme. Sti. Alt. Ton. Exp. Deo.
   Acr. Dia.

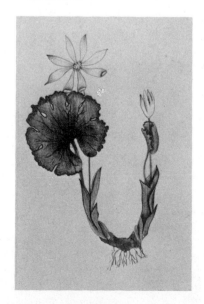

New Lebanon   1836, 1837, 1841, 1851, 1860

Mt. Lebanon   1866, 1872, 1873, 1874, 1851,
1853, 1857, 1860, 1873, 1880

Harvard   1885

Canterbury   1835, 1847, 1848, 1854

Union Village, Ohio   1847, 1850

New Gloucester   1864

Blue Flag

Iris versicolor

Poison Flag. Flag Lily. Water Flag. Fleur
De Lis. Liver Lily. Snake Lily.

ROOT   Diu. Cath. Alt. Sial. Verm. Eme.

A potent remedy in dropsy, scrofula, affections of the liver, spleen and kidneys, and secondary
syphilis.

Watervliet   1850, 1860

New Lebanon   1841, 1851, 1860

Mt. Lebanon   1866, 1872, 1873, 1874

Harvard   1857, 1860, 1873, 1880, 1885

Canterbury   1847, 1848, 1854

Union Village, Ohio   1847, 1850

New Gloucester   1864

Boneset

Eupatorium perfoliatum

Thoroughwort. Feverwort. Through-
stem. Vegetable Antimony. Cross-
wort. Sweating Plant. Indian Sage.
Ague Weed. Eupatorium.

HERB   Sud. Eme. Ton. Ape. Dia. Feb.

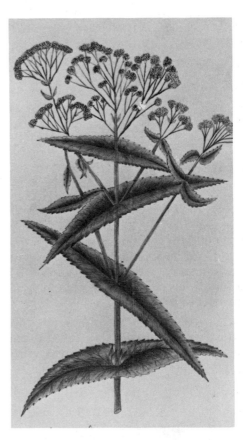

Excellent in colds, fevers, dyspepsia, jaundice and general debility of the system,
fever, and ague. The cold infusion or extract
is tonic and aperient. The warm infusion is
diaphoretic and emetic. A strong tea of
boneset sweetened with honey will break up
an ordinary head cold. Also, can be made
into an ointment or syrup.

CHS: "A common plant on low grounds,
meadows. U.S. and Can. Abundant. The
plant is bitter and used in medicine. Aug."

Watervliet   1830, 1833, 1834, 1837, 1843,
1845, 1847, 1850, 1885, 1860, 1861, 1862

New Lebanon   1836, 1837, 1841, 1849, 1851,
1860

Mt. Lebanon   1866, 1872, 1873, 1874

Harvard   1854, 1857, 1873, 1880

Canterbury   1835, 1847

Union Village, Ohio   1847, 1850

New Gloucester   1864

BORAGE   HERB   Sto. Dia. Ape. Ref.

Borago officinalis

Burrage. Bugloss.

Used in catarrh, rheumatism, and diseases of the skin. It is made into a cordial and is pectoral and aperient. Also used as a culinary herb.

Watervliet   1830, 1833, 1837, 1843, 1845, 1847, 1850

New Lebanon   1836, 1837, 1841, 1851, 1860

Mt. Lebanon   1866, 1872, 1873, 1874

Canterbury   1835

Union Village, Ohio   1847, 1850

BOXBERRY   LEAVES   Aro. Diu. Sto.

Gaultheria procumbens

Wintergreen.

This is a diuretic. Small doses stimulate the stomach; large doses have an extreme effect and cause vomiting.

CHS: "In old woods and on mountains. N.E. to Newfoundland. May. June."

Harvard   1857, 1873, 1880

Canterbury   1835

New Gloucester   1864

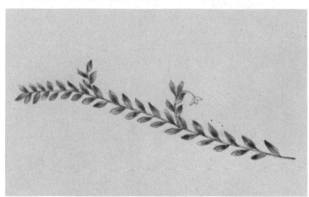

BOXWOOD   BARK   Ton. Ast. Stim.

Cornus florida   FLOWERS   Emm. Sud.

Dogwood. Flowering Cornel. Bud-
    wood.

An excellent substitute for Peruvian bark. Valuable in jaundice and liver complaint. The flowers are used for accelerating the discharge of the menses. The bark should only be used in its dried state. Cornine, its active principle, seems to have been used occasionally as a substitute for quinine.

Watervliet   1830, 1833, 1837, 1843, 1845, 1847, 1850, 1860, 1861, 1863

New Lebanon   1836, 1837, 1841, 1851, 1860

Mt. Lebanon   1866, 1872, 1873, 1874

Harvard   1851, 1853, 1857, 1860, 1873, 1880, 1885

Canterbury   1835, 1847, 1848, 1854

Union Village, Ohio   1850.

New Gloucester   1864

BROOKLIME   HERB   A-scorb. Diu. Emm. Feb. Dis. Alt.
Veronica beccabunga
Water Pimpernel. Water Purslain.
   Beccabunga.

Beneficial in obstructed menstruation, scurvy, fevers, skin diseases, and coughs.

New Lebanon   1851, 1860   Mt. Lebanon   1866, 1873, 1874

BROOM   HERB   Eme. Cath. Diu.
Cytisus scoparius
Link. Genista. Banal.

Especially beneficial in dropsy. Said never to fail in increasing the flow of urine. Broom tops are purgative and act on the kidneys. This tea is of great service. It is often used in equal parts with the root of dandelion for diuretic purpose.

Mt. Lebanon   1873   Harvard   1849, 1880

BUCHU   LEAVES   Diu. Dia. Sti.
Barosma betulina
Bookoo. Bucku. Diosma Betulina.

Useful in derangement [dysfunction] of the urinary organs. Native to southern Africa, the Shakers imported or bought it.

New Lebanon   1851, 1860
Mt. Lebanon   1866, 1872, 1873, 1874

BUCKBEAN   ROOT   Ton. Diu. Anthel.
Menyanthes trifoliata   HERB   Ton. Diu. Anthel. Cath. Deo.
Bogbean. Trefoil. Water Shamrock.
   Wind Shamrock. Bitterworm. Marsh
   Trefoil. Bog Myrtle.

Used in the treatment of scurvy, rheumatism, jaundice, dyspepsia, hepatics, and worms. A tea of buckbean improves digestion and promotes and improves gastric juices.

Watervliet   1830, 1833, 1837, 1843, 1850
New Lebanon   1836, 1837, 1841, 1851, 1860
Mt. Lebanon   1866, 1872, 1873, 1874
Harvard   1851, 1853, 1854, 1857, 1860, 1873, 1880, 1885
Canterbury   1835, 1847, 1848, 1854
New Gloucester   1864

BUCKHORN BRAKE

Osmunda regalis

Male Fern. Royal Fern. King's Fern.

ROOT   Ton. Muc. Dem. Styp. Ver. Ast.

Very valuable in female weakness, cough, and dysentery; said to be a certain cure for rickets, spine complaint, and debility of the muscles.

CHS: "A large and beautiful fern in swamps and meadows. The fronds are 3 feet high. June."

New Lebanon   1851, 1853, 1857, 1860

Mt. Lebanon   1866, 1873, 1874

Harvard   1880, 1885

Canterbury   1835, 1847, 1848, 1854

New Gloucester   1864

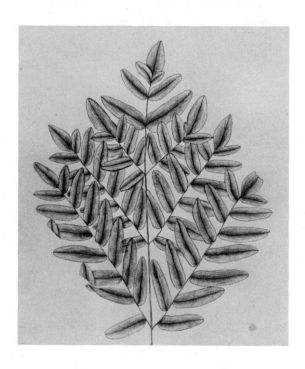

BUCKTHORN

Rhamnus cathartica

Purging Berries. Red Root. New Jersey
  Tea. Arrow Wood. Alder Dogwood.
  Bird Cherry.

BARK   Hydr. Cath. Ver.
BERRIES   Hydr. Cath. Alt.

The bark should be at least one year old before using. It is purgative, its action similar to that of rhubarb. Used in rheumatism, gout, dropsy, and eruptive diseases. An ointment made of the fresh bark is excellent for skin irritation. (The syrup is made from bark and berries.)

Watervliet   1830, 1833, 1837, 1850, 1860

New Lebanon   1836, 1837, 1851, 1860

Mt. Lebanon   1866, 1872, 1873, 1874

Harvard   1851, 1853, 1857, 1860, 1873, 1880, 1885

Canterbury   1835, 1847, 1848, 1854

BUGLE, BITTER   HERB   Sty. Ast. Ton. Nar. Pec. Deo.
Lycopus europaeus
Bugle Weed. Gipseywort.

Recommended in intermittent fever, hemorrhage of lungs, bowels, or stomach.

Watervliet   1850
Mt. Lebanon   1873
Harvard   1851, 1853, 1854, 1857, 1860, 1873, 1880, 1885
Canterbury   1835, 1847, 1848, 1854
Union Village, Ohio   1850
New Gloucester   1864

BUGLE, SWEET   HERB   Sud. Ton. Ast. Deo. Sty. Pec.
Lycopus americanus   Sed. Nar.
Water Bugle. Paul Betony. Water Hore-
   hound. Green Archangel.

Useful in phthisis, hemorrhage of the lungs, diabetes, and chronic diarrhea. It is sedative and
mildly narcotic.

Watervliet   1830, 1832, 1833, 1834, 1837, 1843, 1845, 1847, 1850, 1860
New Lebanon   1836, 1837, 1841, 1851, 1860
Mt. Lebanon   1866, 1872, 1873, 1874
Harvard   1851, 1853, 1854, 1857, 1860, 1873, 1880, 1885
Canterbury   1835, 1847, 1848, 1854
Union Village, Ohio   1850
New Gloucester   1864

BURDOCK   LEAVES   Sud. Emo. Dia. Ape.
Arctium lappa   ROOT   Sud. Herp. A-scor. Alt.
Clotbur. Bardana.   SEEDS   Car. Ton. Diu.

Used in gout and scorbutic, syphilitic, scrofulous, and leprous diseases; the leaves are used as a
cooling poultice. The root should be dug in the fall or early spring. Only year-old roots should be
used. Externally, it is valuable in salves or as a wash for burns, wounds, and skin irritations.

Watervliet   1830, 1833, 1837, 1843, 1845, 1847, 1850, 1860
New Lebanon   1836, 1837, 1841, 1849, 1851, 1860
Mt. Lebanon   1866, 1872, 1873, 1874
Harvard   1849, 1851, 1853, 1854, 1857, 1860, 1873, 1880, 1885
Canterbury   1835, 1847, 1848, 1854
Union Village, Ohio   1847, 1850
New Gloucester   1864

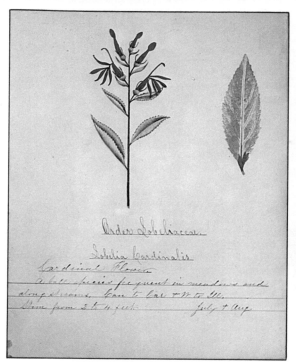

Order Lobeliaceae.

Lobelia Cardinalis

Cardinal Flower

A tall species frequent in meadows and along streams. Can. to Car. & N. to Ill.

Stem from 2 to 4 feet.   *July & Aug.*

Red Cardinal

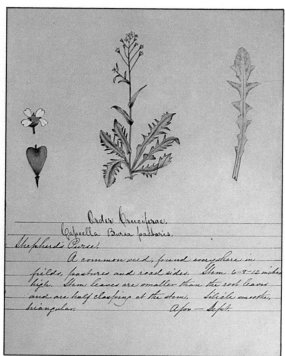

Order Cruciferae.

Capsella Bursa pastoris.

Shepherd's Purse!

A common weed, found everywhere in fields, pastures and road sides. Stem 6-8-12 inches high. Stem leaves are smaller than the root leaves and are half clasping at the stem. Silicle smoother, triangular.   *Apr — Sept.*

Shepherd's Purse

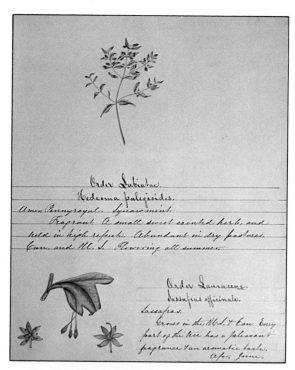

Order Labiatae.

Hedeoma pulegioides.

American Pennyroyal. Squaw mint.

Fragrant. A small sweet scented herb, and held in high repute. Abundant in dry pastures. Can. and Ill. S. Flowering all summer.

Order Lauraceae.

Sassafras officinale.

Sassafras.

Grows in the Ill. S. & Can. Every part of the tree has a pleasant fragrance & an aromatic taste.   *Apr. June.*

Top, Pennyroyal; *bottom,* Sassafras

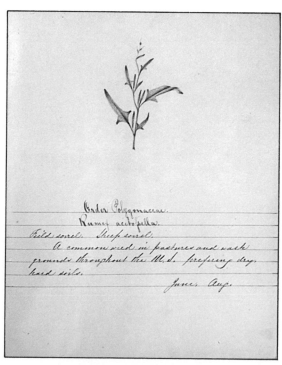

Order Polygonaceae.

Rumex acetosella.

Field sorrel. Sheep sorrel.

A common weed in pastures and waste grounds throughout the Ill. S. preferring dry hard soils.

June. Aug.

Field Sorrel (Sheep Sorrel)

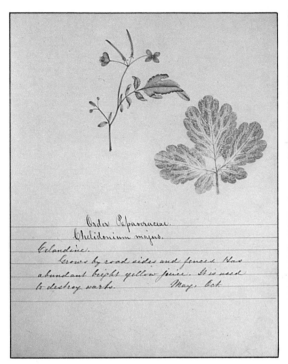

Celandine

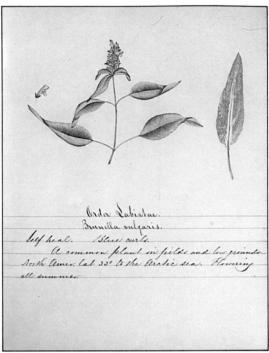

Self-heal

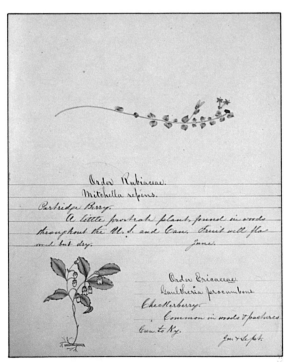

Top, Partridge Berry (Squaw Vine);
bottom, Checkerberry

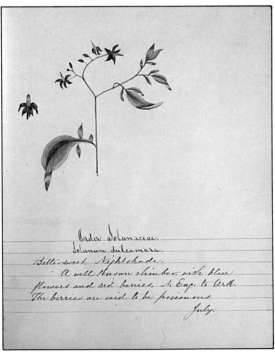

Bittersweet

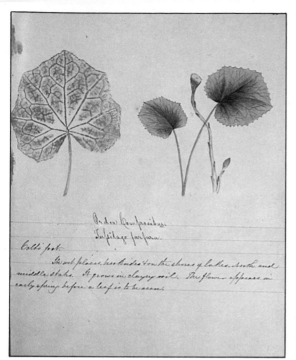

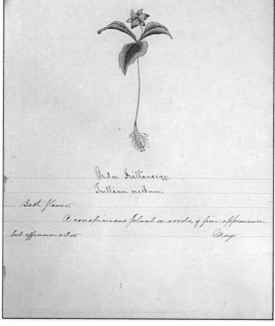

Coltsfoot

Goldthread

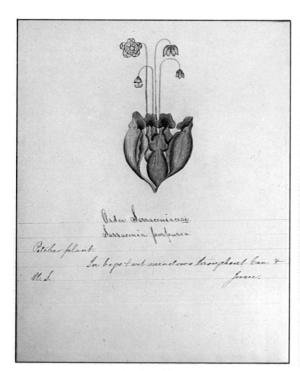

Pitcher Plant

Bathflower (Purple Trillium)

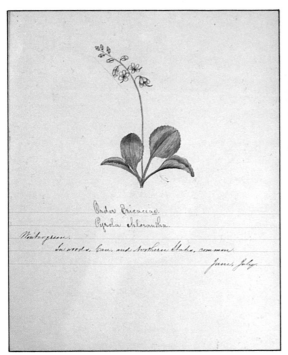

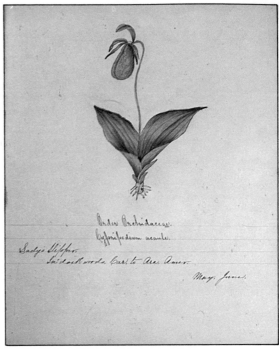

Wintergreen

Lady's Slipper

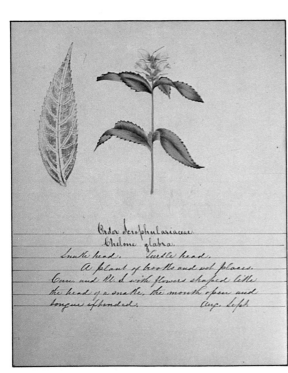

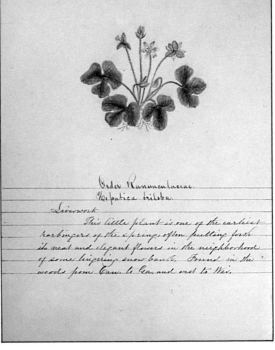

Snakehead

Liverwort

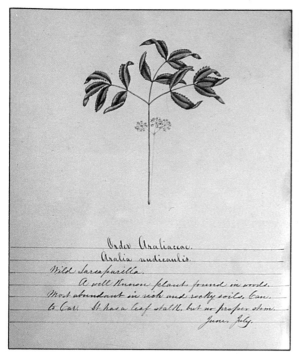

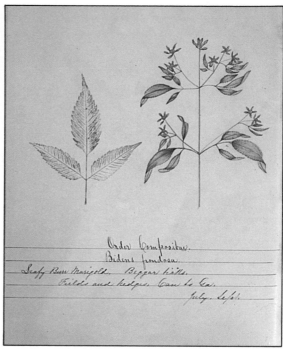

Wild Sarsaparilla (American Sarsaparilla)

Beggar's Tick (Cuckold)

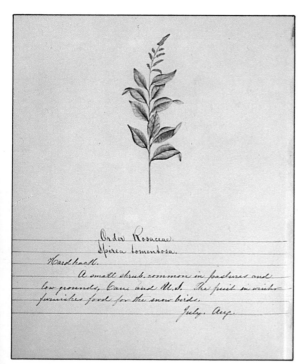

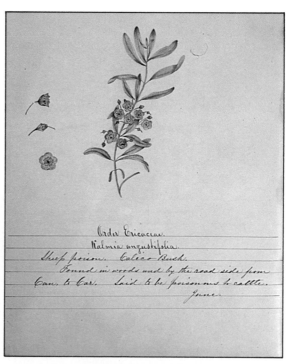

Hardhack

Sheep Poison (Laurel)

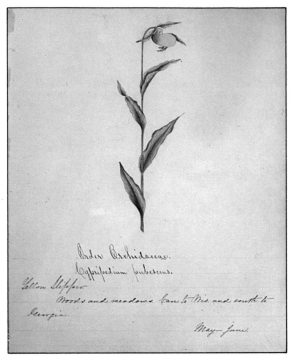

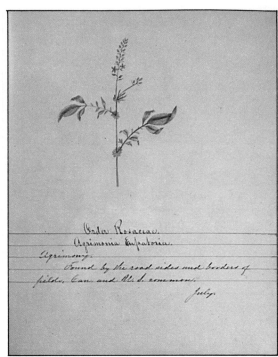

Yellow Lady's Slipper

Agrimony

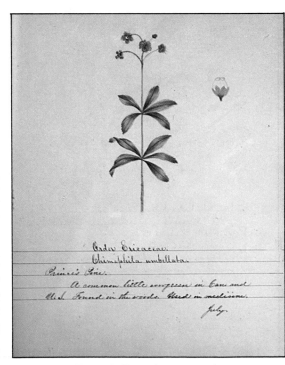

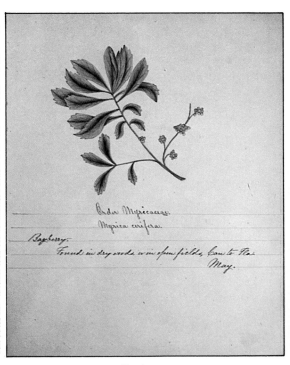

Prince's Pine (Pipsissewa)

Bayberry

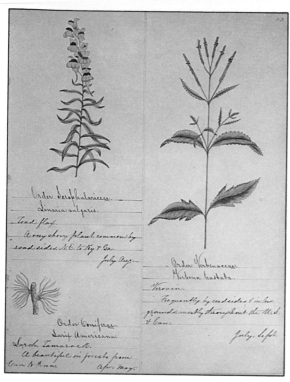

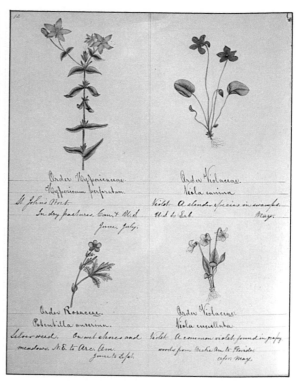

Top left, Toad Flax (Flax); *right,* Vervain; *bottom left,* Larch Tamarack (Tamarack)

Top left, St. Johnswort (Johnswort); *top right,* Violet; *bottom left,* Silverweed; *bottom right,* Violet

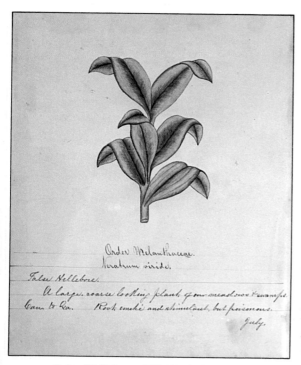

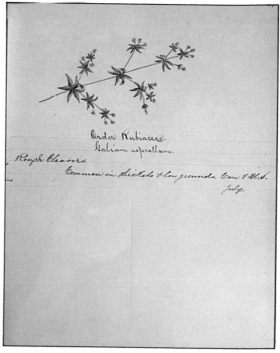

False Hellebore (White Hellebore)

Rough Cleavers (Cleavers)

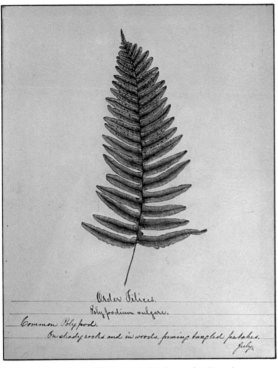

Common Polypod (Polypody Fern)

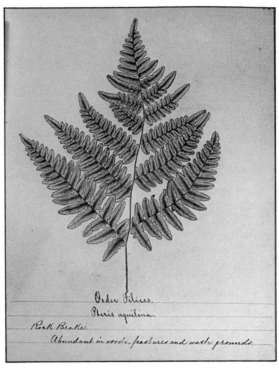

Rockbrake

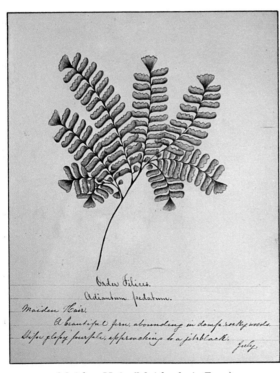

Maiden Hair (Maidenhair Fern)

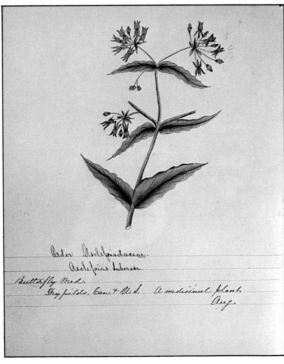

Butterfly Weed (Pleurisy Root)

BURNET, GREAT
Sanguisorba officinalis
Garden or Common Burnet.

WHOLE PLANT   Ast. Ton.

Both herb and root are administered internally in all abnormal discharges in diarrhea, dysentery, and leucorrhea. Dried and powdered, it has been used to stop purgings. A decoction of the whole herb has been found useful in arresting hemorrhage.

Hancock   1821

BUTTERCUP
Ranunculus acris
Crowfoot.

HERB   Acr. A-sep.

This plant is too acrid to be used internally, especially when fresh. When applied externally, it may be employed where conditions of counterirritation are indicated. Its action, however, is generally so violent that it is seldom used.

CHS: "This is the most common species in the N.E. and Can. In fields and pastures. June. Sept."

Canterbury   1835
Union Village, Ohio   1850

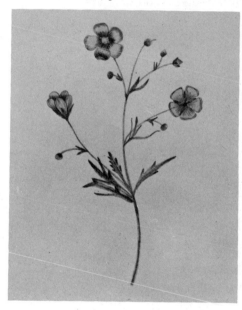

BUTTERNUT
Juglans cinerea
White Walnut. Oil Nut. Lemon Walnut.

BARK (INNER)   Cath. Alt. Deo. Ton.
LEAVES   Cath. Alt. Deo. Ton.

Used in habitual constipation as a gentle and agreeable cathartic, acting like rhubarb; also in intermittent and remittent fevers. The bark was used in the preparation of vegetable dyes and candied butternut meats were an item in most of the Shaker Sisters' shops.

Watervliet   1830, 1843, 1845, 1847, 1850, 1860
New Lebanon   1841, 1849, 1851, 1860
Mt. Lebanon   1866, 1872, 1873, 1874

CANCER ROOT
Orobanche virginiana
Beech Drops. Broom Rape.

ROOT   Ast.
WHOLE PLANT   Ast. Ton.

Beneficial in hemorrhage of the bowels, uterus, and in diarrhea. Valuable in erysipelas, and, as a local application, to arrest the tendency of ulcers and wounds to gangrene. This is a plant that is parasitic upon the roots of beech trees. It flowers in August and September.

Watervliet 1837, 1843, 1845, 1860	Harvard 1851, 1853
New Lebanon 1836, 1837, 1841, 1851, 1860	Canterbury 1835, 1847, 1848, 1854
Mt. Lebanon 1866, 1872, 1873, 1874	Union Village, Ohio 1850

CANELLA   BARK   Ano. Sto.

Canella alba

White Wood. Wild Cinnamon.

An aromatic bitter useful in enfeebled conditions of the stomach, and often given with other medicines.

NOTE: The Shakers bought this, as it is native only in the West Indies and Florida.

Mt. Lebanon   1874

CANKER ROOT   ROOT   Ast. Ton.

Prenanthes alba

Rattlesnake Root.

Used in diarrhea and relaxed and debilitated conditions of the bowels.

Mt. Lebanon   1873

CANKER WEED   HERB   Ast. Ton.

Prenanthes serpentaria

Useful as a mouthwash or gargle.

Watervliet   1837, 1843, 1845, 1860
New Lebanon   1836, 1837, 1841, 1849, 1851, 1860
Mt. Lebanon   1866, 1872, 1874

CARAWAY   SEED   Aro. Carm. Ton. Sto.

Carum carvi

Used in flatulent colic of children, as a corrective to nauseous purgatives, and to improve the flavor of disagreeable medicines. Used also as a potherb and as a spice in breads and cakes.

Watervliet 1830, 1833, 1837, 1843, 1845, 1847, 1850, 1860	Harvard 1851, 1853, 1854, 1857, 1860
New Lebanon 1836, 1837, 1841, 1851, 1860	Canterbury 1847, 1848, 1854
Mt. Lebanon 1866, 1872, 1873, 1874, 1888	Union Village, Ohio 1847, 1850
	New Gloucester 1864

CARDAMOM   SEED   Car. Sti. Aro.
Elettaria cardamomum

The seeds are useful in flatulency because of their warmth, but are rarely used alone. Used as a spice and also as a breath sweetener. Imported by the Shakers to resell.

Watervliet   1860
New Lebanon   1851, 1860
Mt. Lebanon   1866, 1872, 1874

CARDINAL, BLUE   HERB   Diu. Eme. Cath. Her. Deo. Sud.
Lobelia syphilitica
Blue Lobelia.

Used in gonorrhea, dropsy, diarrhea, and dysentery.

Watervliet   1830, 1833, 1837, 1843, 1845, 1847, 1850, 1860
New Lebanon   1836, 1837, 1841, 1851, 1860
Mt. Lebanon   1872, 1873, 1874
Union Village, Ohio   1847, 1850

CARDINAL, RED   HERB   Anthel. Ner. A-spas. Cath. Diu.
Lobelia cardinalis   Eme. Ver.
Hog Physic. Red Lobelia. Cardinal
   Flower. Indian Pink.

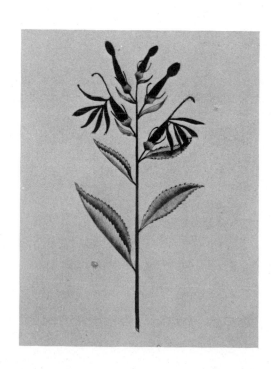

Used in early days as a dye. Said to be useful in removing worms from the bowels.

CHS: "A fall species frequent in meadows and along streams. Can. to Car. [Carolinas] and west to Illinois. Stem from 2 to 4 feet. July and August."

Watervliet   1860
New Lebanon   1851, 1860
Mt. Lebanon   1866, 1872
Union Village, Ohio   1850

CARDUS, SPOTTED   HERB   Ton. Dia. Emet. Dia. Diu.
Cnicus benedictus   ROOT   Ton. Dia. Emet.
Blessed Thistle. Holy Thistle. Milk
   Thistle.

Used as a tonic in loss of appetite, dyspepsia, and body coldness. Useful in producing copious perspiration when taken hot, for intermittent fevers. Taken double or triple strength, it becomes an emetic. The seeds also considered therapeutic.

Watervliet   1830, 1833, 1837, 1843, 1845, 1847, 1850
New Lebanon   1836, 1837, 1841, 1851, 1860
Mt. Lebanon   1866, 1872, 1873, 1874
Harvard   1851, 1853, 1857, 1860
Canterbury   1835, 1847, 1848, 1854
Union Village, Ohio   1850
New Gloucester   1864

CARPENTER'S SQUARE   LEAVES   Deo. Ton. Alt.
Scrophularia marilandica   ROOT   Deo. Ton. Alt.
Heal-All. Square Stalk. Figwort.

Used externally, in the form of an ointment, on bruises and scratches; internally as an alterative.

Union Village, Ohio   1847, 1850

CARROT, WILD   LEAVES   Stim. Diu. Carm. Emm. Deo.
Daucus carota   ROOT   Stim. Diu.
Bee's Nest Seed. Queen Anne's Lace.   SEED   Stim. Diu. Carm. Emm. Deo.

Used in dropsy, gravel, strangury, and as a poultice in foul and indolent ulcers.

Watervliet   1860
New Lebanon   1851, 1860
Mt. Lebanon   1866, 1872, 1873, 1874

CASTOR OIL PLANT   SEED   Cath.
Ricinus communis
Castor Bean.

The seeds are cathartic and yield castor oil.

Mt. Lebanon   1888

CATMINT   HERB Sud. A-spas. Diaph. Carm.
Nepeta cateria   Emm. Sto.
Catnip. Catnep.

Useful in febrile, nervous, and infantile diseases; also to restore the menstrual secretions. Useful in flatulency and upset stomach. Cats eat it ravenously, being fond of it for its effect.

Watervliet   1830, 1833, 1834, 1837, 1843, 1845, 1847, 1850, 1860
New Lebanon   1836, 1837, 1841, 1849, 1851, 1860
Mt. Lebanon   1866, 1872, 1873, 1874, 1888
Harvard   1851, 1853, 1854, 1857, 1860, 1873, 1880, 1885
Canterbury   1835, 1847, 1848, 1854
Union Village, Ohio   1848, 1850
New Gloucester   1864

CAYENNE   POWDER Sti. Rub. Err.
Capsicum annuum
Bird Pepper Chillies.

A stimulant that produces heat and redness of the skin and causes discharge at the nostrils. Used only in conjunction with other material, not alone. Grown in Africa, it was bought by the Shakers for use and resale.

Mt. Lebanon   1874
Hancock   1821
Harvard   1851, 1853, 1857, 1860
Canterbury   1847, 1848, 1854
Union Village, Ohio   1850
New Gloucester   1864

CEDAR, RED   APPLES Anthel.
Juniperus virginiana   LEAVES Stim. Diu.

Used in kidney complaints, suppression of urine, and obstructed menstruation.

Union Village, Ohio   1850

CELANDINE, GARDEN
Chelidonium majus
Tetterwort. Turmeric. Great Celandine.

HERB Cath. Acr. Alt. Stim. Diu. Diaph. Herp.

Used in scrofula, cutaneous diseases, piles, and affections of the spleen. The juice is used to cure warts, ringworms, and fungus growths.

CHS: "Grows by road sides and fences. Hast abundant bright yellow juice. It is used to distroy warts. May–Oct."

Watervliet   1843, 1845, 1847, 1850, 1860

New Lebanon   1849, 1851, 1860

Mt. Lebanon   1866, 1872, 1873, 1874

Harvard   1851, 1853, 1854, 1857, 1860, 1873, 1880, 1885

Canterbury   1835, 1847, 1848, 1854

Union Village, Ohio   1847, 1850

New Gloucester   1864

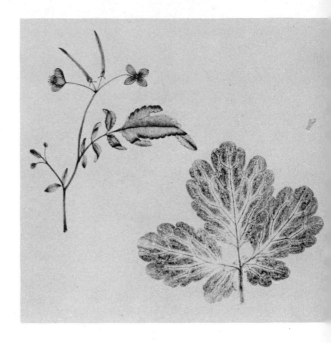

CELANDINE, WILD
Impatiens pallida
Jewelweed. Touch-Me-Not. Balsam-
  weed. Slipperweed.

HERB Aper. Diu. A-bil. Sto.

Recommended in jaundice, dropsy, liver complaint, salt rheum, and to cleanse foul ulcers. Used internally as decoction or tincture and externally as poultice or ointment.

Watervliet   1830, 1833, 1837, 1843, 1845, 1847, 1850, 1860
New Lebanon   1836, 1837, 1841, 1851, 1860
Mt. Lebanon   1866, 1872, 1873, 1874
Canterbury   1835
Union Village, Ohio   1847, 1850

CENTAURY, AMERICAN
Sabatia angularis
Red Centaury. Rose Pink. Bitter Clover.
  Eyebright. Bitter Bloom. Wild
  Succory.

HERB Ton. Ast. Sto.

Useful in autumnal fevers, dyspepsia, worms, and to restore the menstrual secretion. Should be gathered during flowering season. An excellent tonic; serviceable as a bitter tonic in dyspepsia and convalescence. Should be administered in warm infusion.

Watervliet 1860

New Lebanon 1851, 1860

Mt. Lebanon 1872, 1873, 1874

Canterbury 1835

Harvard 1873, 1880, 1885

Union Village, Ohio 1850

New Gloucester 1864

CHAMOMILE
Anthemis nobilis
Roman Chamomile. Mayweed.

FLOWERS Ton. Aro. Stim. Eme. Feb. Sud.

Used in dyspepsia, weak stomach, intermittent and typhus fevers, hysteria, and nervousness. When used as a tea, it is the flower which is used. The cold infusion is used as a hair rinse, not a dye but a brightener.

Watervliet 1860

New Lebanon 1851, 1860

Mt. Lebanon 1866, 1872, 1873, 1874

Union Village, Ohio 1847, 1850

CHAMOMILE, LOW
Anthemis arvensis
Garden Chamomile. Corn Chamomile.

HERB Ton. Stom.

Employed in fevers, colds, and to produce perspiration.

Watervliet 1830, 1832, 1833, 1837, 1843, 1845, 1847, 1850, 1860

New Lebanon 1836, 1837, 1841, 1851, 1860

Mt. Lebanon 1866, 1872, 1873, 1874

Harvard 1851, 1853, 1857, 1860, 1873, 1880, 1885

Canterbury 1835, 1847, 1848, 1854

New Gloucester 1864

CHECKERBERRY
Gaultheria procumbens
Mountain Tea. Deer Berry. Tea Berry.
  Box Berry.

LEAVES Stim. Aro. Ast. Diu. Sto. Eme.

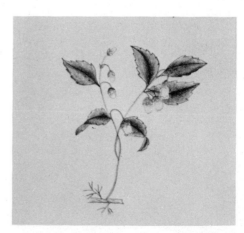

Valuable in dropsy and diarrhea. The oil was used to flavor other medicines. The essence was used for colic in infants.

CHS: "Common in woods and pastures. Can. to Ky. June and Sept."

Mt. Lebanon 1873

CHERRY, WILD   CHERRIES   Feb. Ast. Ton. A-sep. Pec.
Prunus serotina   Sto. Sed.
Black Cherry. Choke-Cherry. Virginia   BARK   Ast. Ton. A-sep.
    Prune.

Valuable in all cases where it is desirable to give tone and strength to the system; also in fever, cough, diarrhea, jaundice, dyspepsia, scrofula, and general debility. The inner bark is the part used medicinally. The outside layer of the bark should be removed; the green layer is then stripped off and carefully dried. Young thin bark is the best.

Watervliet   1830, 1833, 1837, 1843, 1845, 1847, 1850, 1860
New Lebanon   1836, 1837, 1841, 1851, 1860
Mt. Lebanon   1866, 1872, 1873, 1874
Harvard   1851, 1853, 1854, 1857, 1860, 1873, 1880, 1885
Canterbury   1835, 1847, 1848, 1854
New Gloucester   1864

CHESTNUT   LEAVES   Ast. Ton. Feb.
Cerastium vulgatum

Used a remedy in fevers and for its tonic and astringent properties. The Shakers also used chestnut leaves in the preparation of vegetable dyes and sold them for this purpose.

Harvard   1880, 1885

CHICKWEED   HERB   Ref. Emo. Dem.
Stellaria media
Mouse Ear.

Used as a poultice for old and indolent ulcers and with benefit also in ophthalmia,
erysipelas, and cutaneous diseases. It is a
cooling demulcent. The fresh leaves are
bruised and applied as a poultice. An ointment may be made by bruising young
leaves in fresh lard, and used for skin
irritations.

CHS: "Grows in fields and wash grounds.
Can. and U.S. Flowering all summer."

Watervliet   1860
New Lebanon   1851, 1860
Mt. Lebanon   1866, 1872, 1873, 1874

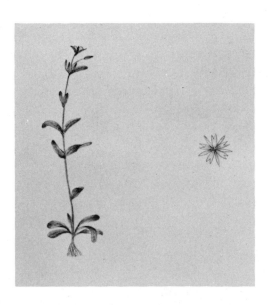

CHICORY   ROOT   Ton. Diu. Lax. Sto.
Cichorium intybus   HERB   Ton. Diu. Lax.
Succory. Wild Succory. Endive. Cen-
    taury.

Used in jaundice and liver complaints. A tea made of the dried root is good for sour stomach. It
may be taken whenever the stomach has been upset by any kind of food.

Watervliet   1860
New Lebanon   1851, 1860
Mt. Lebanon   1866, 1872, 1873, 1874

CHOLIC ROOT   ROOT   A-spas. Diu. Exp.
Dioscorea villosa
Colic Root. Rheumatism Root.

Used in biliary colic. In large doses, it seems to be diuretic and to act as an expectorant.

Union Village, Ohio   1850

CICELY, SWEET   ROOT   Aro. Stom. Carm. Expec. Stom.
Osmorhiza longistylis
Anise Root. Sweet Anise. Sweet Javril

Useful in coughs, flatulence, and as a gentle stimulant tonic to debilitated stomachs.

Watervliet   1830, 1833, 1837, 1843, 1845, 1847, 1850, 1860
New Lebanon   1836, 1837, 1841, 1851, 1860
Mt. Lebanon   1866, 1872, 1873, 1874
Union Village, Ohio   1847

CICUTA   LEAVES   Nar. Ano. A-spas. Dis. Deo.
Conium maculatum   SEED   Nar. Ano. A-spas. Dis.
Spotted Cowbane. Beaver Poison. Mus-
    quash Root. Poison Hemlock. Poison
    Parsley. Water Hemlock. Poison Root.
    Spotted Hemlock.

Used in chronic rheumatism, neuralgia, asthma, and excited condition of the nervous system. Use
cautiously, it is a virulent poison suitable for use only by a skilled physician.

Watervliet   1830, 1832, 1833, 1837, 1843, 1845, 1847, 1850, 1860
New Lebanon   1836, 1837, 1841, 1849, 1851, 1860

Mt. Lebanon   1866, 1872, 1873, 1874
Harvard   1851, 1853, 1854, 1857, 1860, 1873, 1880, 1885
Canterbury   1835, 1847, 1848, 1854
Union Village, Ohio   1847, 1850
New Gloucester   1864

CINCHONA   BARK   Ton. A-per. Ast. Feb.
Cinchona succirubra
Peruvian Bark. Foso Bark. Red Bark.
   Crown Bark.

Useful as a tonic and antiperiodic; moderately astringent and eminently febrifuge. Used freely as a mouthwash and gargle and given internally as a remedy for malaria. Taken internally, it imparts a sensation of warmth to the stomach and fights fevers.

Mt. Lebanon   1874

CINNAMON   OIL   Germicide
Cinnamomum zeylanicum   POWDERED SPICE   Food preservative

Imported or bought by the Shakers for use as a flavoring and as an antiseptic to prevent food rancidity.

Several Shaker societies used it, but did not list it in their catalogs.

CLARY   HERB   A-spas. Bals. Sto. Dia.
Salvia sclarea   Diu. Sti.
Clammy Sage. Clarry.

Used in night sweats, hectic fever, and flatulence. Also used in the making of wine and beer, especially the fresh flowers, which give a distinctive flavor to raisin wine and sweeten it. The leaves and flowers are more highly scented than common sage, and are used in sachets and potpourri.

Watervliet   1830, 1833, 1837, 1843, 1845   Canterbury   1835, 1847, 1848, 1854
New Lebanon   1836, 1837, 1841, 1851, 1860   Union Village, Ohio   1847, 1850
Mt. Lebanon   1866, 1872, 1873, 1874

CLEAVERS   HERB   Ref. Diu. Sud.
Galium aparine
Goose Grass. Clivers. Catch Weed. Bed
   Straw. Rough Cleavers.

Valuable in curing suppression of urine, and to cure inflammation of kidney and bladder. As a wash it was used to remove freckles.

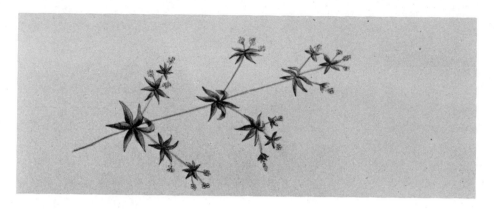

CHS: "Common in thickets and low ground. Can. and U.S. July."

Watervliet   1830, 1833, 1837, 1843, 1845, 1847, 1850, 1860
New Lebanon   1836, 1837, 1841, 1851, 1860
Mt. Lebanon   1866, 1872, 1873, 1874
Harvard   1851, 1853, 1854, 1857, 1860, 1873, 1880, 1885
Canterbury   1835, 1847, 1848, 1854
Union Village, Ohio   1847, 1850
New Gloucester   1864

CLOVER, RED   BLOSSOMS   Acr. Pec. Exp. Diu.
Trifolium pratense
Sweet Clover. King's Clover. Clover
   Blows.

An extract of the blossoms is an excellent remedy for cancerous ulcers, corns, and burns.

Watervliet   1860   Harvard   1873, 1880, 1885
New Lebanon   1849, 1851, 1860   Union Village, Ohio   1850
Mt. Lebanon   1866, 1872, 1873, 1874

CLOVER, WHITE   BLOSSOMS   Exp. Diu.
Melilotus alba
Sweet White Clover. Sweet Melilot.

Used in chest complaints. Also used to flavor cheese and tobacco.

Mt. Lebanon   1872
Harvard   1880, 1885
Union Village, Ohio   1850

CLOVER, YELLOW
Trifolium filiforme

BLOSSOMS Exp. Diu.

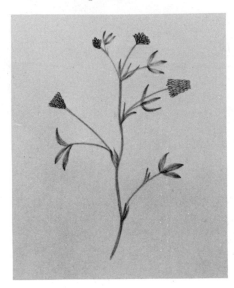

Used for the same purposes as white clover.
Very sweet and pleasant in sachets and potpourri mixtures.

CHS: "In dry soils. N.H. [New Hampshire]
to Va. [Virginia]. Flowers at length reflexed.
June, July."

Canterbury   1887

CLOVES
Eugenia caryophyllata

BUD Ast.

Imported or bought from importers by Shakers and offered for sale. Used in cooking and for
preparing foods for storage and for astringent purposes. (See Cinnamon.)

Mt. Lebanon   1874

COCASH
Aster puniceus
Squaw Weed. Life Root. Cocash Weed.
   Red Stalked Aster. Cold Water Root.
   September Weed.

ROOT Sud. Sto. Stim. Diaph. Ton. Ast.
Diu. Car.

The warm infusion is used for colds, rheumatism, nervous debility, headache, and menstrual
irregularities.

Watervliet   1860
New Lebanon   1851, 1860
Mt. Lebanon   1866, 1872, 1873, 1874

COHOSH, BLACK
Cimicifuga racemosa
Rattle Root. Black Snake Root. Bugbane.
  Rattle Weed. Squaw Root. Baneberry.

ROOT Deo. Alt. A-per. Nar. Ner. Dia.
Diu. Sed. A-spas.

Useful for rheumatism, dropsy, epilepsy, and spasmodic affections. Valuable in female complaints and as a postpartum accelerator. Its leaves are said to drive away bugs. Boiling water absorbs the properties of the root only partially, but alcohol absorbs them completely. A purifying tea and pectoral syrup.

Groveland, N.Y.   1842
Watervliet   1830, 1833, 1837, 1843, 1845, 1847, 1850, 1860
New Lebanon   1836, 1837, 1841, 1851, 1860
Mt. Lebanon   1866, 1872, 1873, 1874
Harvard   1851, 1853, 1857, 1860, 1873, 1880, 1885
Canterbury   1835, 1847, 1848, 1854
New Gloucester   1864

COHOSH, BLUE
Caulophyllum thalictrioides
Squaw Root. Papoose Root. Blue Berry.

ROOT Sti. A-spas. Diu. Dia. Part. Emm.
Anthel.

A favorite remedy in chronic uterine diseases. As a parturient it has proved invaluable. Also used in rheumatism, dropsy, cramps, colic, and hysterics. The seeds, which ripen in August, make a decoction which closely resembles coffee.

New Lebanon   1851, 1860
Mt. Lebanon   1866, 1872, 1873, 1874
Harvard   1880, 1885
Union Village, Ohio   1850

COHOSH, RED
Actea rubra

ROOT Diu. Dia. Anthel. Deo. Nar.

Used in uterine diseases, rheumatism, dropsy, and colic.

Watervliet   1830, 1833, 1837, 1843
New Lebanon   1836, 1837, 1841, 1851, 1860
Mt. Lebanon   1866, 1872, 1874
Harvard   1851, 1853, 1857, 1860, 1873

COHOSH, WHITE   ROOT   Purg. Emm. Deo. Nar. Car.
Actea alba
Necklace Weed. Bane Berry. Noah's Ark.

A decoction useful for the itch. Also used in rheumatism, flatulence, and nervous irritability.

Watervliet   1830, 1833, 1837, 1843
New Lebanon   1836, 1837, 1841, 1851, 1860
Mt. Lebanon   1866, 1872, 1873, 1874
Harvard   1851, 1853, 1857, 1860, 1873, 1880, 1885
Canterbury   1847, 1848, 1854
New Gloucester   1864

COHOSH, YELLOW   ROOT   Alt. Deo. Nar.
Flavus pulvus

Slightly narcotic, useful as a mild sedative. It exerts a tonic influence over mucous tissues.

Canterbury   1847, 1848, 1854

COLCHICUM   ROOT   Acr. Nar. Sed. Cath. Diu. Eme.
Colchicum autumnale   SEED   Acr. Nar. Sed. Cath. Diu. Eme.
Meadow Saffron. Autumn–Crocus.

Used in gout, rheumatism, palpitation of the heart, gonorrhea, and enlarged prostrate. Should be used cautiously.

Mt. Lebanon   1873, 1874

COLOCYNTH   THE FRUIT DIVESTED OF ITS RIND.   Car.
Cucumis colocynthis
Bitter Cucumber. Bitter Apple.

Strong cathartic, should *never* be used alone—with henbane it loses its irritant properties.

Mt. Lebanon   1874
Union Village, Ohio   1850

COLOMBO   ROOT   Ton. Chol.
Cocculus palmatus

Employed in dyspepsia, chronic diarrhea and dysentery, cholera morbus and cholera infantum, and for convalescence from fevers. An African climbing plant, imported by the Shakers.

Mt. Lebanon   1873, 1874

COLOMBO, AMERICAN   ROOT   Ton. Cath. Eme.
Cocculus carolinis
Indian Lettuce. Pyramid Flower. Mea-
    dow Pride. Yellow Gentian.

An excellent tonic, which may be used in all cases where a mild cathartic or emetic is required.

New Lebanon   1851, 1860
Mt. Lebanon   1866, 1872, 1873
Union Village, Ohio   1850

COLTSFOOT   LEAVES AND FLOWERS   Emo. Dem. Ton.
Tussilago farfara   Pec. Dem. Exp.
Bullsfoot. Ginger Root. Coughwort.   ROOT   Emo. Dem. Ton.

In coughs, asthma, whooping cough and pulmonary affections, scrofula, and scrofulous tumors. Used as snuff in headaches. Used externally in the form of a poultice. The leaves should be collected at full size, the flowers as soon as they open, and the root immediately after the leaves mature.

CHS: "In wet places, brooksides and on the shore of lakes, North and Middle States. It grows in clayey soil. The flower appears in early spring before a leaf is to be seen. Early Spring."

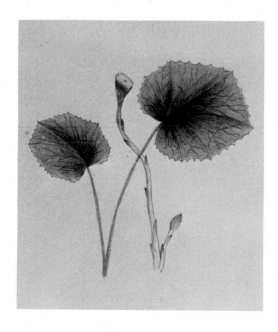

Watervliet   1830, 1833, 1837, 1843, 1845,
    1847, 1850, 1860
New Lebanon   1836, 1837, 1841, 1851, 1860
Mt. Lebanon   1866, 1872, 1873, 1874
Harvard   1851, 1853, 1857, 1860, 1873, 1880,
    1885
Canterbury   1835, 1847, 1848, 1854
Union Village, Ohio   1850
New Gloucester   1864

COMFREY   ROOT   Dem. Ast. Bal. Pec.

Symphytum officinale

Gum Plant. Healing Herb. Slippery
   Root.

Useful in diarrhea, dysentery, coughs, leucorrhea, and female debility. As an application to
bruises, fresh wounds, sores and burns, and in nasal congestion or catarrh.

Watervliet   1830, 1833, 1837, 1843, 1845, 1847, 1850, 1860

New Lebanon   1836, 1837, 1841, 1851, 1860

Mt. Lebanon   1866, 1872, 1873, 1874

Harvard   1851, 1853, 1854, 1857, 1860, 1873, 1880, 1885

Canterbury   1835, 1847, 1848, 1854

Union Village, Ohio   1847, 1850

New Gloucester   1864

COMPOSITION POWDERS

Any combination of pulverized or powdered herbs made to order and put up in 2– and 4–ounce
packages.

Watervliet   1850

Mt. Lebanon   1872, 1874

CONSUMPTION BRAKE   ROOT   Ast. Sti. Ton.

Botrychium lunaria

Moonwort.

Used in diarrhea and dysentery, and to prevent mucus discharges.

New Lebanon   1851, 1860

Mt. Lebanon   1866, 1872, 1873, 1874

COOLWORT   HERB   Dia. Ton. Diu.

Mitella cordifolia

Mitrewort. Bishops-Cap.

Valuable in strangury, diabetes, and all kidney complaints.

New Lebanon   1849, 1851, 1860

Mt. Lebanon   1866, 1872, 1873, 1874

CORIANDER   SEED   Sto. Stim. Carm.
Coriandrum sativum

Used to flavor and correct the action of other medicines. In syrup, used for pain in the stomach and side. The Shakers imported it or bought it for resale.

Groveland, N.Y.   1842
Watervliet   1830, 1833, 1837, 1843, 1845, 1847, 1850, 1860
New Lebanon   1836, 1837, 1841, 1860
Mt. Lebanon   1866, 1872, 1873, 1874, 1888
Union Village, Ohio   1847, 1850

COTTON ROOT   BARK OF ROOT   Emm. Part. Abo.
Gossypium herbaceum

Said to promote uterine contractions as efficiently as the herb ergot, and with perfect safety. The seed is used in fever and ague. It should not be employed by the unskilled. Although a native of Asia, it was cultivated in the southern portion of America more successfully than anywhere else.

Mt. Lebanon   1873, 1874
Harvard   1880, 1885

COWPARSNIP   LEAVES   Ner. Car. Diu. Aro. Sto.
Heracleum lanatum   ROOT   Car. Diu. Ner. Nar. Sto.
                                        SEED   Car. Aro. Ner. Sto. Diu.

Useful as a diuretic and to expel wind.

Watervliet   1830, 1837, 1843, 1845, 1847, 1850, 1860
New Lebanon   1837, 1841, 1849, 1851, 1860
Mt. Lebanon   1866, 1872
Harvard   1851, 1853, 1857, 1860, 1873, 1880
Canterbury   1835, 1847, 1848, 1854
Union Village, Ohio   1847, 1850

COWPARSNIP, ROYAL   LEAVES   A-spas. Ton.
Imperatoria ostruthium   ROOT   A-spas. Ton.
Masterwort. Golden Alexanders.   SEED   Car. Aro.

Used in asthma, colic, palsy, and apoplexy. The Shakers produced the extract in vast quantities.

Harvard   1851, 1853, 1857, 1860, 1873, 1880
Canterbury   1835, 1847, 1848, 1854

CRAMP BARK
Viburnum opulus
High Cranberry. Squawbush.

Very effective in relaxing cramps and spasms in asthma, hysteria, pains incident to females during pregnancy, convulsions, etc. A poultice of the fruit is said to be efficacious when applied to the throat for minor irritations.

CHS: "A handsome shrub, in woods and borders of fields. Northern States and British Am. June."

Watervliet　1860
New Lebanon　1851, 1860
Mt. Lebanon　1866, 1872, 1873, 1874
Harvard　1880, 1885
Union Village, Ohio　1850

BARK　A-spas.

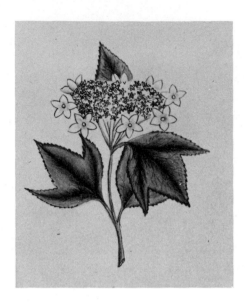

CRANESBILL
Geranium maculatum
Spotted Geranium. Crowfoot [not to be confounded with crowfoot of the *Ranunculus* family]. Alumroot. Dovefoot. American Tormentilla. Storksbill.

A powerful astringent used in dysentery, diarrhea, cholera infantum, hemorrhage, canker, and also as a gargle.

CHS: "In dry rocky places. Can. to Va. Stem reddish. It has a disagreeable smell. May to Sept."

Watervliet　1830, 1833, 1837, 1843, 1845, 1847, 1850, 1860
New Lebanon　1836, 1837, 1841, 1851, 1860
Mt. Lebanon　1866, 1872, 1873, 1874
Harvard　1851, 1853, 1857, 1860, 1873, 1880, 1885

ROOT　Ast. Sty. Ton.

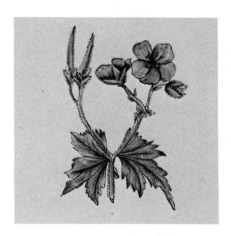

Canterbury　1835, 1847, 1848, 1854
Union Village, Ohio　1847, 1850
New Gloucester　1864

CRAWLEY   ROOT   Sed. Feb. Diaph. Bal. Sto.

Corallorhiza odontorhiza

Dragon's Claw. Coral Root. Fever Root.
    Chickentoe.

Invaluable in low typhoid fever and intermittent fever, pleurisy, and night sweats. One of the most prompt and satisfactory diaphoretics in the materia medica, but its scarcity and high price have tended to keep it from coming into general use. It can be combined with blue cohosh, and also with black root or mayapple to act upon the bowels. Mixed with colicroot, it is helpful in flatulent and bilious colic.

Groveland, N.Y.   1842

Watervliet   1833, 1837, 1843, 1845, 1847, 1850, 1860

New Lebanon   1836, 1837, 1841, 1851, 1860

Mt. Lebanon   1866, 1872, 1873, 1874

Harvard   1880, 1885

Union Village, Ohio   1850

CUBEBS   BERRIES   Exp. Stom. Carm.

Piper cubeba

Tail Pepper. Java Pepper.

Useful in bronchitis, cough, and diseases of the urinary organs. A native of Java and other islands in the Indian Ocean. Imported by the Shakers for resale.

Mt. Lebanon   1873, 1874

CUCKOLD   HERB   Ast. Diu. Car. Emm. Exp.

Bidens frondosa

Swamp Beggar's Tick. Beggar Lice. Har-
    vest Lice.   Spanish Needles.   Cow
    Lice. Leafy Burr Mangold.

Used in palpitation of the heart, cough, and uterine derangement. Roots or seeds are also used as an expectorant in throat irritation.

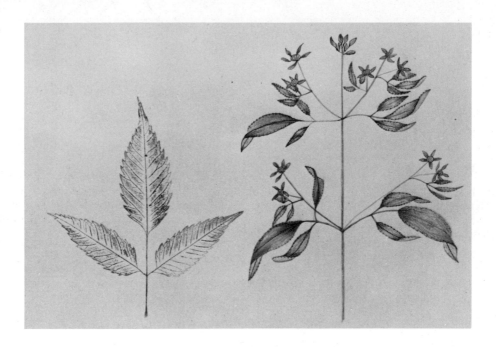

Watervliet   1860
New Lebanon   1851, 1860
Mt. Lebanon   1866, 1874

CULVER'S ROOT   ROOT   Cath. Deo. Ton. Diu.
Leptandra virginica
Blackroot. Tall Speedwell. Culver's Phy-
   sic. Tall Veronica. Leptandra.

The fresh root is too irritating to be employed, but the dried root is laxative, cholagogic, and tonic.
Its medicinal virtues are stronger when the roots are dug from plants growing in limestone areas.
It should be gathered in the fall of the second year.

Watervliet   1830, 1833, 1837, 1843, 1845, 1847, 1850, 1860
New Lebanon   1836, 1837, 1841, 1851, 1860
Mt. Lebanon   1866, 1872, 1873, 1874
Harvard   1851, 1853, 1854, 1857, 1860, 1873, 1880, 1885
Canterbury   1847, 1848, 1854
Union Village, Ohio   1847, 1850
New Gloucester   1864

DAFFODIL   ROOT   Eme. Cath.
Narcissus pseudo-narcissus
Daffy-Downdillies.

Powdered, the roots act as an emetic and afterwards as a purge, and are excellent for use in all obstructions.

Union Village, Ohio   1850

DAISY, WHITE   FLOWERS   Ton. Diu. A-spas. Eme. Vul.
Leucanthemum vulgare
White Weed. Ox-eye Daisy.

Used in whooping cough, asthma, nervousness, leucorrhea, and as a local application to wounds and cutaneous diseases.

Watervliet   1850, 1860   Mt. Lebanon   1866, 1872, 1873, 1874
New Lebanon   1851, 1860

DANDELION   HERB   A-bil.   Stom.   Alt.   Ton.   Diu.
Taraxacum officinale   Cath. Deo.
Blow Ball. Cankerwort.   ROOT   Ast. Stom. Alt. Ton. Diu. Cath.
                                                      Deo.

Recommended in diseases of the liver, and in constipation, dropsy, diseases of the skin, and uterine obstructions. Should be collected when the plant is in flower. The young plant possesses some slight narcotic properties. The dried root, when fresh, is a stomachic and tonic with slightly diuretic and aperient actions.

Watervliet   1830, 1833, 1837, 1843, 1845, 1847, 1850, 1860
New Lebanon   1836, 1837, 1841, 1849, 1851, 1860
Mt. Lebanon   1866, 1872, 1873, 1874
Harvard   1851, 1853, 1857, 1860, 1873, 1880, 1885
Canterbury   1835, 1847, 1848, 1854
Union Village, Ohio   1847, 1850
New Gloucester   1864

DILL   SEED   Car. Aro. Stom. Exp.
Anethum graveolens
Dillseed. Dilly.

Used in flatulency, colic, to stop hiccups, and expel gas. Also used in cooking.

Watervliet   1860
New Lebanon   1851, 1860
Mt. Lebanon   1866, 1872, 1873, 1874, 1881, 1885, 1888
Union Village, Ohio   1847, 1850

DITTANY   LEAVES Diap. Stim. Ner. Carm. A-
Cunila mariana   spas. Aro. Ton. Sud.
Stone Mint. Mountain Dittany. Ameri-   FLOWERS Diap. Stim. Ner. Carm. A-
    can Dittany. Wild Basil.   spas. Aro. Ton. Sud.

Used in a warm infusion for colds, headache, fevers, colic, and nervous affections. Warm tea is
diaphoretic.

Watervliet   1860
New Lebanon   1851, 1860
Mt. Lebanon   1866, 1872, 1873, 1874

DOCK, BROADLEAF   ROOT Ton. Cath. Deo. Her.
Rumex obtusifolius

A purge and tonic. Useful when blood needs purifying.

Watervliet   1850, 1860
Canterbury   1847, 1848, 1854

DOCK, WATER   ROOTS Det. Alt. Deo. Her. Ast. Dia.
Rumex aquaticus
Great Water Dock. Sour Dock. Narrow
    Dock.

Useful in diseases of an eruptive nature; used in ointment form for itching.

Watervliet   1860
New Lebanon   1851, 1860
Mt. Lebanon   1866, 1872, 1873
Harvard   1851, 1853, 1857, 1860, 1880, 1885
New Gloucester   1864

DOCK ROOT, YELLOW   ROOTS Det. Alt. Deo. Her. Ton. Ast.
Rumex crispus
Sour Dock. Narrow Dock. Curled Dock.
    Rumex.

Useful in scrofula, syphilis, leprosy, diseases of an eruptive nature; as an ointment for itching and indolent glandular tumors; and in all cases where the blood needs purifying. There are two other varieties of dock, *Rumex aquaticus* (water dock) and *Rumex obtusifolius* (broadleaf dock), but yellow dock is the only one entitled to extensive consideration. It is a very rich source of digestible plant iron.

Watervliet   1830, 1833, 1837, 1843, 1845, 1847, 1850, 1860

New Lebanon   1836, 1837, 1841, 1849, 1851, 1860

Mt. Lebanon   1866, 1872, 1873, 1874

Harvard   1851, 1853, 1854, 1857, 1860, 1873, 1880, 1885

Canterbury   1835, 1847, 1848, 1854

Enfield, N.H.   1889

Union Village, Ohio   1847, 1850

New Gloucester   1864

DOG GRASS

Agropyron repens

Witch Grass. Quick Grass. Couch Grass. Scratch Grass. Triticum. Durfa Grass.

ROOT   Diu. Ape. Dem. Ton. Cath. Feb.

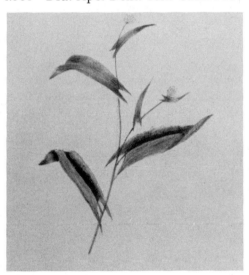

Useful in conditions in which it is desirable to promote or increase the flow of urine. Large and frequent doses are considered a good tonic in the spring. Kills worms in children.

CHS: "A rough species. Flowers white. Can. and U.S. June."

Harvard   1880, 1885

DOGWOOD

Cornus sericea

Boxwood. Green Ozier. Flowering Cornel. Rose Willow.

BARK   Ast. Stim. Ton.

FLOWERS   Ast. Stim. Ton.

The bark should be used in its dried state. Cornine, the active principle, is used occasionally as a substitute for quinine. Dogwood exerts its best virtues in the form of an ointment.

Canterbury   1835

Union Village, Ohio   1847

DRAGON ROOT   ROOT   Dia. Sti. Acr. Nar. Exp.
Arum triphyllum
Jack-in-the-Pulpit. Wild Turnip. Indian
   Turnip. Wake Robin.

It is acrid, and used as an expectorant; it is also diaphoretic. It is used as well for lung diseases. The root should be used fresh, but must be partially dried, as it loses its strength with age.

Harvard   1851, 1853, 1854, 1857, 1860, 1873, 1880, 1885
Canterbury   1835, 1847, 1848, 1854
New Gloucester   1864

ELDER   BARK   Cath. Deo. Diu. Sud. Her. Ner.
Sambucus canadensis   BERRIES Cath. Alt. Ape.
Sweet Elder. American Elder. Panicle   FLOWERS Dia. Stim. Diu. Sud. Herp.
   Elder Sambucus.   Alt.

The bark is used in dropsy, erysipelas, and as an alterative in various chronic complaints; the berries are used in rheumatism and gouty affections. The flowers are used in erysipelas, fevers, and constipation.

CHS: "A common shrub 6 to 10 ft. high in hilly pastures and woods, U.S. and Can. Berries dark purple. May. July."

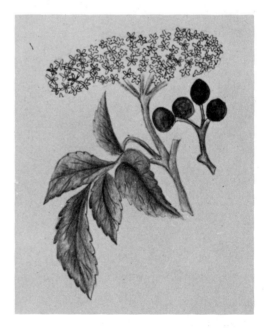

Watervliet   1830, 1833, 1837, 1843, 1845, 1847, 1850, 1860
New Lebanon   1836, 1837, 1841, 1849, 1851, 1860
Mt. Lebanon   1866, 1872, 1874
Harvard   1851, 1853, 1854, 1857, 1860, 1873, 1880, 1885
Canterbury   1835, 1847, 1848, 1854
Union Village, Ohio   1847, 1850
New Gloucester   1864

ELDER, DWARF   ROOT   Diu. Alt. Dem. Ton. Dia.
Aralia hispida
Wild Elder. Bristlestem Sarsaparilla.

Very valuable in dropsy, gravel, suppression of urine, and other urinary disorders.

Watervliet   1830, 1833, 1837, 1843, 1847, 1850, 1860

New Lebanon   1836, 1841, 1851, 1860

Mt. Lebanon   1866, 1872, 1873, 1874

Harvard   1851, 1853, 1857, 1860, 1873, 1880, 1885

Canterbury   1835, 1847, 1848, 1854

Union Village, Ohio   1850

New Gloucester   1864

ELECAMPANE   ROOT Dia. Diu. Exp. Ast. Sto. Ton.
Inula helenium   Stim.
Scabwort.

Much used in cough, colds, lung diseases, weakness of the digestive organs, and dyspepsia; also in tetter, itching, and cutaneous diseases. The root should be gathered in its second year, during the fall months.

Groveland, N.Y.   1842

Watervliet   1830, 1833, 1837, 1843, 1845, 1847, 1850, 1860

New Lebanon   1836, 1837, 1841, 1851, 1860

Mt. Lebanon   1866, 1872, 1873, 1874

Harvard   1851, 1853, 1854, 1857, 1860, 1873, 1880, 1885

Canterbury   1835, 1847, 1848, 1854

Union Village, Ohio   1847, 1850

New Gloucester   1864

ELM, SLIPPERY   BARK, INNER Emo. Diu. Dem. Exp.
Ulmus fulva   Ton.
Red Elm. Indian Elm. Sweet Elm.   GROUND Emo. Diu. Dem. Exp. Ton.
  Moose Elm.   FLOUR Emo. Diu. Dem. Exp. Ton.

Highly beneficial in dysentery, diarrhea, inflammation of the lungs, bowels, stomach, bladder or kidneys, also as poultices for skin irritation. The bark is chewed for sore throat. (The tree is not to be confused with American elm.)

Watervliet   1830, 1833, 1837, 1843, 1845, 1847, 1850, 1860

New Lebanon   1836, 1837, 1841, 1849, 1851, 1860

Mt. Lebanon   1866, 1872, 1874

Harvard   1851, 1853, 1857, 1860, 1873, 1880

Canterbury   1847, 1848, 1854

Union Village, Ohio   1847, 1850

New Gloucester   1864

ERGOT
Secale cornatum
Spurred Rye. Smut Rye.

SEED (DEGENERATED SEEDS OF COM-
MON RYE) Acr.

Used to promote uterine contractions.

Mt. Lebanon   1872, 1874

EUPHORBIA
Euphorbia ipecacuanha
Spreading Spurge. Dysentery-Weed.
  Milk Purslane. American Ipecac.

ROOT Ast. Eme. Cath. Ton. Dia. Exp.

Valuable in bilious colic, dropsical affections, dyspepsia, jaundice, and sluggishness of the liver.

Watervliet 1860
New Lebanon   1851, 1860
Mt. Lebanon   1866, 1872, 1873

FENNEL
Foeniculum vulgare
Wild Fennel. Sweet Fennel. Large
  Fennel.

SEED Aro. Carm. Stim. Stom. Diu.
Pec.

Used to expel wind from the bowels. A good aromatic; used to flavor other medicines.

Watervliet   1830, 1833, 1837, 1843, 1845, 1847, 1850, 1860
New Lebanon   1836, 1837, 1841, 1851, 1860
Mt. Lebanon   1866, 1872, 1873, 1874, 1881, 1885, 1888
Enfield, Conn.   1790, 1800
Canterbury   1835
Union Village, Ohio   1847, 1850

FERN, MAIDENHAIR
Adiantum pedatum

HERB Car. Ref. Exp. Ton. Sud. Ast.
Pec. Sto.

Valuable in cough, asthma, hoarseness, influenza, pleurisy, jaundice, febrile diseases, and erysipelas. A decoction of the plant is cooling and of benefit in coughs resulting from colds, nasal congestion, catarrh, and hoarseness. It can be used freely.

CHS: "A beautiful fern, abounding in damp rocky woods. Stalk glossy purple, approaching to a jet black. July."

Watervliet   1830, 1833, 1837, 1843, 1845, 1847, 1850, 1860

New Lebanon   1836, 1837, 1841, 1849, 1851, 1860

Mt. Lebanon   1866, 1872, 1873, 1874

Harvard   1849, 1851, 1853, 1854, 1857, 1860, 1873, 1880, 1885

Canterbury   1835, 1847, 1848, 1854

Union Village, Ohio   1847, 1850

New Gloucester   1864

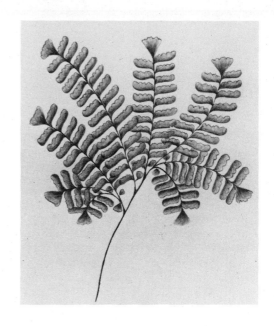

FERN, MALE   ROOT   Ver. Ton. Ast.
Dryopteris filix-mas
Male Shield Fern.

Valuable to expel tapeworm.

Watervliet   1830, 1833, 1837, 1843, 1847, 1860
New Lebanon   1837, 1851, 1860
Mt. Lebanon   1866, 1872, 1873, 1874

FERN, POLYPODY   ROOT AND TOP   Pec. Dem. Purg. Anthel.
Polypodium vulgare   Cath.
Rock Polypod. Rock Brake. Brake Root. Female Fern.

Used in pulmonary and hepatic complaints; also used to expel worms.

CHS: "On shady rocks and in woods forming tangled patches. July."

New Lebanon   1851, 1860
Mt. Lebanon   1866, 1872, 1873, 1874

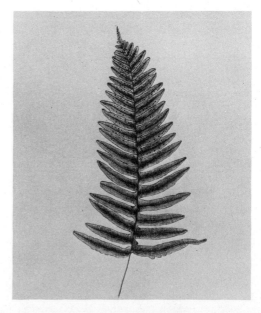

FERN, SWEET
Comptonia asplenifolia
Spleenwort Bush. Fern Gale. Sweet
Fern. Sweet Bush.

HERB Ton. Ast. Alt. Sto.

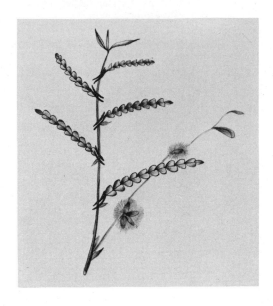

Useful in cholera infantum, dysentery,
leucorrhea, debility following fevers,
bruises, and rheumatism. Also, because of
its tonic and astringent properties, it is successful in diarrhea.

CHS: "A well known handsome aromatic
shrub common in pastures and on hillsides.
The main stem is covered with a rusty
brown bark which becomes reddish in the
branches, and white downy in the young
shoots. Leaves numerous. Fertile flowers in
a dense rounded burr or head situated
below the barren ones. May."

Watervliet   1830, 1833, 1837, 1843, 1845,
1847, 1850, 1860
New Lebanon   1836, 1837, 1841, 1851, 1860
Mt. Lebanon   1866, 1873, 1874
Harvard   1851, 1853, 1854, 1857, 1860, 1873,
1880, 1885

Canterbury   1835, 1847, 1848, 1854
Union Village, Ohio   1850
New Gloucester   1864

FEVERBUSH
Lindera benzoin
Wild Allspice. Spice Bush. Snap
Wood. Fever Wood. Benjamin Bush.

LEAVES Aro. Ton. Sti. Verm. Feb.
Ner. Sto.
TWIGS Aro. Ton. Sti. Verm. Feb. Ner.
Sto.

Recommended in fever and ague, colds, coughs, and as an anthelmintic.

Watervliet   1837, 1843, 1845, 1847, 1850, 1860
New Lebanon   1837, 1841, 1849, 1851, 1860
Mt. Lebanon   1866, 1872, 1873, 1874
Canterbury   1835

FEVERFEW
Chrysanthemum parthenium
Featherfew.

HERB Ton. Carm. Emm. Ver. Stim.
Ner. Sto.

A warm infusion is used for recent colds, flatulency, worms, irregular menstruation, hysterics, and suppression of urine.

Watervliet   1830, 1833, 1834, 1837, 1843, 1845, 1847, 1850, 1860
New Lebanon   1836, 1837, 1841, 1851, 1860
Mt. Lebanon   1866, 1872, 1874
Harvard   1851, 1853, 1854, 1857, 1860, 1873, 1880, 1885
Canterbury   1835, 1847, 1848, 1854
Union Village, Ohio   1850
New Gloucester   1864

FEVERROOT   ROOT   Ton. Cath. Eme. Diu.
Triosteum perfoliatum
Wild Ipecac. Horse Gentian. Tinker's
  Weed. Wild Coffee.

Used in fever and ague, pleurisy, dyspepsia, and rheumatism.

Watervliet   1830, 1833, 1837, 1843, 1845, 1847, 1850, 1860
New Lebanon   1836, 1837, 1841, 1851, 1860
Mt. Lebanon   1866, 1872, 1873, 1874
Union Village, Ohio   1847, 1850

FIREWEED   HERB   Ast. Eme. Cath. Ton. Alt. Vul.
Erechtites hieracifolia   Deo.
Pilewort.   ROOT   Ast. Eme. Cath. Ton. Alt. Vul.
  Deo.

Excellent in diseases of the mucous tissues of the lungs, stomach, and bowels, summer gastric complaint of children, piles, hemorrhage, and dysentery.

Watervliet   1850
New Lebanon   1851, 1860
Mt. Lebanon   1866, 1872, 1873, 1874
Harvard   1885

FITROOT   ROOT   A-spas. Ton. Sed. Ner.
Monotropa uniflora
Pipe Plant. Bird's Nest. Ice Plant. In-
  dian Pipe. Fit Plant. Dutchman's
  Pipe. Ghostflower. Ova Ova.

The whole plant is ivory white, resembling frozen jelly, and when handled, melts away like ice.

Watervliet 1860

Mt. Lebanon 1866, 1872, 1873, 1874

New Lebanon 1851, 1860

FIVE-FINGER GRASS
Potentilla canadensis
Cinquefoil.

LEAVES Ton. Ast. Emm.
ROOT Ton. Ast. Emm.

Useful in fevers, bowel complaints, night sweats, spongy gums, sore mouth, and hemorrhages, and can be brewed as a tea. Excellent as a mouthwash and gargle. The root is used for a red dye.

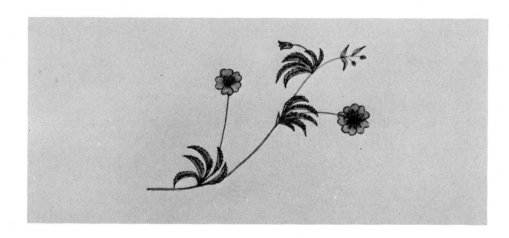

CHS: "Common in fields and in thickets U.S. and Canada. Apr. Aug."

Watervliet 1860

Mt. Lebanon 1866, 1872, 1873, 1874

New Lebanon 1849, 1851, 1860

Union Village, Ohio 1847, 1850

FLAX
Linum usitatissimum
Linseed. Lint Bells. Toad Flax.

SEED Dem. Emo.

Useful internally in coughs resulting from colds. The ground seed, used in combination with elm bark, makes an excellent poultice for general use. The flowers are used for yellow dye.

CHS: "A very showy plant common by road sides, N. Eng. to Ky. and Ga. 1 to-2 ft. high, very leafy. July. Aug."

Harvard   1851, 1853
Canterbury   1835, 1847, 1848, 1854

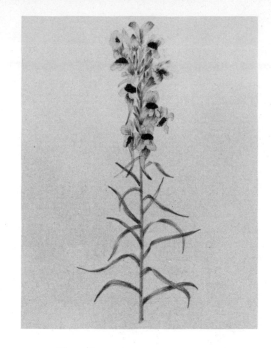

FLEABANE

Erigeron canadense

Colt's Tail. Pride Weed. Scabious. Horse Weed. Butter Weed.

HERB   Ton. Diu. Sty. Ast. Aro. Nar.

Efficient in diarrhea, gravel, diabetes, urine scald, and in hemorrhage of bowels or uterus, and bleeding of wounds. Should be gathered when in bloom.

CHS: "By roadsides and in fields throughout North America. Aug. Nov."

Watervliet   1830, 1832, 1833, 1837, 1843, 1845, 1847, 1850, 1860
New Lebanon   1836, 1837, 1841, 1851, 1860
Mt. Lebanon   1866, 1872, 1873, 1874
Harvard   1849, 1851, 1853, 1854, 1857, 1860, 1873, 1880
Canterbury   1835, 1847, 1848, 1854
Union Village, Ohio   1847, 1850
New Gloucester   1864

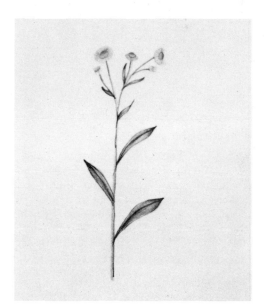

FLOWER DE LUCE

Iris sambucina

Fleur-De-Lis. Blue Flag. Water Flag.

ROOT   Diu. Deo. Dia. Nar. Alt. Cath.

A useful cathartic and used as an alterative, often combined with mandrake, poke, or black cohosh. It will sometimes cause salivation, but need cause no apprehension.

Watervliet   1837, 1860
New Lebanon   1837, 1851, 1860

Mt. Lebanon   1866, 1872
Union Village, Ohio   1847, 1850

FOXGLOVE   HERB Nar. Diu. Sed. Dia.

Digitalis purpurea

An active remedy in neuralgia, insanity, febrile diseases, acute inflammatory complaints, dropsy, palpitation of the heart, or asthma. Should be used only on the advice of a physician.

CHS: "A showy plant 2 to 4 ft. high. In woods throughout the U.S. Aug. and Sept."

Watervliet   1830, 1833, 1837, 1843, 1845, 1847, 1850, 1860

New Lebanon   1836, 1837, 1841, 1849, 1851, 1860

Mt. Lebanon   1866, 1872, 1874

Harvard   1849, 1851, 1853, 1857, 1860, 1873, 1880

Canterbury   1835, 1847, 1848, 1854

Union Village, Ohio   1847, 1850

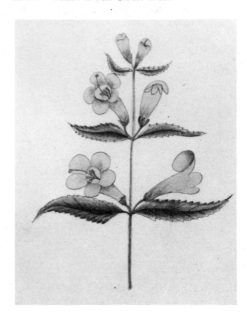

FROSTWORT   HERB Ton. Ast. A-scro.

Helianthemum canadense

Rock Rose. Frost Plant. Scrofula Weed.

A valuable remedy in scrofula, syphilis, cancerous affections, and as a gargle in scarlatina and canker; as a wash in ophthalmia, itching, and cutaneous diseases. Used in the form of a decoction, syrup, or fluid extract. In combination with the herb stillingia it is more valuable.

Watervliet   1830, 1833, 1834, 1837, 1843, 1845, 1847, 1850, 1860

New Lebanon   1836, 1837, 1841, 1851, 1860

Mt. Lebanon   1866, 1872, 1873, 1874

Harvard   1849, 1851, 1853, 1857, 1860, 1873, 1880

Canterbury   1835, 1847, 1848, 1854

Union Village, Ohio   1850

New Gloucester   1864

FUMITORY   HERB Ton. Dia. Aper. Alt. Diu. Lax.

Fumaria officinalis   Deo.

Hedge Fumitory. Earth Smoke. Fumatory.

Used in jaundice, obstruction of the bowels, scurvy, and in general debility of the digestive organs. A wineglass of an infusion of the leaves is usually given every four hours.

New Lebanon   1851, 1860

Mt. Lebanon   1866, 1872, 1873, 1874

Harvard   1851, 1853, 1854, 1857, 1860, 1873

Canterbury   1847, 1848, 1854

Union Village, Ohio   1847, 1850

GALANGAL   ROOT   Aro. Sti.

Alpinia galangal

East India Catarrh Root. Catarrh Root.
   Kassamak Root.

An aromatic stimulant. Has been used as a snuff in catarrh and nervous headache. Somewhat similar to ginger.

Mt. Lebanon   1873

GARGET   BERRIES   Eme. Nar. Cath. Alt. Acr. Deo.

Phytolacca decandra   LEAVES   Eme. Nar. Cath. Alt. Acr. Deo.

Pigeon Berry. Poke. Poke Root. Skoke.   ROOT   Eme. Nar. Cath. Alt. Acr. Deo.
   Scoke Root. Coakum.

Valuable in chronic rheumatism, syphilis, scrofula, and as an ointment in itching and scab head.

Watervliet   1830, 1833, 1837, 1843, 1845, 1847, 1850, 1860

New Lebanon   1836, 1837, 1841, 1849, 1851, 1860

Mt. Lebanon   1866, 1872, 1873, 1874

Harvard   1851, 1853, 1854, 1857, 1860, 1873, 1880, 1885

Canterbury   1835, 1847, 1848, 1854

Union Village, Ohio   1847

New Gloucester   1864

GARLIC   BULBS   Stim. Diu. Exp. Rub. Ton.

Allium sativum

Recommended in cough, asthma, catarrh, hoarseness; promotes activity of the excretory organs. Externally it is used as a counterirritant in pulmonary affections.

Watervliet   1860

New Lebanon   1851, 1860

Mt. Lebanon   1866, 1872, 1873, 1874

Union Village, Ohio   1850

GELSEMIUM   ROOT   Sed. A-spas. Dia. Feb.
Gelsemium sempervirens
Yellow Jasmine. Wild Woodbine.
   False Jasmine.

A powerful spinal depressant. A poison.

Mt. Lebanon   1874

GENTIAN, BLUE-FRINGED   ROOT   Ton. Stom. Aro.
Gentiana crinita

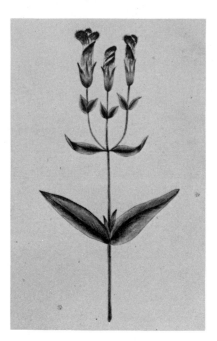

A powerful tonic; improves the appetite,
aids digestion, and gives force to the circulation. Used in dyspepsia, jaundice, gout,
scrofula, and fever and ague.

CHS: "Not uncommon in cool, low
grounds. Can. to Car. August."

Watervliet   1860
New Lebanon   1851, 1860
Mt. Lebanon   1866, 1872, 1873, 1874

GINGER   LEAVES   Stim. Aro. Diu. Eme. Cath.
Asarum canadense   ROOT   Stim. Aro. Diu. Purg.
Wild Ginger. Canada Snakeroot.

The root is useful to flavor meats and fish. Ground, it is a reliable digestive, which also increases
the flow of urine. The leaves and roots act upon the bowels.

Mt. Lebanon   1874   Union Village, Ohio   1847, 1850

GINGER, AFRICAN   ROOT   Stom. Ton. Stim. Rub. Err. Sial.
Zingiber officinale
Jamaica. Ginger.

Valuable in diarrhea, dysentery, cholera, cholera morbus, habitual flatulency, dyspepsia, and to relieve pains in the bowels and stomach. Also to prevent the griping of cathartic medicines.

Mt. Lebanon   1873

GINSENG   ROOT   Ton. Stim. Ner. Sial.
Panax quinquefolium
Ninsin. Chinese Seng. Five Fingers.
   Garantogen.

Useful in loss of appetite, nervous debility, weak stomach, asthma, and gravel. Also, it increases the flow of saliva.

Watervliet   1860
New Lebanon   1851, 1860
Mt. Lebanon   1866, 1872, 1873, 1874

GOLDENROD   HERB   Stim. Carm. Diaph. Aro. Diu.
Solidago odora
Sweet Scented Goldenrod. Blue Mountain
   Tea.

Used in flatulent colic, stomach sickness, convalescence from severe diarrhea, dysentery, cholera morbus, dropsy, gravel, and urinary difficulties. As a tea it is diaphoretic when taken warm. It is excellent to use to disguise the taste of medicinal herbs.

Watervliet   1850, 1860   Canterbury   1835, 1847, 1848
New Lebanon   1851, 1860   Union Village, Ohio   1850
Mt. Lebanon   1866, 1872, 1873, 1874   New Gloucester   1864
Harvard   1851, 1853, 1854, 1857, 1860, 1873,
   1880, 1885

GOLDENSEAL   ROOT   Ton. Sto. Ape. A-bil. Cath.
Hydrastis canadensis
Yellow Puccoon. Ohio Curcuma. Ground
   Raspberry. Eye Balm. Orange Root.
   Turmeric Root.

Invaluable in dyspepsia, erysipelas; in remittent, intermittent, and typhoid fevers; torpor of the liver, ulceration of the mouth, ophthalmia, and spermatorrhea. A good mouthwash. The powder may be boiled in water and sniffed up into the nostrils for nasal congestion. As a dye, goldenseal imparts a rich durable light yellow of great brilliancy, which, when used with different mordants, gives all the shades of yellow from pale to orange. With indigo it imparts a fine green to wool, silk, and cotton.

Watervliet   1837, 1843, 1845, 1847, 1850, 1860   Canterbury   1835, 1847, 1848, 1854

New Lebanon   1836, 1837, 1841, 1851, 1860   Union Village, Ohio   1847, 1850

Mt. Lebanon   1866, 1872, 1873, 1874   New Gloucester   1864

Harvard   1851, 1853, 1857, 1860, 1873, 1880, 1885

GOLDTHREAD   ROOT   Ton. Ast. Sto.

Coptis trifolia

Mouth Root. Canker Root. Yellow Root.

Valuable as a gargle in ulceration of the mouth; used in dyspepsia, inflammation of the stomach, and with goldenseal to destroy the appetite for intoxicating liquors. A pure, bitter tonic.

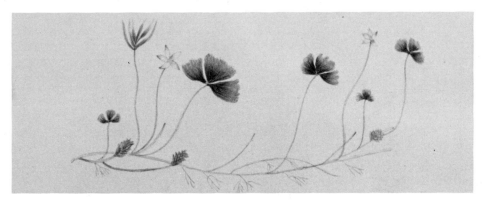

CHS: "Found from Arctic Amer. to Penn. in shady woods. Stem creeping, golden yellow very bitter. Peduncle bears a single, white star like flower. May."

Watervliet   1833, 1837, 1843, 1845, 1847, 1850,   Canterbury   1835, 1847, 1848, 1854
     1860   Union Village, Ohio   1850

New Lebanon   1836, 1837, 1841, 1849, 1851,   New Gloucester   1864
     1860

Mt. Lebanon   1866, 1872, 1873, 1874

Harvard   1851, 1853, 1857, 1860, 1873, 1880,
     1885

GRAVEL PLANT   HERB   Diu. Ast. Dem.

Epigaea repens

Trailing Arbutus. Winter Pink. Gravel
     Weed. Mountain Pink. Mayflower.
     Ground Laurel.

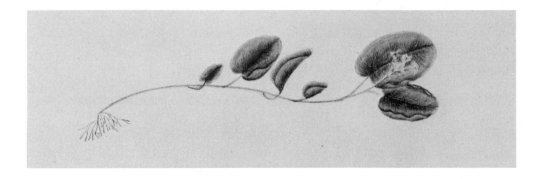

A superior remedy to buchu in gravel and all diseases of the urinary organs. The whole plant is used, but the leaves are especially useful.

CHS: "Found in the woods from Newfoundland to Ky. A little shrubby plant, grows flat on the ground. Flowers are very fragrant. Apr. May."

Watervliet   1837, 1843, 1845, 1847, 1850, 1860

New Lebanon   1836, 1837, 1841, 1851, 1860

Mt. Lebanon   1866, 1872, 1873, 1874

Harvard   1880, 1885

Canterbury   1835

Union Village, Ohio   1850

HARDHACK

Spiraea tomentosa

Meadow Sweet. White Leaf. Steeple Bush.

ROOT   Ast. Ton. Diu.

LEAVES   Ast. Ton. Diu.

Valuable in cholera infantum, dysentery, diarrhea, and debility of the bowels, and to improve the digestion. Useful as an astringent tonic in diarrhea.

CHS: "A small shrub, common in pastures and low grounds, Can. and U.S. The fruit in winter furnishes food for the snow-birds. July. Aug."

Watervliet   1830, 1833, 1837, 1843, 1845, 1847, 1850, 1860

New Lebanon   1836, 1837, 1841, 1849, 1851, 1860

Mt. Lebanon   1866, 1872, 1873, 1874

Harvard   1849, 1851, 1853, 1854, 1857, 1860, 1873, 1880

Canterbury   1835, 1847, 1848, 1854

Union Village, Ohio   1850

New Gloucester   1864

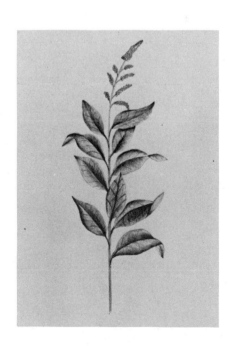

HARVEST-LICE   HERB   Ast. Ton.
Bidens connata
Cockhold Herb. Beggar's Tick. Swamp
   Beggar's Tick.

Root and seeds are employed domestically as an emmenagogue to some extent, as well as for the
purposes of an expectorant in throat irritation.

Harvard   1849, 1851, 1853, 1857, 1860, 1873, 1880
Canterbury   1835, 1847, 1848, 1854
New Gloucester   1864

HEAL-ALL   HERB   Ast.
Prunella vulgaris
Self-Heal. Figwort. Stone Root.

Valuable in hemorrhages, and for gargle in canker and sore throat.

Watervliet   1860   Mt. Lebanon   1866, 1872, 1873, 1874
New Lebanon   1851, 1860

HEART'S EASE   HERB   Sud. Feb. Diu.
Polygonum persicaria
Ladies' Thumb. Spotted Knot Weed.

Said to be useful in asthma, colds, and fevers. Useful as a diuretic.

Watervliet   1860   Mt. Lebanon   1866, 1872, 1873, 1874
New Lebanon   1851, 1860

HELLEBORE, BLACK   ROOT   Dras. Cath. Diu. Emm. Anthel.
Helleborus niger
Christmas Rose.

Used in palsy, insanity, apoplexy, dropsy, epilepsy, chlorosis, amenorrhea. In large doses it is a
powerful poison.

New Lebanon   1851, 1860   Mt. Lebanon   1866, 1872, 1873, 1874

HELLEBORE, WHITE   ROOT   Nar. Sed. Dia. Eme. Ner. Acr.
Veratrum viride
Swamp Hellebore. American Hellebore.
   False Hellebore. Itch Weed. Indian
   Poke.

Valuable as an arterial sedative in pneumonia, typhoid fever, and itching, but only on the advice of a physician. The powder or decoction is useful to destroy insects on plants.

CHS: "A large, coarse looking plant, of our meadows and swamps. Can. to Ga. Root emetic and stimulant, but poisonous. July."

Watervliet   1837, 1843, 1845, 1847, 1850

New Lebanon   1836, 1837, 1841, 1851, 1860

Mt. Lebanon   1866, 1873, 1874

Harvard   1849, 1851, 1853, 1857, 1860, 1873, 1880

Canterbury   1835, 1847, 1848, 1854

Union Village, Ohio   1850

New Gloucester   1864

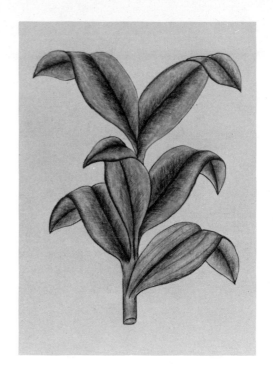

HEMLOCK
Abies canadensis
Hemlock Spruce.

BARK   Ast. Ton.
LEAVES   Sud. Emm. Dia. Alt.

The bark is used in leucorrhea, prolapsus uteri, diarrhea, and gangrene. The oil is used in liniments, the gum in plasters.

New Lebanon   1851, 1860, 1866

Mt. Lebanon   1873, 1874

Harvard   1849

Canterbury   1847

HEMLOCK
Pinus rigida
Pitch Pine.

BARK   Ast. Ton.
GUM   Ast. Ton.
LEAVES   Dia. Emo. Alt. Sud.

Hemlock pitch (also known as Canada pitch) is a gentle rubefacient. The oil from this tree is used in liniment.

From a manuscript, Watervliet, 1832: "Hemlock Plant grows 6 ft. high or more, good to ease pain in open cancer which it does more powerfully than opium, used also in open tumors, ulcers, consumption, venereal ulcers, epilepsies and convulsions. Produces sweat and urine. But this plant is so very poisonous that it is imprudent to eat it. It ought not to be administered by those unskilled in medicine. Dose of the leaves in powder—or if the extract, a grain or 2. Great care ought to be taken to distinguish this plant from Water Hemlock for the latter is a deadly poison."

Watervliet   1837, 1843, 1845, 1847, 1850, 1860

New Lebanon   1836, 1837, 1841, 1851

Mt. Lebanon   1866, 1872

Harvard   1851, 1853, 1857, 1860, 1873, 1880

Canterbury   1835, 1848, 1854

Union Village, Ohio   1850

New Gloucester   1864

HENBANE, BLACK   HERB   Nar. Ner. A-spas.
Hyoscyamus niger

Used in gout, neuralgia, asthma, chronic rheumatism, and to produce sleep, and remove irregular
nervous action.

Watervliet   1830, 1833, 1837, 1843, 1845, 1847, 1850, 1860
New Lebanon   1836, 1837, 1841, 1849, 1851, 1860
Mt. Lebanon   1866, 1872, 1873, 1874
Harvard   1851, 1853, 1857, 1860, 1873, 1880, 1885
Canterbury   1835, 1847, 1848, 1854

Union Village, Ohio   1847, 1850
New Gloucester   1864

HOLLYHOCK   FLOWERS   Emo. Dem. Diu. Ast.
Althaea rosea

Used in coughs and female weakness, inflammation of the bladder, retention of urine, and affection of the kidneys.

Watervliet   1832, 1833, 1837, 1843, 1845, 1847, 1850, 1860
New Lebanon   1836, 1837, 1841, 1851, 1860
Mt. Lebanon   1866, 1872, 1873, 1874
Harvard   1849, 1851, 1853, 1854, 1857, 1860, 1873, 1880
Canterbury   1835, 1847, 1854
Union Village, Ohio   1847, 1850
New Gloucester   1864

HOPS   FLOWERS   Anthel. Hyp. Feb. A-lith.
Humulus lupulus   Ano. Aro.

Valuable as a sedative to produce sleep and in nervousness or delirium tremens; used externally as
fomentation in cramps, pains, swellings, indolent ulcers, salt rheum, and tumors.

Watervliet   1830, 1833, 1837, 1843, 1845, 1847, 1850, 1860
New Lebanon   1836, 1837, 1841, 1849, 1851, 1860
Mt. Lebanon   1866, 1872, 1873, 1874, 1888
Harvard   1849, 1851, 1853, 1854, 1857, 1860, 1873, 1880
Union Village, Ohio   1847, 1850
New Gloucester   1864

HOREHOUND   HERB   Stim. Ton. Expec. Diu. Sto. Pec.
Marrubium vulgare   Deo.

Useful in coughs, colds, chronic catarrh, asthma, and pulmonary affections; the cold infusion is used for dyspepsia and as a vermifuge.

Watervliet   1830, 1832, 1833, 1834, 1837, 1843, 1845, 1847, 1850, 1860
New Lebanon   1836, 1837, 1841, 1849, 1851, 1860
Mt. Lebanon   1866, 1872, 1873, 1874, 1881, 1888
Harvard   1851, 1853, 1854, 1857, 1860, 1873, 1880, 1885
Canterbury   1835, 1847, 1848, 1854
Union Village, Ohio   1847, 1850
New Gloucester   1864

HORSEMINT   HERB   Stim. Carm. Sud. Diu. Aro. Ton.
Monarda punctata

Used in flatulence, nausea, vomiting, suppression of urine, and as an emmenagogue.

CHS: "An herbaceous, grayish plant 1 to 2 ft. high. Growing in muddy situations, Can. to Ky. Aromatic like pennyroyal, but less so. June. July."

Watervliet   1860
New Lebanon   1851, 1860
Mt. Lebanon   1866, 1872, 1873, 1874
Harvard   1857, 1860, 1873, 1880, 1885
Canterbury   1848, 1854
Union Village, Ohio   1850
New Gloucester   1864

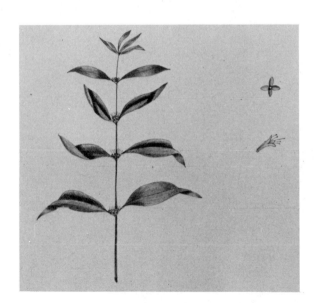

HORSERADISH   LEAVES   Stim. Diu. A-scor. Rub. Emm.
Armoracia lapathifolia   Acr.
                                             ROOT   Stim. Diu. A-scor. Rub. Emm.
                                                    Acr.

Used with advantage for paralysis, rheumatism, dropsy, scurvy. Grated with sugar and used for hoarseness. The grated fresh root is used in cooking.

Watervliet   1837, 1843, 1845, 1847, 1850, 1860
New Lebanon   1836, 1837, 1841, 1851, 1860
Mt. Lebanon   1866, 1872, 1873, 1874
Harvard   1851, 1853, 1854, 1857, 1860, 1873, 1880, 1885
Canterbury   1835, 1847, 1848, 1854
Union Village, Ohio   1847, 1850
New Gloucester   1864

HYDRANGEA   ROOT   Diu.
Hydrangea aborescens
Seven Barks. Wild Hydrangea.

Valuable to remove gravel and brick-dust deposits from the bladder, and to relieve excruciating
pains caused thereby. A mild and soothing diuretic. It is reputed to be an old Cherokee Indian
remedy.

Mt. Lebanon   1873, 1874

HYSSOP   HERB   Stim. Aro. Carm. Ton. Dia. Sto.
Hyssopus officinalis   Exp. Ceph.

Valuable in quinsy, asthma, and chest diseases; the leaves applied to bruises remove pain and
discoloration.

Watervliet   1830, 1832, 1833, 1837, 1843, 1845, 1847, 1850, 1860
New Lebanon   1836, 1837, 1841, 1851, 1860
Mt. Lebanon   1866, 1872, 1873, 1874, 1881, 1888
Harvard   1851, 1853, 1854, 1857, 1860, 1873, 1880, 1885
Canterbury   1835, 1847, 1848, 1854
Union Village, Ohio   1847, 1850
New Gloucester   1864

ICELAND MOSS   WHOLE PLANT   Pec. Dem. Ton.
Cetraria islandica
Eryngo-Leaved Liverwort.

It is demulcent, tonic, and nutritious. Boiled with milk, it forms an excellent nutritive and tonic.

Harvard   1851, 1853, 1857, 1860, 1873, 1880, 1885
Canterbury   1835, 1847, 1848, 1854
New Gloucester   1864

IGNATIA BEAN   SEEDS
Ignatius amara
St. Ignatius' Bean.

Very similar to nux-vomica seeds, but more dangerous. They should not be used domestically.
    The Mt. Lebanon Shakers purchased it for resale.

Mt. Lebanon   1874

INDIAN CUP   PLANT   Dia. Sti. Alt.
Silphium perfoliatum
Indian Cupweed.

Ragged Cup. Prairie Dock. Compass Plant. Rosin Weed. Used in coughs and painful affections of
the chest.

Mt. Lebanon   1873
Union Village, Ohio   1850

INDIAN HEMP, BLACK   ROOT   Nau. Cath. Diaph. Diu. Ver. Ton.
Apocynum cannabinum   Eme.
Canadian Hemp. Indian Physic. Indian
    Hemp.

Used in dropsy, remittent and intermittent fevers, pneumonia, and obstructions of the kidneys,
liver, and spleen.

Watervliet   1833, 1837, 1843, 1845, 1847, 1850, 1860
New Lebanon   1836, 1837, 1841, 1849, 1851, 1860
Mt. Lebanon   1866, 1872, 1873, 1874
Harvard   1885
Canterbury   1835, 1847, 1848, 1854
Union Village, Ohio   1847, 1850

INDIAN HEMP, WHITE   ROOT   Ape. Diu. Eme. Anthel. Ver.
Asclepias incarnata   Cath. Alt.
Swamp Milk Weed. Rose-Colored Silk
    Weed. Water Nerve Root.

Recommended in rheumatic, asthmatic, catarrhal, and syphilitic affections, and as a vermifuge.

Watervliet   1860
New Lebanon   1849, 1851, 1860
Mt. Lebanon   1866, 1872, 1873, 1874
Harvard   1851, 1853, 1854, 1857, 1860, 1873, 1880
Canterbury   1847, 1848, 1854
New Gloucester   1864

INDIAN PHYSIC   ROOT   Eme. Cath. Sud. Ton.
Gillenia trifoliata
Bowman's Root. Dropwort.

Valuable in amenorrhea, rheumatism, dropsy, costiveness, dyspepsia, worms, and intermittent
fevers.

Mt. Lebanon   1873, 1874

INDIAN TURNIP   ROOT   Acr. Expec. Diaph. Sti. Nar.
Arum triphyllum   Aro.
Wake Robin. Wild Turnip. Dragon Root.
   Dragon Turnip. Jack-in-the-Pulpit.
   Pepper Turnip. Bog Onion. Marsh
   Turnip.

Recommended internally in croup, low typhoid, and externally in scrofulous tumors, and scald
head (a Shaker term meaning scabs on the scalp).

Watervliet   1860
New Lebanon   1851, 1860
Mt. Lebanon   1866, 1872, 1873, 1874
Union Village, Ohio   1847, 1850

INDIGO, WILD   HERB   Purg. Eme. Stim. A-sep. Ton.
Baptisia tinctoria   Dia.
Horsefly Weed. Rattle Bush. Indigo   ROOT   Purg. Eme. Stim. A-sep. Ton.
   Weed. Indigo Broom. Yellow Broom.   Dia.

Valuable as a wash in all species of ulcers, such as malignant sore mouth and throat, mercurial
sore mouth, scrofulous or syphilitic ophthalmia, fetid leucorrhea and discharges.

Watervliet   1830, 1833, 1837, 1843, 1845, 1847, 1850, 1860
New Lebanon   1836, 1837, 1841, 1851, 1860
Mt. Lebanon   1866, 1872, 1873, 1874

Harvard   1851, 1853, 1857, 1860, 1873, 1880, 1885
Canterbury   1835, 1847, 1848, 1854
Union Village, Ohio   1847, 1850
New Gloucester   1864

IPECAC, AMERICAN   ROOT   Eme. Cath. Ton. Exp.
Euphorbia ipecacuanha
Indian Physic. Bitter Root. Ipecac Milk.
    Fever Root. Emetic Root. Blooming
    Spurge.

Watervliet   1860
New Lebanon   1851, 1860
Mt. Lebanon   1866, 1872, 1874

IRIS   ROOT   Aro. Cath.
Iris florentina
Orris Root.

Used mostly as a sachet for its violet like odor. The fresh root is a powerful cathartic; its juice is used in dropsy.

Mt. Lebanon   1874
Union Village, Ohio   1850

IRONWEED   ROOT   Ton.
Vernonia fasciculata

A bitter tonic used to improve the blood.

Union Village, Ohio   1850

IVY, GROUND   LEAVES   Dem. Sto. Ton. Emm.
Nepeta glechoma
Gill Run. Alehof. Cat's-Paw. Gill-Go-
    Over-the-Ground. Field Balm. Turn-
    hoof. Ground Joy.

A stimulant, tonic, and pectoral. An infusion of the leaves is very beneficial in lead-colic and painters very often make use of it. The fresh juice sniffed up the nose often relieves nasal congestion and headache. Used in diseases of the lungs and kidneys, asthma, and jaundice.

Watervliet   1830, 1837
Mt. Lebanon   1872
Harvard   1834, 1853, 1857, 1860, 1873, 1880, 1885
Canterbury   1835
Union Village, Ohio   1847
New Gloucester   1864

JACOB'S LADDER   HERB   A-lith. Diu. Emm. Ner. Sial.
Polemonium coeruleum

Valuable in kidney diseases, stones in the bladder, and falling of the womb.

Watervliet   1860
New Lebanon   1851, 1860
Mt. Lebanon   1866, 1872, 1873, 1874
Union Village, Ohio   1850

JALAP   ROOT   Cath.
Ipomoea jalapa
Bindweed.

This is irritant and cathartic, operating energetically.

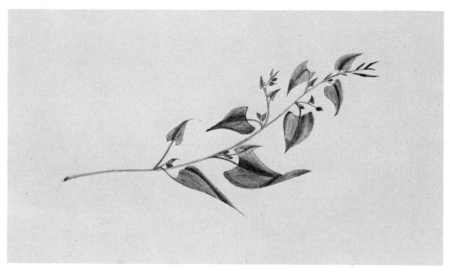

CHS: "Thickets. Can. and U.S. Climbing over bushes. July and Sept."

Mt. Lebanon   1872, 1874

JOB'S TEARS   SEED Diu.
Onosmodium virginianum
Gromwell. False Gromwell.

Said to dissolve calculi; used also in dropsy and incontinence of urine.

Watervliet   1860
New Lebanon   1851, 1860
Mt. Lebanon   1866, 1872, 1873

JOHNSWORT   HERB Ast. Sed. Diu. Bal.
Hypericum perforatum
St. Johnswort.

Used to cure suppression of urine, chronic
urinary affections, diarrhea, dysentery,
worms, and jaundice. As an ointment, used
for wounds, ulcers, caked breast, and
tumors.

CHS: "In dry pastures. Can. and U.S. June,
July."

Watervliet   1830, 1833, 1834, 1837, 1843,
   1845, 1847, 1850, 1860
New Lebanon   1836, 1837, 1841, 1849, 1851,
   1860
Mt. Lebanon   1866, 1872, 1873, 1874
Harvard   1851, 1853, 1854, 1857, 1860, 1873,
   1880, 1885
Canterbury   1835, 1847, 1848, 1854
Union Village, Ohio   1847, 1850
New Gloucester   1864

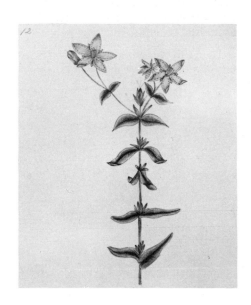

JUNIPER   BERRIES Stim. Car. Diu.
Juniperus communis
Juniper Bush.

Efficacious in gonorrhea, gleet, leucorrhea, affections of the skin, scorbutic diseases, dropsy, and
many kidney complaints.

Watervliet   1860
New Lebanon   1851, 1860   Harvard   1851, 1853, 1885
Mt. Lebanon   1866, 1872, 1873, 1874   Canterbury   1847, 1848, 1854

KING'S CLOVER   HERB Emo. Diu. Dis.
Melitotus officinalis
Melilot. Sweet Clover.

The leaves and flowers boiled in lard are useful in all kinds of ulcers, inflammations, and burns.

New Lebanon 1851, 1860
Mt. Lebanon 1866, 1873

KNOT GRASS   ROOT Diu. Aper. Ner. Car.
Triticum repens
Dog Grass. Couch Grass. Quickens.
 Witch Grass.

Valuable in kidney diseases, irritation of the bladder, and spasmodic affections. The juice is used to heal wounds, cuts, and bruises.

CHS: "Found in wet grounds. Can. to Ga. It has very large halbert shaped leaves. June. July."

Watervliet 1860
New Lebanon 1851, 1860, 1866
Mt. Lebanon 1872, 1873, 1874

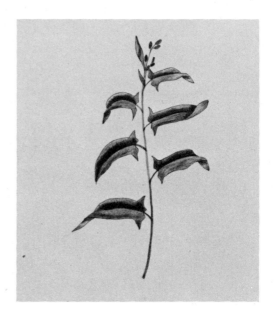

LABRADOR TEA   HERB Diu. Bal. Pec. Ton.
Ledum latifolium

Useful in coughs, dyspepsia, dysentery, and skin diseases. It is sometimes used as a table tea.

Watervliet 1837, 1843   Mt. Lebanon 1866, 1872, 1873, 1874
New Lebanon 1837, 1841, 1851, 1860 Union Village, Ohio 1850

LADY'S SLIPPER   ROOT Ton. Dia. Anti-spas. Ner. Ano.
Cypripedium acaule
Pink Lady's Slipper. Pink Moccasin
 Flower. Nerve Root.

Beneficial in cases of nervous headache when administered with other remedies such as catnip or sweet balm in equal parts, taken as a tea about every half hour when needed.

CHS: "In dark woods. Car. to Arc. Amer. May. June."

Harvard   1851, 1853, 1857, 1860, 1873, 1880
Canterbury   1835
New Gloucester   1864

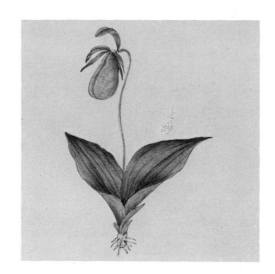

LADY'S SLIPPER   ROOT   Ner. Ano.
Cypripedium flavum

Preparations made from these roots are tonic, diaphoretic, and antispasmodic. They have been referred to as gentle nervous stimulants.

Watervliet   1837, 1843, 1845, 1847, 1850   Mt. Lebanon   1872
New Lebanon   1836, 1837, 1841   Canterbury   1847

LADY'S SLIPPER, YELLOW   ROOT   Ner. Ano. Ton. Dia. Anti-spas.
Cypripedium pubescens   Sti. Sed.
Nerve Root. American Valerian. Umbel.
   Yellow Moccasin Flower. Noah's Ark.

Useful in ordinary nervous headache. A gentle nervous stimulant or antispasmodic. The roots should be gathered in August or September and carefully cleansed.

CHS: "Woods and meadows. Can. to Wis. and south to Georgia. May. June."

Watervliet   1860
New Lebanon   1849, 1851, 1860
Mt. Lebanon   1866, 1874
Canterbury   1848, 1854
Union Village, Ohio   1850

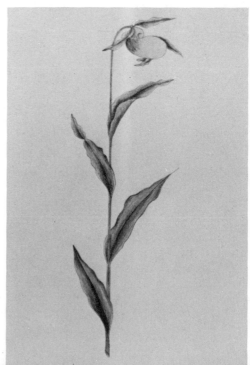

LARKSPUR   HERB   Eme. Cath. Diu. Nar. Acr.
Delphinium consolida   SEED   Diu. Nar. Acr.
Stave's Acre.

Used externally as an ointment in cutaneous diseases and to destroy insects on the body, such as lice.

Watervliet   1830, 1833, 1837, 1843, 1845, 1847, 1850, 1860
New Lebanon   1836, 1837, 1841, 1851, 1860
Mt. Lebanon   1866, 1872, 1873, 1874
Union Village, Ohio   1847, 1850

LAUREL, SHEEP   LEAVES   A-syph. Sed. Ast. Her. A-sep.
Kalmia angustifolia
Laurel. Lambkill.

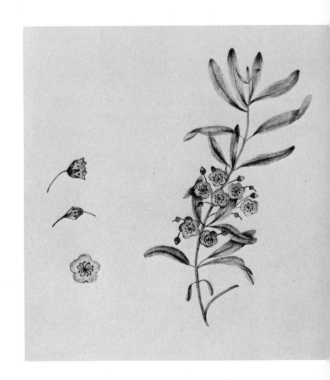

Used in syphilitic diseases, scalp scabs, cutaneous affections, hemorrhages, diarrhea, flux, and neuralgia. When stewed with lard, it is serviceable as an ointment for various skin irritations.

CHS: "Sheep poison—Calico bush. Found in woods and by the road side from Can. to Car. Said to be poisonous to cattle. June."

Watervliet   1860
New Lebanon   1851, 1860
Mt. Lebanon   1866, 1872, 1873, 1874
Canterbury   1835
Union Village, Ohio   1850

LAVENDER, ENGLISH   FLOWERS   Car. Ton. Stim. Aro. Pec. Ner.
Lavandula vera

Valuable in flatulency, fainting, and to arrest vomiting; usually combined with other medicines.

Watervliet   1860
New Lebanon   1851, 1860
Mt. Lebanon   1866, 1872, 1873, 1874, 1881, 1888

LEATHERWOOD   BARK   Eme. Acr. Rub. Sud. Exp.
Dirca palustris
Moosewood. American Mezereon.

A poultice of the bark will produce vesication. It is used in combination with alteratives.

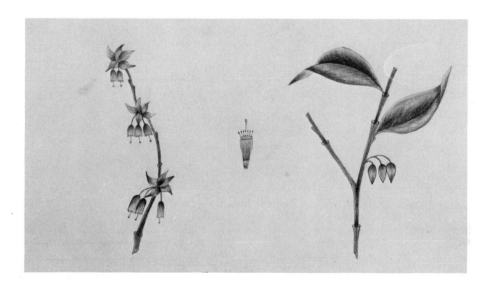

CHS: "Grows near mountain streams or rivulets. U.S. and Can. Every part of the shrub is very tough. Apr. May."

Mt. Lebanon   1873
Union Village, Ohio   1850

LETTUCE, GARDEN   HERB   Diu. Nar. Hyp. Ano.
Lactuca sativa

Used as a narcotic where opium is objectionable.

Watervliet   1830, 1860
New Lebanon   1851, 1860
Mt. Lebanon   1866, 1873, 1874

LETTUCE, WILD   HERB   Diu. A-scor. Nar.
Lactuca virosa
Poison Lettuce. Acrid Lettuce.

Similar to garden lettuce in effect.

Watervliet   1830, 1860   Mt. Lebanon   1866, 1872, 1873, 1874
Groveland, New York   1842   Union Village, Ohio   1850
New Lebanon   1849, 1851, 1860

LIFE EVERLASTING   HERB   Ast. Dia. Sto. Sud.
Gnaphalium polycephalum
White Balsam. Indian Posey. Field
   Balsam. Sweet Balsam.

Used for bowel complaints, coughs, colds, bleeding of the lungs, and to produce perspiration.
(Note in Watervliet manuscript, 1832: "Made into a tea good for ulcers in mouth.")

Watervliet   1830, 1832, 1833, 1834, 1837, 1843, 1845, 1847, 1850, 1860
New Lebanon   1836, 1837, 1841
Mt. Lebanon   1873, 1874
Harvard   1851, 1853, 1854, 1857, 1860, 1873, 1880, 1885
Canterbury   1835, 1847, 1848, 1854
New Gloucester   1864
Union Village, Ohio   1850

LIFE ROOT   HERB AND ROOT   Aro. Sto. Diu. Dia. Ton.
Senecio aureus   Feb.
Ragwort. Golden Senecio. Uncum. Squaw
   Weed. Female Regulator. Cocash
   Weed. False Valerian.

Valuable in profuse menstruation, gravel, and strangury.

Watervliet   1830, 1833, 1837, 1843, 1845, 1847, 1850
New Lebanon   1836, 1837, 1841, 1851, 1860
Mt. Lebanon   1866, 1872, 1873, 1874
Harvard   1880, 1885
Union Village, Ohio   1847, 1850

LILY, WHITE WATER   THE FRESH ROOT   Ast. Dem. Alt. Pec.
Nymphaea odorata   Ton. Emo.
Toad Lily. Pond Lily. Sweet-Scented   FLOWERS
   Water Lily.

Useful in dysentery, diarrhea, leucorrhea, and scrofula. Combined with cherry bark, it is used for bronchial affections. Used externally as a poultice for boils, tumors, and scrofulous ulcers.

Watervliet   1837, 1843, 1845, 1847, 1850, 1860
New Lebanon   1836, 1837, 1841, 1851, 1860
Mt. Lebanon   1866, 1872, 1873, 1874
Harvard   1851, 1853, 1854, 1857, 1860, 1873, 1880, 1885
Canterbury   1835, 1847, 1848, 1854
Union Village, Ohio   1847, 1850
New Gloucester   1864

LILY, YELLOW WATER   THE FRESH ROOT   Ast. Dem. Alt. Pec.
Nuphar advena   Emo. Ton.
Spatterdock. Frog Lily. Beaver Root.

The properties are very similar to those of the white water lily.
It is mucilaginous, demulcent, tonic, and astringent. Boiled in milk, it is also useful for external purposes.

CHS: "Found in meadows and wet places. Can. and U.S. July."

Watervliet   1860
New Lebanon   1851, 1860
Mt. Lebanon   1872, 1873, 1874
Harvard   1849, 1851, 1853, 1854, 1857, 1860,
   1873, 1880
Canterbury   1835, 1847, 1848, 1854
New Gloucester   1864

LIQUORICE   ROOT   Nut. Dem. Exp. Lax.
Glycyrrhiza glabra   EXTRACT   Nut. Dem. Exp. Lax.
Licorice.

Useful in coughs, catarrh, irritation of the urinary organs, pain of the intestines in diarrhea, and bronchial affections.

Groveland, N.Y.   1842   Mt. Lebanon   1866, 1872, 1873, 1874
Watervliet   1860   Union Village, Ohio   1850
New Lebanon   1851, 1860

LIVERWORT   HERB   Muc. Ast. Pec. Deo. Nar. Dem.

Hepatica americana

Noble Liverwort. Kidney Liver Leaf.
   Liver Leaf.

Used in fevers, hepatic complaints, bleeding
of the lungs, and coughs.

CHS: "This little plant is one of the earliest
harbingers of the spring often putting forth
its neat and elegant flowers in the neighborhood of some lingering snow bank.
Found in the woods from Can. to Ga. and
west to Wis."

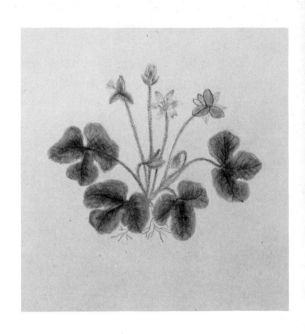

Watervliet   1830, 1833, 1834, 1837, 1843,
   1845, 1847, 1850, 1860

New Lebanon   1836, 1837, 1841, 1851, 1860

Mt. Lebanon   1866, 1872, 1873, 1874

Harvard   1851, 1853, 1854, 1857, 1860, 1873,
   1880, 1885

Canterbury   1835, 1847, 1848, 1854

Union Village, Ohio   1847, 1850

New Gloucester   1864

LOBELIA   HERB   Anti-spas. Eme. Exp. Diaph. Nar. Diu.
                                                            SEED   Anti-spas. Eme. Exp. Diaph.
Lobelia inflata

Wild or Indian Tobacco. Emetic Root.
   Puke Weed. Eye-Bright. Asthma Weed.

Invaluable in spasmodic asthma, croup,
pneumonia, catarrh, epilepsy, hysteria,
cramps, and convulsions. Externally it is
used as a poultice in sprains, bruises,
ringworm, erysipelas, insect stings, and
poison ivy.

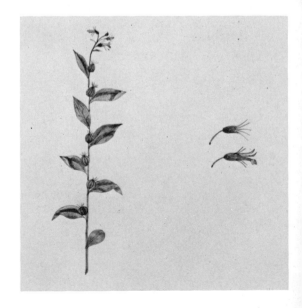

CHS: "In fields and woods. Can. and U.S.
The species of Lobelia are more or less
poisonous. The milky juice is narcotic, producing effects similar to those of tobacco.
July. Sept."

Watervliet   1833, 1834, 1837, 1843, 1845,
   1847, 1850, 1860

New Lebanon   1836, 1837, 1841, 1851, 1860

Mt. Lebanon   1866, 1872, 1874

Harvard   1851, 1853, 1854, 1857, 1860, 1873,
   1880, 1885

Canterbury   1835, 1847, 1848, 1854
Union Village, Ohio   1847, 1850

LOGWOOD   BARK   Ast.
Haematoxylon campechianum
Peachwood. Bloodwood.

A mild astringent, especially useful in the weakness of the bowels following cholera infantum.
May be used in chronic diarrhea.

Mt. Lebanon   1874

LOVAGE   LEAVES   Aro. Car. Diaph. Sto. Nar.
Levisticum officinale   Emm.
                                           ROOT   Car. Diaph. Sto.
Smellage. Lavose.   SEED   Aro. Car. Diaph. Sto.

Combined with other drugs, it is used as a corrective and for its flavor. Sometimes used in female
complaints and nervousness.

Watervliet   1830, 1833, 1837, 1843, 1845, 1847, 1850, 1860
New Lebanon   1836, 1837, 1841, 1851, 1860
Mt. Lebanon   1866, 1872, 1873, 1874
Harvard   1851, 1853, 1857, 1860, 1873, 1880, 1885
Canterbury   1835, 1847, 1848, 1854
Union Village, Ohio   1847, 1850
New Gloucester   1864

LUNGWORT   PLANTS   Pec. Sto. Dem. Sto. Ton.
Pulmonaria virginica
Virginia Cowslip. Maple Lungwort.

Used in diseases of the lungs, coughs, influenza, and catarrh.

Watervliet   1860
New Lebanon   1851, 1860
Mt. Lebanon   1866, 1872, 1873, 1874
Harvard   1851, 1853, 1857, 1860, 1873, 1880, 1885
Canterbury   1835, 1847, 1848, 1854
New Gloucester   1864

MALLOW, LOW   LEAVES   Diu. Dem. Pec.
Malva rotundifolia   ROOT   Diu. Dem. Pec.
Cheeses. Cheese Plant. Maller.

Used for cough, irritation of the bowels, kidneys and urinary organs, and as poultice for boils.

Watervliet   1830, 1833, 1834, 1837, 1843, 1850, 1860
New Lebanon   1836, 1837, 1841, 1849, 1851, 1860
Mt. Lebanon   1866, 1872, 1873, 1874
Harvard   1851, 1853, 1857, 1860, 1873, 1880, 1885
Canterbury   1835, 1847, 1848, 1854
Union Village, Ohio   1847, 1850

MALLOW, MARSH   FLOWERS   Ast. Dem. Diu.
Altheae officinalis   LEAVES   Dem. Diu.
                                              ROOT   Dem. Diu. Emo.

Valuable in hoarseness, catarrh, pneumonia, gonorrhea, irritation of the veins, dysentery, strangury, gravel, and all kidney complaints; used as a poultice in all painful swellings.

Watervliet   1830, 1833, 1834, 1837, 1843, 1845, 1847, 1850, 1860
New Lebanon   1836, 1837, 1841, 1849, 1851, 1860
Mt. Lebanon   1866, 1872, 1873, 1874
Harvard   1851, 1853, 1854, 1857, 1860, 1873, 1880, 1885
Canterbury   1835, 1847, 1848, 1854
Union Village, Ohio   1847, 1850
New Gloucester   1864

MANDRAKE   ROOT   Deo. Cath. Alt. Anthel.
Podophyllum peltatum   Hydr. Sial. A-bil. Diu. Nar.
May Apple. Wild Lemon. Raccoon
   Berry. Wild Mandrake.

Valuable in jaundice, bilious and intermittent fevers, scrofula, syphilis, liver complaint, rheumatism, and where a powerful cathartic is required.

Watervliet   1830, 1833, 1837, 1843, 1845, 1847, 1850, 1860
New Lebanon   1836, 1837, 1841, 1849, 1851, 1860
Mt. Lebanon   1866, 1872, 1873, 1874
Harvard   1851, 1853, 1857, 1860, 1873, 1880, 1885
Canterbury   1835, 1847, 1848, 1854
Union Village, Ohio   1847, 1850
New Gloucester   1864

MAN ROOT
Convolvulus panduratus
Wild Jalap. Man-in-the-Ground. Man-
   in-the-Earth. Wild Potatoe. Bind
   Weed. Wild Scammony.

ROOT   Cath. Diu. Pec.

Has been recommended in dropsy, strangury, calculus affections, and diseases of the lungs, liver, and kidneys.

New Lebanon   1851, 1860
Mt. Lebanon   1866, 1872, 1873, 1874

MAPLE, RED
Acer rubrum
Soft Maple. Whistle Wood.

BARK   Ton. Ast. Anthel. Ver.

Used for worms, as a gentle tonic, and as a wash for sore eyes.

CHS: "Common in the woods of New England. Flowers are crimson. Apr."

Watervliet   1860
New Lebanon 1851, 1860
Mt. Lebanon   1866, 1872, 1873, 1874

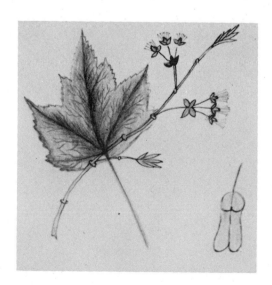

MAPLE, STRIPED   BARK   Ver. Ton. Sti.
Acer pensylvanicum
Canada Maple. Moosewood.

Used for worms and as an eyewash.

CHS: "A small tree 10 or 15 ft. high. In
woods. May."

Watervliet 1860
New Lebanon   1851, 1860
Mt. Lebanon   1866, 1874

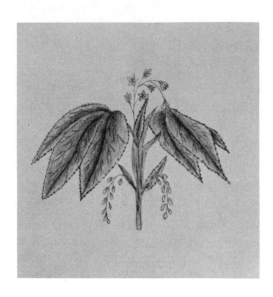

MARIGOLD   FLOWERS   Stim. Diaph. Sto. Aro.
Calendula officinalis
Pot Marigold. Marygold.

Valuable in controlling eruptions; the tincture is used for cuts, bruises, sprains, wounds, etc. It is
unequaled in preventing gangrene.

Watervliet   1830, 1833, 1837, 1843, 1845, 1847, 1850, 1860
New Lebanon   1836, 1837, 1841, 1849, 1851, 1860
Mt. Lebanon   1866, 1872, 1873, 1874
Harvard   1851, 1853, 1857, 1860, 1873, 1880, 1885
Canterbury   1835, 1847, 1848, 1854
Union Village, Ohio   1847, 1850
New Gloucester   1864

MARJORAM, SWEET   HERB   Stim. Ton. Emm. Sto. Aro. Diu.
Origanum marjorana   Sud.

Promotes perspiration, menstruation when recently stopped, and relieves eruptive disease.

Watervliet   1830, 1832, 1833, 1834, 1837, 1843, 1845, 1847, 1850, 1860
New Lebanon   1836, 1837, 1841, 1849, 1851, 1860
Mt. Lebanon   1866, 1872, 1873, 1874, 1888
Harvard   1851, 1853, 1857, 1860, 1873, 1880, 1885

Canterbury   1835, 1847, 1848, 1854
Union Village, Ohio   1847, 1850
New Gloucester   1864

MARSH ROSEMARY   ROOT   Ast. Ton. A-sep.
Statice caroliniana
Sea Lavender. Ink Root. Meadow Root.
   American Thrift. Sea Thrift.

A domestic remedy for dysentery, diarrhea, canker, leucorrhea, and gleet.

Watervliet   1860
New Lebanon   1851, 1860
Mt. Lebanon   1866, 1872, 1873, 1874
Harvard   1851, 1853, 1857, 1860, 1873, 1880, 1885
Canterbury   1835, 1847, 1848, 1854
Union Village, Ohio   1850
New Gloucester   1864

MASTERWORT   ROOT   Stim. A-spas. Carm. Diu. Ton.
Imperatoria ostruthium   Aro. Ner.
Cowparsnip. Royal Cow Parsnip.   SEED   Stim. A-spas. Carm. Diu. Ton.
                                        LEAVES   Stim. A-spas. Carm. Diu. Ton.
                                               Aro. Ner.

Used in flatulency, dyspepsia, epilepsy, asthma, amenorrhea, colic, dysmenorrhea, palsy, and apoplexy.

Watervliet   1860
New Lebanon   1851, 1860
Mt. Lebanon   1866, 1872, 1873, 1874
Canterbury   1854

MATICO   LEAVES   Aro. Stim. Ast.
Piper angustifolium
Soldier's Herb.

An aromatic stimulant with astringent properties for internal use in arresting hemorrhages and treating diarrhea. Externally it is used in local applications to ulcers. Bought by Shakers for resale.

Mt. Lebanon   1874

MAYWEED   HERB   Ton. Eme. A-spas. Emm. Dia. Sto.

Anthemis cotula

Wild Chamomile. Dog Fennel.

Used in colds to induce perspiration; also
used for sick headache, amenorrhea, and
convalescence from fevers.

CHS: "Found in waste places in hard soils,
especially by road sides in large patches.
The plant is ill scented. June and Sept."

Watervliet   1830, 1833, 1837, 1843, 1845,
   1847, 1850, 1860

New Lebanon   1836, 1837, 1841, 1851, 1860

Mt. Lebanon   1866, 1872, 1873, 1874

Harvard   1851, 1853, 1854, 1857, 1860, 1873,
   1880, 1885

Canterbury   1835, 1847, 1848, 1854

Union Village, Ohio   1847, 1850

New Gloucester   1864

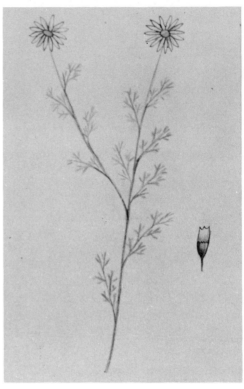

MEADOW SAFFRON   CORMS   Ner. Emet. Cath.

Colchicum autumnale   SEEDS   Ner. Emet. Cath.

Colchicum.

It is a sedative, cathartic, diuretic, and an emetic, but great care should be used in its employment as serious results such as violent purging may follow an overdose.

Union Village, Ohio   1847

MELILOT   FLOWERS   Dem. Ton. Exp. Diu.

Melilotus officinalis

Sweet Clover. Yellow Clover. Sweet
   Melilot.

An expectorant and a diuretic. Used to flavor tobacco, cheese, and other products. Used also in
sachets and potpourri mixtures.

Harvard   1851, 1853, 1857, 1860, 1873, 1880

Canterbury   1835, 1847, 1848, 1854

New Gloucester   1864

MEZEREON

Daphne mezereum

Spurge Olive. American Mezereon.
  Leather Wood.

BARK OF ROOT AND STEM   Sti. Alt. Diu. Nar.
Dia.
BERRIES, ROOTS

In small doses used in syphilis, scrofula, chronic rheumatism, and diseases of the skin.

New Lebanon   1851, 1860
Mt. Lebanon   1866, 1872, 1873

MILKWEED

Asclepias syriaca

Silk Weed.

ROOT   Ano. Emm. Diu. Alt. Aro. Sud.
  Ton. Lax. Exp.

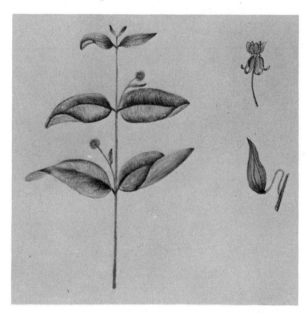

Valuable in amenorrhea, dropsy, retention of urine, dyspepsia, asthma, and scrofulous diseases. Capable of producing vomiting; promotes moderate perspiration. It is tonic and acts upon the bowels.

CHS: "A common, very milky herb, 3 to 4 ft. high on hedges and road sides. Pods full of seeds with their long-silk. July."

Watervliet   1837, 1843, 1845, 1847, 1850, 1860
New Lebanon   1837, 1841, 1851, 1860
Mt. Lebanon   1866, 1872, 1874
Harvard   1851, 1853, 1857, 1860, 1885
Union Village, Ohio   1847, 1850

MILKWORT

Polygala vulgaris

European Seneca.

ROOT   Dia. Exp. Pec.

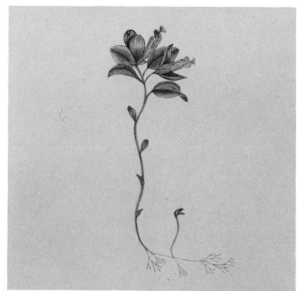

This is a bitters and used in coughs and chest ailments.

CHS: "In woods and swamps from Can. to Ga. Stem from 3 to 4 inches high. Bears from 2 to 4 flowers. May."

Mt. Lebanon   1872

MONARDA   HERB   Diu. Sto. Ton. Aro.
Monarda punctata
Horsemint.

Aromatic and pungent, it contains volatile oil. Useful as a carminative and diuretic in flatulent colic, upset stomach, and nausea.

New Lebanon   1851, 1860
Mt. Lebanon   1866, 1874
Canterbury   1847

MOSS, HAIRCAP   WHOLE PLANT   Diu. Cath.
Polytrichum juniperinum
Robin's Eye. Ground Moss. Bear's Bud.

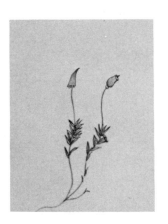

Relieves urinary distress and used to advantage with the hydragogue cathartics.

CHS: "Shady places common. Plant 6 inches high."

Mt. Lebanon   1872

MOTHERWORT   HERB   Emm. Ner. A-spas. Lax. Sto.
Leonurus cardiaca   Dia.
Roman Motherwort. Lion's Tail.
    Throwwort.

Valuable in female complaints, nervousness, colds, delirium, wakefulness, disturbed sleep, liver affections.

Watervliet   1830, 1832, 1833, 1837, 1843, 1845, 1847, 1850, 1860
New Lebanon   1836, 1837, 1841, 1851, 1860
Mt. Lebanon   1866, 1872, 1873, 1874
Harvard   1851, 1853, 1854, 1857, 1860, 1873, 1880, 1885
Canterbury   1835, 1847, 1848, 1854
Union Village, Ohio   1847, 1850
New Gloucester   1864

MOUNTAIN DITTANY
Cunila origanoides
Wild Basil. Stone Mint. American
Dittany.

LEAVES   Sti. Ton. Ner. Sud. Dia.
FLOWERS   Sti. Ton. Ner. Sud. Dia.

The warm tea is diaphoretic.

Watervliet   1860
New Lebanon   1851, 1860
Mt. Lebanon   1866, 1872, 1874

MOUNTAIN MINT
Pycnanthemum montanum
Basil. Wild Marjoram.

HERB   Sti. Ton. Emm. Sto. Aro. Sud.

Used for obstructed menstruation, to produce perspiration, and in colds, fevers, and eruptions.

Watervliet   1830, 1833, 1834, 1837, 1843, 1845, 1847, 1850, 1860
New Lebanon   1836, 1837, 1841, 1851, 1860
Mt. Lebanon   1866, 1872, 1873, 1874
Harvard   1851, 1853, 1857, 1860, 1873, 1880, 1885
Canterbury   1835, 1847, 1848, 1854
Union Village, Ohio   1850
New Gloucester   1864

MOUSE EAR*
Gnaphalium uliginosum
Dysentery Weed. Cud Weed. Everlast-
ing.

HERB   Sud. Sto. Muc. Diu.

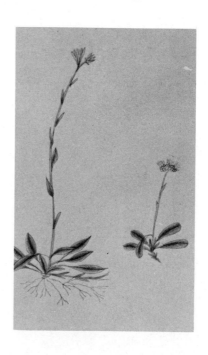

Used in coughs, diarrhea, and obstructions.

CHS: "Fields and pastures. U.S. and Can.
May."

New Lebanon   1851, 1860
Mt. Lebanon   1866, 1872, 1873, 1874

* This Mouse Ear is not to be confused with the
Hawkweed which is called Mouse Ear.

MUGWORT   HERB   Dia. Emm. Ner. A-bil. Deo. Ton.
Artemisia vulgaris   ROOT   Dia. Emm. Ner. A-bil. Deo. Ton.

Useful in epilepsy, hysteria, amenorrhea, promotes perspiration, and increases the flow of urine and menses.

Watervliet   1830, 1833, 1837, 1843, 1845, 1847, 1850, 1860
New Lebanon   1836, 1837, 1841, 1851, 1860
Mt. Lebanon   1866, 1872, 1873, 1874
Harvard   1851, 1853, 1854, 1857, 1860, 1873, 1880, 1885
Canterbury   1835, 1847, 1848, 1854
Union Village, Ohio   1847, 1850
New Gloucester   1864

MULBERRY   BARK   Verm. Cath.
Morus rubra
Red Mulberry.

The infusion of pulverized bark is useful as a cathartic and to dispel worms.

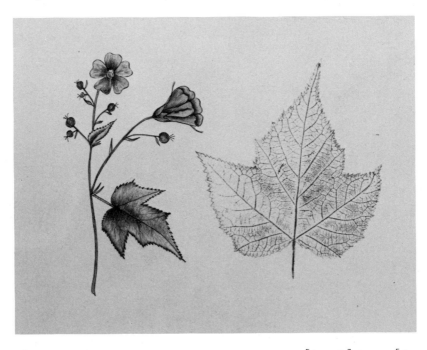

CHS: "A fine flowering shrub, in upland woods, U.S. and Brit. [British] Amer. [America] common. Fruit bright red, sweet. Fruit ripe in Aug. Flowers in June and July."

Mt. Lebanon   1872

MULLEIN   FLOWERS Ast. Dem. Emo.
Verbascum thapsus   HERB Dem. Diu. Ano. A-spas. Emo.
                                              Ast.
                                            ROOT Dem. Diu. Ano. A-spas. Emo.
                                              Ast.
                                            SEED Nar.

Used in cough, catarrh, diarrhea, dysentery, piles, etc. Also as a poultice in white swellings, mumps, and sore throat.

Watervliet   1830, 1833, 1837, 1843, 1845, 1847, 1850, 1860
New Lebanon   1836, 1837, 1841, 1849, 1851, 1860
Mt. Lebanon   1866, 1872, 1873, 1874
Harvard   1851, 1853, 1854, 1857, 1860, 1873, 1880, 1885
Canterbury   1835, 1847, 1848, 1854
Union Village, Ohio   1847, 1850
New Gloucester   1864

MUSTARD, BLACK   SEED Diu. Ves. Sti. Rub. Eme.
Brassica nigra

It is used in large doses as an emetic. In cases of poison, should be administered immediately in lukewarm water. Ground, it is used as a condiment.

Watervliet   1860   Mt. Lebanon   1866, 1872, 1873, 1874
New Lebanon   1851, 1860   Union Village, Ohio   1850

MUSTARD, WHITE   SEED Stim. Rub. Ves. A-scor.
Brassica alba

The whole seed was used as a tonic in dyspepsia, in large doses acts as an emetic, externally, as a poultice, to rouse the system to activity, relieve pain and mitigate inflammation; ground, it is used as a condiment.

Watervliet   1860   Mt. Lebanon   1866, 1872, 1873, 1874
New Lebanon   1851, 1860   Union Village, Ohio   1847, 1850

NANNY BUSH   BARK Ton.
Viburnum lentago
Sheep Berry. Sweet Viburnum. Nanny
   Berry.

New Lebanon   1851, 1860   Mt. Lebanon   1866, 1872, 1873, 1874

NETTLE   FLOWERS   Ton.
Urtica dioica   HERB   Ast. Ton. Diu.
Stinging Nettle.   ROOT   Ast. Ton. Diu.

Valuable in diarrhea, dysentery, hemorrhoids, hemorrhages, gravel, and scorbutic affections. The seeds reduce corpulence.

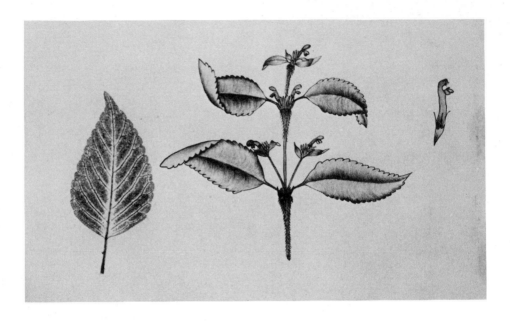

CHS: "A common weed in waste and cultivated grounds in Southern States. Stem covered with deflexed bristles. Internodes thickened upwards. June, July."

New Lebanon   1851, 1860   Union Village, Ohio   1850
Mt. Lebanon   1866, 1872, 1873, 1874

NIGHTSHADE, BLACK   LEAVES   Nar. Ano. A-spas.
Solanum nigrum
Black Cherry. Garden Nightshade.

This is an energetic narcotic. It is anodyne, antispasmodic, calmative, and relaxant. It is too powerful for general or domestic use and should be confined to the hands of skilled herbal physicians only.

Watervliet   1830, 1837, 1843, 1850, 1860   Harvard   1851
New Lebanon   1837, 1841, 1849, 1851, 1860   Canterbury   1835, 1847, 1848, 1854
Mt. Lebanon   1866, 1874   Union Village, Ohio   1847, 1850

Nux Vomica   SEEDS
Strychnos nux-vomica
Poison Nut. Ratsbane.

This is an energetic poison, principally affecting the spinal cord. A poisonous dose produces spasms like tetanus or lockjaw. Should be employed *only* by an educated physician.

Mt. Lebanon   1874

Oak Bark, Black   BARK   Ast. Ton.
Oak Bark, Red   BARK   Ast. Ton. Sti.
Oak Bark, White   BARK   Ton. Ast. A-sep.
Quercus tinctoria
Quercus rubra
Quercus alba

Used in sore throat, offensive ulcers, obstinate chronic diarrhea, hemorrhage, in gargles and injections, in leucorrhea, prolapsus ani, and piles.

Watervliet   1830, 1833, 1837, 1843, 1845, 1847, 1850, 1860
New Lebanon   1836, 1837, 1841, 1851, 1860
Mt. Lebanon   1866, 1872, 1873, 1874
Harvard   1851, 1853, 1857, 1860, 1873, 1880, 1885
Canterbury   1835, 1847, 1848, 1854
Union Village, Ohio   1847, 1850
New Gloucester   1864

Oak of Jerusalem   HERB   Anthel. A-spas. Ver. Sto. Emm.
Chenopodium botrys and *Chenopodium*   SEED   Anthel. A-spas. Ver. Sto. Emm.
    anthelminticum
Worm Seed. Jesuit Tea. Jerusalem Tea.
    Jerusalem Oak.

Used to expel worms in children; also reputed beneficial in amenorrhea.

Watervliet   1830, 1833, 1837, 1843, 1845, 1847, 1850
New Lebanon   1836, 1837, 1841, 1849, 1851, 1860
Mt. Lebanon   1866, 1872, 1873, 1874
Harvard   1849, 1851, 1853, 1854, 1857, 1860, 1873, 1880, 1885
Canterbury   1835, 1847, 1848, 1854
Union Village, Ohio   1850
New Gloucester   1864

ORANGE   FLOWERS   Aro. A-spas.
Citrus aurantium   PEEL   Aro. Ton. Sto.

Used to cover the taste of disagreeable medicines and lessen their tendency to nauseate. The fruit is given after fevers where acids are craved, as in scurvy.

New Lebanon   1851, 1860
Mt. Lebanon   1866, 1872, 1873, 1874

OSIER, GREEN   BARK   Ast. Ton. Sto. Herp. Diu. Deo.
Cornus circinata
Broad-Leaved Dogwood. Dogachamus.
   Alder-Leaved Dogwood. Round-
   Leaved Cornel.

Useful in diarrhea, dysentery, as gargle in sore throat, also in typhoid fever and ague.

Groveland, N.Y.   1842   Harvard   1873, 1880, 1885
Watervliet   1837, 1843, 1860   Canterbury   1835
New Lebanon   1837, 1841, 1851, 1860   Union Village, Ohio   1850
Mt. Lebanon   1866, 1872, 1873, 1874

OSWEGO TEA   HERB   Feb. Sti. Car. Sud. Diu. Sto. Aro.
Monarda didyma   Ton.
Mountain Balm. High Balm. Bee Balm.
   Bergamot Monarda.

The infusion is used in flatulence, nausea, vomiting, and in suppression of urine and menstruation.

Watervliet   1837, 1843   Mt. Lebanon   1866, 1872, 1873, 1874
New Lebanon   1836, 1837, 1841, 1849, 1851, 1860   Union Village, Ohio   1850

PAPOOSEROOT   ROOT   Deo. Nar. Emm.
Caulophyllum thalictrioides
Blue Cohosh. Blueberry Root, Squaw root.

A favorite remedy in chronic uterine diseases, and as a parturient it has proved invaluable. Also used in rheumatism, dropsy, colic, and hysterics.

Watervliet   1830, 1833, 1837, 1843, 1845, 1847, 1850
New Lebanon   1836, 1837, 1841, 1851, 1860
Mt. Lebanon   1866, 1872, 1874

PAREIRA BRAVA   ROOT   Ton. Diu. Aper.
Chondrodendron tomentosum
Velvet Leaf. Ice Vine. Cissampelos
   Pareira.

Used in chronic inflammation of the bladder, disorders of the urinary organs, leucorrhea, dropsy, and jaundice.

Mt. Lebanon   1873, 1874

PARILLA, YELLOW   ROOT   Ton. Lax. Alt.
Menispermum canadense
Canadian Moonseed. Vine Maple.

A superior laxative bitter, used in scrofula, syphilis, rheumatism, gout, and cutaneous diseases.

New Lebanon   1851, 1860   Mt. Lebanon   1866, 1872, 1873, 1874

PARSLEY   LEAVES   Dem. Diu. Dia.
Petroselinum sativum   ROOT   Dem. Diu. Dia.
Rock Parsley.   SEED   Dem. Carm. Dia.

Root useful in dropsy, retention of urine, strangury, and gonorrhea. Leaves were bruised to use as fomentation for bites and stings of insects. Seed used to destroy vermin in the hair.

Hancock   1821
Watervliet   1830, 1833, 1837, 1843, 1845, 1847, 1850, 1860
New Lebanon   1836, 1837, 1841, 1843, 1851, 1860
Mt. Lebanon   1866, 1872, 1873, 1874
Harvard   1851, 1853, 1857, 1860, 1873, 1880, 1885
Canterbury   1835, 1847, 1848, 1854
Union Village, Ohio   1847, 1850
New Gloucester   1864

PEACH   BARK   Ton. Stom. Cath.
Amygdalis persica   KERNELS   Ton. Sto.
                                       LEAVES   Ton. Ver. Lax.

Bark and kernels recommended in intermittent fever, leucorrhea, dyspepsia, and jaundice. The leaves were used in irritability of the bladder and urethra, and inflammation of the stomach and abdomen.

Watervliet   1860   Mt. Lebanon   1866, 1872, 1874
New Lebanon   1849, 1851, 1860   New Gloucester   1854

Pennyroyal

HERB Stim. Diaph. Emm. Carm. Sto. Aro.

Hedeoma pulegioides
Tick Weed. Squaw Mint.

Promotes perspiration, restores suppressed lochia, excites the menstrual discharge.

CHS: "Fragrant, a small sweet scented herb, and held in high repute. Abundant in dry pastures. Can. and U.S. Flowering all summer."

Watervliet 1830, 1832, 1833, 1837, 1843, 1845, 1847, 1850, 1860

New Lebanon 1836, 1837, 1841, 1849, 1851, 1860

Mt. Lebanon 1866, 1872, 1873, 1874

Harvard 1851, 1853, 1854, 1857, 1860, 1873, 1880, 1885

Canterbury 1835, 1847, 1848, 1854

Union Village, Ohio 1847, 1850

New Gloucester 1864

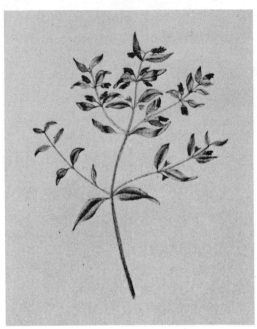

Peony
Paeonia officinalis

FLOWERS A-spas. Ton. Ner. Ver.
ROOT A-spas. Ton. Ner. Ver.

Valuable in St. Vitus's dance, epilepsy, spasms, nervous diseases, and whooping cough. Seeds reputed effective in preventing nightmares of dropsical persons.

Watervliet 1830, 1833, 1837, 1843, 1845, 1847, 1850, 1860
New Lebanon 1836, 1837, 1841, 1851, 1860
Mt. Lebanon 1866, 1872, 1873, 1874
Harvard 1851, 1853, 1857, 1860, 1873, 1880
Canterbury 1835, 1847, 1848, 1854
Union Village, Ohio 1847, 1850
New Gloucester 1864

Peppermint
Mentha piperita

HERB Sti. A-spas. Car. Sto. Sud. Aro.

Used in flatulent colic, hysterics, spasm cramps in the stomach; to allay nausea and vomiting; also to flavor other medicines.

Watervliet   1830, 1832, 1833, 1834, 1837, 1843, 1845, 1847, 1850, 1860
New Lebanon   1836, 1837, 1841, 1849, 1851, 1860
Mt. Lebanon   1866, 1872, 1873, 1874
Harvard   1851, 1853, 1854, 1857, 1860, 1873, 1880, 1885
Canterbury   1835, 1847, 1848, 1854
Union Village, Ohio   1847, 1850
New Gloucester   1864

PILEWORT   HERB   Ast. Herp.
Amaranthus hypochondriacus
Prince's Feather. Lovely Bleeding. Red
   Cockscomb.

Recommended in severe menorrhagia, diarrhea, dysentery, hemorrhage of the bowels, leucorrhea, and ulcers.

Watervliet   1837, 1843, 1845, 1847, 1850   Mt. Lebanon   1866, 1872, 1873, 1874
New Lebanon   1836, 1837, 1841, 1851, 1860   Union Village, Ohio   1850

PINE, WHITE   BARK   Sti. Diu. Pec. Lax. Dia. Dem. Bal.
Pinus strobus   PITCH   Sti. Diu. Pec. Lax. Dia. Dem. Bal.
Spanish Pine.

Used in cough, rheumatism, scurvy, kidney complaints. The pitch is used in gonorrhea, gleet, fluor albus, and kidney and bladder complaints. Bark and sprigs should be mixed with wild cherry, sassafras, and spikenard when used as an expectorant.

Groveland, N.Y.   1842
Watervliet   1850, 1860
New Lebanon   1851, 1860
Mt. Lebanon   1866, 1872, 1873, 1874
Harvard   1851, 1853, 1857, 1860, 1873, 1880, 1885
Canterbury   1835, 1847, 1848, 1854
New Gloucester   1864

PINK ROOT   ROOT   Sud. Anthel.
Spigelia marylandica
Carolina-Maryland Pink. Wormgrass.
   Starbloom.

An active and certain vermifuge combined with senna and manna.

Mt. Lebanon   1872, 1873, 1874

PIPSISSEWA

Chimaphila umbellata

Prince's Pine. Noble Pine. Ground
Holly. Pyrola. Rheumatic Weed. False
Wintergreen.

Useful in scrofula, chronic rheumatism,
kidney diseases, strangury, gonorrhea,
catarrh of the bladder, and cutaneous diseases.

CHS: "A common little evergreen in Can.
and U.S. Found in the woods. Used in
medicine. July."

Groveland   1842

Watervliet   1830, 1833, 1834, 1837, 1843,
1845, 1847, 1850, 1860

New Lebanon   1836, 1837, 1841, 1849, 1851,
1860

Mt. Lebanon   1866, 1872, 1873, 1874

Harvard   1849, 1880, 1885

Canterbury   1835

Union Village, Ohio   1850

HERB   Diu. Ton. Alt. Ast. Sti.

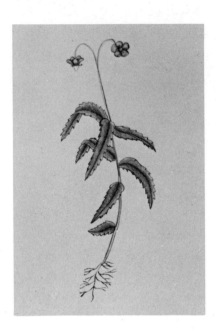

PITCHER PLANT

Sarracenia purpurea

Huntsman's Cup. Eve's Cup. Fly Trap.

Useful for its tonic and beneficial action on
the stomach.

CHS: "In bogs & wet meadows throughout
Can. and U.S. June."

New Lebanon   1851, 1860
Mt. Lebanon   1866, 1872, 1874

WHOLE PLANT   Cath. Deo. Ton. Sto.

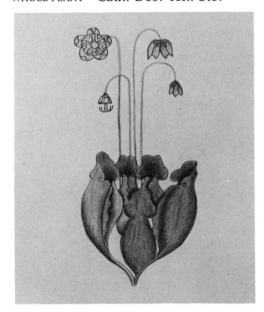

PLANTAIN

Plantago major

Common Plantain, Greater Plantain.
  Bitter Plantain.

LEAVES Alt. Diu. A-sep. Ref. Deo. Ast.
ROOT Alt. Diu. A-sep.

Beneficial in syphilitic, mercurial, and scrofulous diseases, leucorrhea, diarrhea. The leaves are used in ointments.

Watervliet 1860
New Lebanon 1851, 1860, 1866
Mt. Lebanon 1872, 1873, 1874, 1851, 1853, 1854,
  1857, 1860, 1873, 1880, 1885

Canterbury 1835, 1847, 1848, 1854
Union Village, Ohio 1847, 1850
New Gloucester 1864

PLANTAIN, DOWNEY RATTLESNAKE

Goodyera pubescene

Adder's Violet. Rattlesnake Leaf.
  Spotted Plaintain. Rattlesnake Root.

HERB Det.
ROOT Det.

Reputed to have cured scrofula; also used in leucorrhea, prolapsus uteri, and as a wash in scrofulous ophthalmia.

Watervliet 1860
New Lebanon 1851, 1860

Mt. Lebanon 1866, 1872, 1873, 1874

PLEURISY ROOT

Asclepias tuberosa

Butterfly Weed. Wind Root. Tuber Root.

ROOT Dia. Diu. Carm. Ton. Eme.
  Cath. Sud. Ano. Exp.

Used in pleurisy, febrile diseases, flatulency, indigestion, acute rheumatism, dysentery, coughs, inflammation of the lungs, etc. Most often used in decoction or infusion for the purpose of promoting perspiration and expectoration.

CHS: "Dry fields. Can. and U.S. A medicinal plant. Aug."

Watervliet 1830, 1833, 1837, 1843, 1845,
  1847, 1850, 1860
New Lebanon 1836, 1837, 1841, 1851, 1860
Mt. Lebanon 1866, 1872, 1873, 1874
Harvard 1851, 1853, 1854, 1857, 1860, 1873,
  1880, 1885
Canterbury 1835, 1847, 1848, 1854
Union Village, Ohio 1847, 1850
New Gloucester 1864

POISON IVY   LEAVES   Irritant Poison
Rhus toxicodendron
Poison Vine.

Has been used in chronic paralysis, chronic rheumatism, cutaneous diseases, paralysis of the bladder.

Mt. Lebanon   1873

POKE   BERRIES   Deo. Alt. Acr.
Phytolacca decandra   LEAVES   Deo. Alt.
Garget. Pigeon Berry. Scoke. Coakum.   ROOT   Deo. Cath.
   Inkberry. Scokeroot.

Poke is cathartic, alterative, and slightly narcotic. It is a slow-acting emetic, but is not favored for this purpose. It has superior power as an alterative, if properly gathered and prepared.

New Lebanon   1841, 1849, 1851, 1860
Mt. Lebanon   1866, 1874
Canterbury   1835, 1847

POMEGRANATE   RIND OF FRUIT   Ast. Ton.
Punica granatum

Reputed valuable in removing tapeworm, and in intermittent fever, night sweats, passive hemorrhages, diarrhea, and canker in the mouth.

New Lebanon   1851, 1860, 1866
Mt. Lebanon   1866, 1872, 1873, 1874

POPLAR   BARK   Ton. Feb. Ast. Aro. Alt. Sto.
Populus tremuloides   A-scor.
White Poplar. Aspen. American Poplar.   BUDS   Ton. Feb. Ast. Aro. Alt.
   Trembling Poplar.

The active principle of the bark is salicin and populin. Used in intermittent fever, emaciation and debility, impaired digestion, chronic diarrhea, worms, gleet, etc. Used as a vermifuge by veterinaries.

Watervliet   1837, 1843, 1845, 1847, 1850, 1860   Canterbury   1835, 1847, 1848, 1854
New Lebanon   1836, 1837, 1841, 1851, 1860   Union Village, Ohio   1847, 1850
Mt. Lebanon   1866, 1872, 1873, 1874   New Gloucester   1864
Harvard   1851, 1853, 1854, 1857, 1860, 1873,
   1880, 1885

POPPY   CAPSULES   Emo. Ano. Sti. Nar.
Papaver somniferum   FLOWERS   Nar. Ano. Sti.
Opium Poppy. White Poppy.   LEAVES   Nar. Ano. Sti.

Valuable to promote rest, and as poultice for painful swellings; the syrup given to restless children to induce sleep.

Watervliet   1830, 1832, 1833, 1834, 1837, 1843, 1845, 1847, 1850, 1860
New Lebanon   1836, 1837, 1841, 1849, 1851, 1860
Mt. Lebanon   1866, 1872, 1873, 1874, 1881, 1888
Harvard   1849, 1851, 1853, 1854, 1857, 1860, 1873, 1880
Canterbury   1835, 1847, 1848, 1854
Union Village, Ohio   1847, 1850
New Gloucester   1864

PRIVET   LEAVES   Ast. A-scor.
Ligustrum vulgare
Privy. Prim.

The leaves are astringent and may be used in a decoction as a mouthwash and gargle.

Union Village, Ohio   1847, 1850

PTELEA   BARK OF ROOT   Ton. Anthel.
Ptelea trifoliata
Wingseed. Wafer Ash. Shrubby Trefoil.

Recommended in intermittent and remittent fevers, asthma, pulmonary affections, indigestion, and dyspepsia.

Mt. Lebanon   1873, 1874

PUMPKIN   SEED   Muc. Diu.
Cucurbita pepo

Used in scalding of urine, affections of the urinary passages, and said to remove tapeworm effectually.

Mt. Lebanon   1873

PUSSY WILLOW, see W

QUASSIA   THE WOOD   Ton.
Picraena excelsa

Bitter Wood. Bitter Ash.

Bitter tonic.

New Lebanon   1849, 1874

QUEEN OF THE MEADOW   HERB   Ano. Diu. Sti. Ton. A-lith. Dia.
Eupatorium purpureum   ROOT   Diu. Sti. Ton.
Joepye. Trumpet Weed. Gravel Root.
   Purple Boneset.

A valuable remedy in dropsy, strangury, gravel, and all urinary disorders.

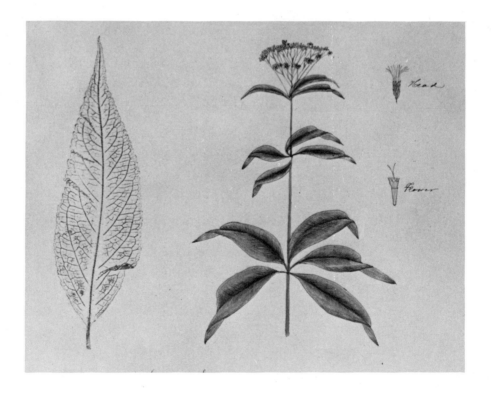

CHS: "Dry fields and woods, common. Stem 3 to 6 ft. high. Aug. Sept."

Watervliet   1837, 1843, 1845, 1847, 1850, 1860   Harvard   1849, 1854, 1857, 1860, 1873, 1880
New Lebanon   1836, 1837, 1841, 1849, 1851,   Canterbury   1835
   1860   Union Village, Ohio   1847, 1850
Mt. Lebanon   1866, 1872, 1873, 1874   New Gloucester   1864

QUEEN'S ROOT   ROOT   Alt. Eme. Cath.
Stillingia sylvatica
Queen's Delight. Yaw Root. Silver Leaf.
   Cock-Up-Hat.

Invaluable in scrofula, syphilis, liver and cutaneous diseases, bronchitis, laryngitis, and lung complaints.

New Lebanon   1851, 1860   Mt. Lebanon   1866, 1872, 1873, 1874

RASPBERRY   LEAVES   Ast. Ton.
Rubus strigosus
Red Raspberry

An excellent remedy in diarrhea, dysentery, cholera infantum, hemorrhage from the stomach, bowels, or uterus, and as an injection in gleet, leucorrhea, and canker.

Watervliet   1837, 1843, 1845, 1847, 1850, 1860
New Lebanon   1836, 1837, 1841, 1851, 1860
Mt. Lebanon   1866, 1872, 1873, 1874
Harvard   1849, 1851, 1853, 1854, 1857, 1860, 1873, 1880
Canterbury   1835, 1847, 1848, 1854
Union Village, Ohio   1847, 1850
New Gloucester   1864

RED ROOT   BARK   Ast. Exp. Sed. A-spas. A-syph.
Ceanothus americanus
New Jersey Tea. Jersey Tea. Wild
Snowball.

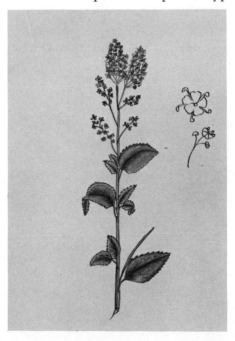

Used in gonorrhea, dysentery, asthma, chronic bronchitis, whooping cough, and as a gargle for canker, sore mouth, etc.

CHS: "A small shrub, found in woods and groves, U.S. and Can. June."

New Lebanon   1849
Mt. Lebanon   1872, 1873
Canterbury   1835

RHATANY   ROOT   Ast.
Krameria triandria

Employed in chronic diarrhea, incontinence of urine, hemorrhages, leucorrhea, profuse menstruation, vomiting blood, and in spongy gums to consolidate them and preserve the teeth.

Mt. Lebanon   1872, 1873, 1874

RHUBARB   ROOT   Cath.
Rheum palmatum

Cathartic principle limited to lower bowel.

Mt. Lebanon   1873, 1874   Union Village, Ohio   1850

RICHWEED   HERB   Diu. Sto. Sti. Ton.
Collinsonia canadensis   ROOT   Diu. Sto. Sti. Ton.
Stone Root. Hardrock. Horseweed.
   Wild Citronella. Oxbalm.

A fair stimulant, and a gentle tonic and diuretic. It is used externally, especially the leaves in
fomentation and poultice for bruises, wounds, blows, sprains, and cuts.

Union Village, Ohio   1847

ROCKBRAKE   HERB   Ast. Anthel.
Pellea atropurpurea   ROOT   Ast. Anthel.
Winter Fern. Cliff Brake. Indian Dream.

Efficacious in diarrhea, dysentery, night
sweats, to remove worms, and as vaginal
injection in leucorrhea, suppression of the
lochia, etc.

CHS: "Abundant in woods, pastures and
waste grounds."

New Lebanon   1851, 1860
Mt. Lebanon   1866, 1873, 1874

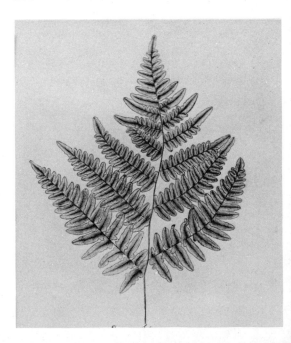

ROMAN WORMWOOD   HERB   Emo. A-sep. Sti. Ton. Ver.
Artemesia pontica
Ragweed. Hogweed.

Used as fomentation in wounds and bruises, and as ointment in piles, ulcers, to reduce painful
swellings, etc.

Watervliet   1860
New Lebanon   1851, 1860
Mt. Lebanon   1866, 1873, 1874
Harvard   1849, 1857, 1860

ROSE   PETALS OF THE FLOWER   Ast. Ton.
Rosa centifolia
Hundred Leaved Rose. Cabbage Rose.

Mildly tonic and astringent.

Union Village, Ohio   1847

ROSE, DAMASK   PETALS OF FLOWERS   Ast. Ton.
Rosa damascena
Pale Rose.

Tonic and mildly astringent. Used in hemorrhages, excessive mucus discharges, and bowel complaints; the infusion with pith of sassafras for inflammation of the eyes, etc. Also used in potpourri and sachets. Considered best source of rose petals as the blossom of the flowers is very full.

Watervliet   1830, 1833, 1837, 1843, 1845, 1860
New Lebanon   1836, 1837, 1841, 1851, 1860
Mt. Lebanon   1866, 1872, 1873, 1874
Canterbury   1835
Union Village, Ohio   1850

ROSE, RED   FLOWERS   Aro. Ton. Ast. Fragrant.
Rosa gallica officinalis

Tonic and mildly astringent. Used in hemorrhages, excessive mucus discharges and bowel complaints; the infusion with pith of sassafras for inflammation of the eyes. This rose was considered
the most useful medically, hence "officinalis." It was also called the apothecary rose and was used
extensively for making rosewater.

Watervliet   1830, 1833, 1834, 1837, 1843, 1845, 1847, 1850, 1860
New Lebanon   1836, 1837, 1841, 1851, 1860
Mt. Lebanon   1866, 1872, 1873, 1874
Harvard   1849, 1851, 1853, 1857, 1860, 1873, 1880
Canterbury   1835, 1847, 1848, 1854
Union Village, Ohio   1850
New Gloucester   1864

ROSE, WHITE   FLOWERS   Ast. Ton.
Rosa alba

Tonic and mildly astringent. Used in hemorrhages, excessive mucus discharges, and bowel complaints; the infusion with pith of sassafras for inflammation of the eyes, etc.

Harvard   1849, 1851, 1853, 1857, 1860, 1873, 1880
Canterbury   1835, 1847, 1848, 1854
Union Village, Ohio   1850
New Gloucester   1864

ROSEMARY   LEAVES AND ROOT   Ast. Ton. Dia. Stim.
Rosmarinus officinalis   A-spas. Emm.

The warm infusion for colds, colic, and nervous conditions; the oil in liniments and plasters as an external stimulant.

Watervliet   1860
New Lebanon   1851, 1860
Mt. Lebanon   1866, 1872, 1873, 1874, 1881, 1888
Union Village, Ohio   1850

ROSIN-WEED   ROOT   Alt. Dia. Diu. Ton.
Silphium laciniatum
Compass Plant. Polar Plant.

The resin has diuretic properties. The root has been used as an expectorant. It is also an emetic.

Mt. Lebanon   1873, 1874

RUE   HERB   Ton. Anthel. Sti. Emm. A-spas.
Ruta graveolens   Diu. Sto.

A narcotic acrid poison, used medically in flatulent colic, hysterics, epilepsy, and as a vermifuge.

Hancock   1821
Watervliet   1830, 1832, 1833, 1834, 1837, 1843, 1845, 1847, 1850, 1860
New Lebanon   1836, 1837, 1841, 1849, 1851, 1860
Mt. Lebanon   1866, 1872, 1873, 1874, 1888
Harvard   1849, 1851, 1853, 1854, 1857, 1860, 1873, 1880
Canterbury   1835, 1847, 1848, 1854
Union Village, Ohio   1847, 1850
New Gloucester   1864

SAFFRON   FLOWERS   Emm. Diaph. Sto. Aro. Dia.

Crocus satirus   Diu.

Has been used beneficially in amenorrhea, dysmenorrhea, chlorosis, hysteria, suppression of the lochial discharges, febrile diseases, scarlet fever, and measles.

Hancock   1821
Groveland, N.Y.   1842
Watervliet   1830, 1833, 1834, 1837, 1843, 1845, 1847, 1850, 1860
New Lebanon   1836, 1837, 1841, 1843, 1851, 1855, 1860
Mt. Lebanon   1866, 1872, 1873, 1874, 1881, 1885, 1888
Harvard   1851, 1854, 1857, 1860, 1873, 1880, 1885
Canterbury   1835, 1847, 1848, 1854
Union Village, Ohio   1847, 1850
New Gloucester   1864

SAGE   HERB   Ton. Ast. Exp. Diaph. Sto. Bal.
Salvia officinalis   Sud.

Valuable in cough, colds, night sweats, worms, spermatorrhea, and as a gargle for ulcerated sore throat; also to produce perspiration.

Hancock   1821
Watervliet   1830, 1832, 1833, 1834, 1837, 1843, 1845, 1847, 1850, 1860
New Lebanon   1836, 1837, 1841, 1843, 1849, 1860
Mt. Lebanon   1866, 1872, 1873, 1874, 1881, 1885, 1888
Harvard   1851, 1853, 1857, 1860, 1873, 1880, 1885
Canterbury   1835, 1847, 1848, 1854
Union Village, Ohio   1847, 1850
New Gloucester   1864

SAGE WILLOW   HERB   Muc. Ast. Dem. Aro. Sto. Bal.
Salix tristis
Rainbow Weed. Purple Willow Herb.
   Loosestrife.

Mucilaginous, astringent, demulcent.

Harvard   1851, 1853, 1857, 1860, 1873, 1880, 1885
New Gloucester   1864

SANICLE, BLACK   ROOT   Dia. A-spas. Exp. Aro. Deo. Sto.
Sanicula marilandica   Ton. Ner. Ano.
Pool Root. American Sanicle. Self-Heal.

Used in ague, stomach complaints, dysentery, erysipelas, cholera, inflammation of the bladder, nervous disease, and pulmonary affections. Resembles valerian.

Watervliet   1837, 1843, 1845, 1847, 1850, 1860   Harvard   1854
New Lebanon   1836, 1837, 1841, 1851, 1860   Canterbury   1835
Mt. Lebanon   1866, 1872, 1873, 1874   Union Village, Ohio   1850

SARSAPARILLA, AMERICAN WILD   ROOT   Alt. Diu. Dem. Deo. Dia.
Aralia nudicaulis
Wild Licorice. Small Spikenard. Dwarf
   Elder. Bristly Stem.

Used in chronic diseases of the skin, rheumatic affections, dropsy, venereal complaints, and in all cases where alteratives are required.

CHS: "A well known plant found in woods. Most abundant in rich and rocky soils, Can. to Car. It has a leaf stalk, but no proper stem. June. July."

Groveland   1842

Watervliet   1830, 1833, 1834, 1837, 1843, 1845, 1847, 1850, 1860

New Lebanon   1836, 1837, 1841, 1849, 1851, 1860

Mt. Lebanon   1866, 1872, 1873, 1874

Harvard   1851, 1853, 1857, 1860, 1873, 1880, 1885

Canterbury   1835, 1847, 1848, 1854

New Gloucester   1864

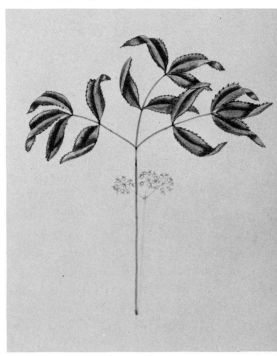

SASSAFRAS
Sassafras officinale

BARK AND BARK OF THE ROOT Diu. Aro. Sti.
Alt. Dia. Sto. Ape. Ton.
PITH Dem. Muc.

Valuable in scrofula and eruptive diseases, and as a flavor. The pith was used as an eyewash in ophthalmia, and as a drink in disorders of the chest, bowels, kidneys, and bladder. Useful as a spring tonic when made into a tea.

CHS: "Grows in the U.S. and Can. Every part of the tree has a pleasant fragrance and an aromatic taste. Apr. June."

Watervliet   1837, 1860

New Lebanon   1837, 1851, 1860

Mt. Lebanon   1866, 1872, 1873, 1874

Harvard   1851, 1853, 1854, 1857, 1860, 1873, 1880, 1885

Canterbury   1835, 1847, 1848, 1854

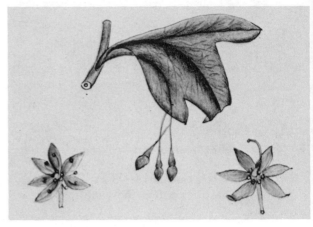

Union Village, Ohio   1847, 1850

New Gloucester   1864

SAVIN
Juniperus sabina

LEAVES Emm. Diu. Diaph. Anthel. Sti.
Acr. Deo.

Used in kidney complaints, suppression of urine, and obstructed menstruation.

Watervliet   1830, 1832, 1833, 1837, 1843, 1845, 1847, 1850, 1860

New Lebanon   1836, 1837, 1841, 1849, 1851, 1860

Mt. Lebanon   1866, 1872, 1873, 1874

Harvard   1851, 1853, 1857, 1860, 1868, 1873, 1880, 1885, 1890

Canterbury   1835, 1847, 1848, 1854

Union Village, Ohio   1850

New Gloucester   1864

SAVORY, SUMMER
Satureia hortensis
Bean Herb. Bohnenkraut.

HERB Sto. Aro. Sti. Car. Emm.

A warm infusion is beneficial in wind colic. Summer savory tea is a good remedy for the nervous headache; drink it hot just before going to bed. Beneficial in colds, menstrual suppression, flatulent colic, and as a gentle stimulating tonic after fevers. The oil is used to relieve toothache.

Hancock   1821
Watervliet   1830, 1832, 1833, 1834, 1837, 1843, 1845, 1847, 1850, 1860
New Lebanon   1836, 1837, 1841, 1843, 1851, 1860
Mt. Lebanon   1866, 1872, 1873, 1874, 1881, 1885, 1888
Harvard   1851, 1853, 1854, 1857, 1860, 1873, 1880, 1885
Canterbury   1835, 1847, 1848, 1854
Union Village, Ohio   1847, 1850
New Gloucester   1864

SAVORY, WINTER   LEAVES   Sto. Sti. Aro. Car.
Satureia montana

Possesses qualities similar to summer savory. The leaves have an aromatic odor and taste like thyme. Both winter and summer savory are cultivated for culinary purposes as well as medicinal.

Mt. Lebanon   1885, 1888

SCABBISH   HERB   Vul. Muc. Dem. Sto.
Oenothera biennis
Tree Primrose. Wild Evening Primrose.

Valuable in cough, tetter, and eruptive diseases.

Watervliet   1830, 1833, 1837, 1843, 1845, 1847, 1850, 1860
New Lebanon   1836, 1837, 1841, 1851, 1860
Mt. Lebanon   1866, 1872, 1873, 1874
Harvard   1851, 1853, 1854, 1857, 1860, 1873, 1880, 1885
Canterbury   1835, 1847, 1848, 1854
Union Village, Ohio   1850
New Gloucester   1864

SCABIOUS   HERB   Diap. Dem. Feb. Diu. Ast. Sud.
Scabiosa succisa   Her.
Sweet Scabious. Devil's Bit. Primrose
   Scabious.

An enduring remedy for promoting moderate perspiration and correcting acrid conditions in the humors. Also abating or driving away fevers.

Watervliet   1833, 1837, 1843, 1845, 1847, 1850,   Mt. Lebanon   1866, 1872
   1860   Union Village, Ohio   1847, 1850
New Lebanon   1836, 1837, 1851, 1860

SCROFULA   HERB   Deo. Alt. Diu. Ano. Ton. Dem.
Scrophularia marilandica   Sto.
Heal-All. Square Stalk. Carpenter's
    Square. Figwort.

Valuable in scrofula, cutaneous diseases, dropsy, and ulcers.

Watervliet   1830, 1833, 1837, 1843, 1845, 1847, 1850, 1860
New Lebanon   1836, 1837, 1841, 1851, 1860
Mt. Lebanon   1866, 1872, 1873, 1874
Union Village, Ohio   1847

SCULLCAP   HERB   Ton. Ner. A-spas. Sud.
Scutellaria lateriflora
Mad-Dog. Hoodwort. Blue Scullcap.
    Virginia Scullcap.

Valuable in all nervous complaints, chorea, wakefulness, delirium tremens, convulsions, and excitability.

Watervliet   1830, 1832, 1833, 1837, 1843, 1845, 1847, 1850, 1860
New Lebanon   1836, 1837, 1841, 1849, 1851, 1860
Mt. Lebanon   1866, 1872, 1873, 1874
Harvard   1851, 1853, 1854, 1857, 1873, 1880, 1885
Canterbury   1835, 1847, 1848, 1854
Union Village, Ohio   1847, 1850
New Gloucester   1864

SCURVEY GRASS   HERB   A-scorb. Stim. Dia. Diu. Ape.
Cochlearia officinalis

Valuable in scurvy, obstructions, dropsy, paralysis, and rheumatism.

Watervliet   1830, 1833, 1837, 1843, 1845, 1847, 1850, 1860
New Lebanon   1836, 1837, 1841, 1849, 1851, 1860
Mt. Lebanon   1866, 1872, 1873, 1874
Canterbury   1835, 1847, 1848, 1854
Union Village, Ohio   1850

SELF-HEAL   HERB Diu.
Prunella vulgaris
Blue Curls. Wound Wort. All Heal. Brown
   Wort. Healall.

Self-heal is pungent and bitter. It increases the secretion of the urine.

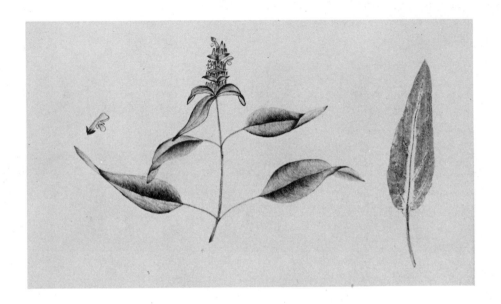

CHS: "It is a member of the mint family. North America. Lat. 33° to the Arctic Sea. Flowering all summer."

Watervliet   1832   New Lebanon   1845

SENNA, AMERICAN   LEAVES Cath. Deo. Diu.
Cassia marilandica
Locust Plant.

A mild cathartic.

Watervliet   1830, 1833, 1837, 1843, 1845, 1847, 1850, 1860
New Lebanon   1836, 1837, 1841, 1849, 1851, 1860
Mt. Lebanon   1866, 1872, 1873, 1874
Harvard   1851, 1853, 1854, 1857, 1860, 1873, 1880, 1885
Union Village, Ohio   1847, 1850
New Gloucester   1864

SHEPHERD'S PURSE
Capsella bursa-pastoris
Shepherd's Heart.

Useful for increasing the secretion of urine, and in controlling scurvy. One of best known specifics for stopping hemorrhages of all kinds.

CHS: "A common weed, found everywhere in fields, pastures and roadsides." Stem 6-8-12 inches high. Stem leaves are smaller than the root leaves and are half clasping at the stems. Silicle smooth, triangular. Apr.-Sept."

Canterbury   1835

HERB. WHOLE PLANT   Diu. A-scor.

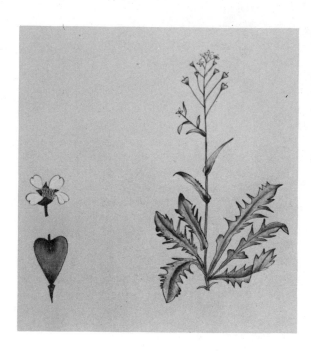

SHIELD FERN
Aspidium spinulosum

Capable of destroying and expelling worms, especially tapeworms.

CHS: "Common in rocky shades. June –Aug."

Canterbury   1835

RHIZOME   Ver. Anthel.

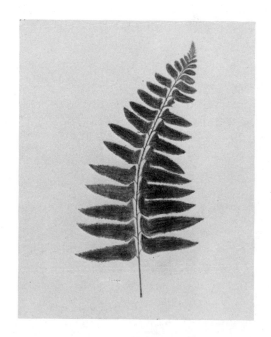

Silver Weed

Potentilla anserina

Silver Cinquefoil. Cramp Weed. Goose
Tansy. Moor Grass.

As a tea it is used for diarrhea. The root is
used as a red dye.

CHS: "A fine species on wet grounds,
meadows and by roadsides. New Eng. to
Arctic Amer. Leaves silvery white beneath.
June. Sept."

Canterbury 1835

HERB Ast.

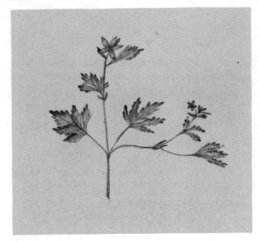

Skunk Cabbage

Symplocarpus foetidus

Meadow Cabbage. Skunk Weed. Polecat
Weed.

ROOT Stim. A-spas. Expec. Ner. Acr.
Ver.

SEED Stim. A-spas. Expec. Ner. Acr.
Ver.

Successfully used in whooping cough, asthma hysteria, chronic rheumatism, spasms, convulsions
during pregnancy, and nervous irritability.

Groveland, N.Y. 1842
Watervliet 1830, 1833, 1837, 1843, 1845, 1847, 1850, 1860
New Lebanon 1836, 1837, 1841, 1851, 1860
Mt. Lebanon 1866, 1872, 1873, 1874
Harvard 1851, 1853, 1857, 1860, 1873, 1880, 1885
Canterbury 1835, 1847, 1848, 1854
Union Village, Ohio 1847, 1850
New Gloucester 1864

Snakehead

Chelone glabra

Balmony. Bitter Herb. Shell Flower.
White Turtlehead. Turtlebloom.

LEAVES A-bil. Ton. Ape. Ver.

A gentle laxative. A tonic with a beneficial effect on the liver. An ointment made from the
fresh leaves is valuable for the itching and irritation of piles.

CHS: "A plant of brooks and wet places. Can. and U.S. with flowers shaped like the head
of a snake, the mouth open and tongue extended. Aug. Sept."

Watervliet 1830, 1833, 1837, 1843, 1845, 1847, 1850, 1860
New Lebanon 1836, 1837, 1841, 1851, 1860
Mt. Lebanon 1866, 1872, 1874
Harvard 1851, 1853, 1854, 1857, 1860, 1873, 1880, 1885
Canterbury 1835, 1847, 1848, 1854
Union Village, Ohio 1847
New Gloucester 1864

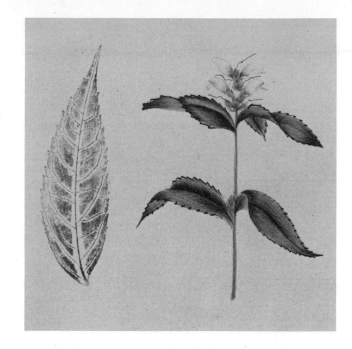

SNAKEROOT, BLACK   ROOT   Nar. Sed. Antispas.
Cimicifuga racemosa
Black Cohosh. Rattleroot.

It is slightly narcotic, sedative, and antispasmodic. Too large doses cause nausea.

Union Village, Ohio 1850

SNAKEROOT, BUTTON   ROOT   Diu. Ton. Emm. Sti. Bal.
Liatris spicata
Gayfeather. Devil's Bit. Blazing Star.
   Colic Root.

Valuable in scrofula, dysmenorrhea, amenorrhea, gleet. Also in Bright's disease, combined with bugle and unicorn.

Watervliet 1860
New Lebanon 1851, 1860
Mt. Lebanon 1866, 1872, 1873, 1874
Union Village, Ohio 1850

SNAKEROOT, CANADA   ROOT   Sti. Aro. Dia. Ner. Her.
Asarum canadense
Indian Ginger. Vermont Snake Root.
   Heart Snake Root.

Valuable in causing perspiration, promotes expectoration, and possesses carminative properties. Used in colic.

Watervliet   1830, 1833, 1835, 1837, 1843, 1845, 1847, 1850, 1860
New Lebanon   1836, 1837, 1841, 1851, 1860
Mt. Lebanon   1866, 1872, 1873, 1874
Harvard   1851, 1853, 1857, 1860, 1873, 1880, 1885
Canterbury   1835, 1847, 1848, 1854
Union Village, Ohio   1847
New Gloucester   1864

SNAKEROOT, SENECA   ROOT   Sial. Exp. Diu. Eme. Cath. Emm.
Polygala senega   Sti. Dia.
Mountain Flax. Seneca Root. Senega
   Root.

Used in chronic catarrh, croup, asthma, and lung diseases, as an expectorant. In large doses it is emetic and cathartic.

Groveland, N.Y.   1849
Watervliet   1850, 1860
New Lebanon   1851, 1860
Mt. Lebanon   1866, 1872, 1873, 1874
Union Village, Ohio   1850

SNAKEROOT, VIRGINIA   ROOT   Stim. Ton. Diaph. Sud.
Aristolochia serpentaria
Snake Root. Snake Weed. Snagrel.

Used to produce perspiration, strengthen the stomach, appetite.

Watervliet   1860
New Lebanon   1851, 1860
Mt. Lebanon   1866, 1872, 1873, 1874

SOAPWORT   HERB   Ton. Dia. Alt. Sud. Aro. Dem.
Saponaria officinalis   Ast.
Bouncing Bet. Old Maid's Pink. London
   Pride.

Valuable in syphilis, scrofula, cutaneous diseases, jaundice, liver complaint.

Watervliet   1847, 1850, 1860
New Lebanon   1851, 1860
Mt. Lebanon   1866, 1872, 1873, 1874
Union Village, Ohio   1847, 1850

SOLOMON'S SEAL, GIANT   ROOT   Ton. Muc. Ast. Dem. Bal. Pec.
Polygonatum multiflorum

Much used in female debility, leucorrhea, piles, pectoral affections, erysipelas, and as a wash to counter the poison from ivy.

Watervliet   1830, 1833, 1837, 1843, 1845, 1847, 1850, 1860
New Lebanon   1836, 1837, 1841, 1851, 1860
Mt. Lebanon   1866, 1872, 1874
Harvard   1851, 1853, 1854, 1857, 1860, 1873, 1880, 1885
Canterbury   1835, 1847, 1848, 1854
Union Village, Ohio   1847, 1850
New Gloucester   1864

SOLOMON'S SEAL, SMALL   ROOT   Tonic. Muc. Ast. Dem.
Smilacina racemosa
Seal Root. Dropberry. False Spikenard.

Much used in female debility, leucorrhea, piles, pectoral affections, erysipelas, and as wash to counter the poison from ivy.

CHS: "A small plant upon the edges of woodlands. Can. and N. Eng. and West to Wis. Berries pale red, speckled with purple. May."

Watervliet   1860
New Lebanon   1851, 1860
Mt. Lebanon   1866

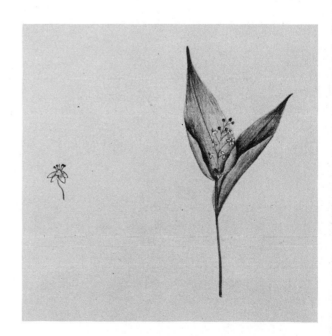

SORREL, LADY'S
Oxalis acetosella
Wood Sorrel. Common Sorrel.

LEAVES Refrig. A-sep. Dia. Diu.

Uses similar to sheep sorrel. Beneficial when eaten green.

CHS: "Woods and shady places, Can. and U.S. June."

New Lebanon   1851, 1860
Mt. Lebanon   1866, 1872, 1873, 1874, 1885, 1888
Union Village, Ohio   1850

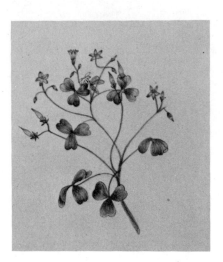

SORREL, SHEEP
Rumex acetosella
Red Top Sorrel. Field Sorrel.

LEAVES Refrig. Diu. A-scor. Ton.

Used in scurvy, scrofula, and skin diseases; as a poultice for tumors, wens, boils; as an extract said to cure cancers and tumors.

CHS: "A common weed in pastures and waste grounds throughout the U.S. preferring dry, hard soils. June, Aug."

Watervliet   1860
New Lebanon   1849, 1851, 1860
Mt. Lebanon   1866, 1872, 1873, 1874

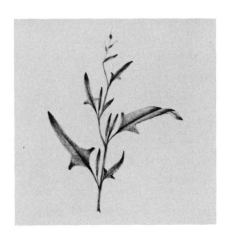

SOUTHERNWOOD
Artemisia abrotanum
Old Man's Tree. Boy's Love.

HERB   Sti. Ner. Ton. Anthel. Det.

Valuable in obstructions, and to remove worms.

Watervliet   1830, 1833, 1837, 1843, 1845, 1847, 1850, 1860
New Lebanon   1836, 1837, 1841, 1851, 1860
Mt. Lebanon   1866, 1872, 1873, 1874

Harvard   1851, 1853, 1857, 1860, 1873, 1880, 1885
Canterbury   1835, 1847, 1848, 1854
Union Village, Ohio   1847, 1850
New Gloucester   1864

SPEARMINT   HERB   Feb. A-spas. Car. Sti. Diu. Aro.
Mentha viridis

Valuable in colic, spasms, dropsy, and to prevent vomiting, gravel, suppression of urine, scalding of urine, and as local application to piles.

Watervliet   1830, 1832, 1833, 1834, 1837, 1843, 1845, 1847, 1850, 1860
New Lebanon   1836, 1837, 1841, 1851, 1860
Mt. Lebanon   1866, 1872, 1873, 1874
Harvard   1851, 1853, 1854, 1857, 1860, 1873, 1880, 1885
Canterbury   1835, 1847, 1848, 1854
Union Village, Ohio   1847, 1850
New Gloucester   1864

SPEEDWELL, COMMON   HERB   Expec. Alt. Ton. Diu. Dia.
Veronica officinalis
Paul Betony.

Recommended in croup, catarrh, renal and skin diseases, jaundice, and scrofula.

CHS: "In meadows, valleys and in grass by the road side. U.S. and Can. May. Aug."

New Lebanon   1851, 1860
Mt. Lebanon   1866, 1872, 1873

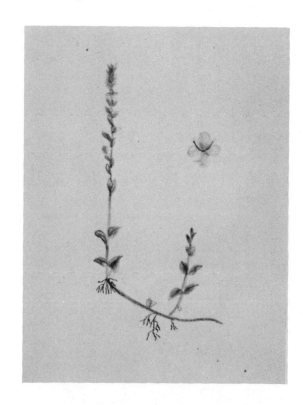

SPICEBUSH   TWIGS   Aro. Feb. Ver. Sti.
Lindera benzoin
Fever Bush. Feverwood.

Useful in reducing fever and expelling worms.

Harvard   1851, 1853, 1854, 1857, 1860, 1873, 1880, 1885
Canterbury   1835, 1847, 1848, 1854
Union Village, Ohio   1847, 1850
New Gloucester   1864

SPIKENARD   ROOT   Pec. Bal. Sto.
Aralia racemosa
Life-of-Man. Petty Morrel. Spignet.

Used in coughs, colds, pulmonary affections, gout, skin diseases, and to purify the blood.

Watervliet   1830, 1833, 1837, 1843, 1845, 1847, 1850, 1860
New Lebanon   1836, 1837, 1841, 1851, 1860
Mt. Lebanon   1866, 1872, 1873, 1874
Harvard   1851, 1853, 1854, 1857, 1860, 1873, 1880, 1885
Canterbury   1835, 1847, 1848, 1854
Union Village, Ohio   1847, 1850
New Gloucester   1864

SPLEENWORT, COMMON   HERB   Dem. Pec. Diu.
Asplenium angustifolium

Used in pectoral and lung diseases and to cure an enlarged spleen.

New Lebanon   1851, 1860
Mt. Lebanon   1866, 1872, 1873

SPURRED RYE   THE DEGENERATED SEEDS   Abo. Nar.
Secale cereale
Smut Rye. Ergot.

Its chief use as a medicine is to promote uterine contractions. It is too powerful and dangerous for domestic use or self-medication.

Watervliet   1860
New Lebanon   1851, 1860
Mt. Lebanon   1866, 1872

Squaw Vine   HERB   Part. Diu. Ast. Emm.
Mitchella repens
Partridge Berry. Winter Clover. Deer
   Berry. One Berry. Checkerberry.

Highly beneficial in diseases of the uterus, parturition, dropsy, suppression of urine; a powerful uterine tonic. Similar in effect to the Pipsissewa.

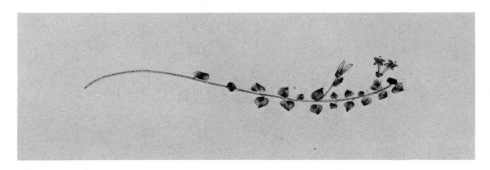

CHS: "A little prostrate plant, found in woods throughout the U.S. and Can. Fruit well flavored but dry. Used by the Indians hence its name. June."

Watervliet   1860   Mt. Lebanon   1866, 1872, 1873, 1874
New Lebanon   1851, 1860   Harvard   1851, 1885

Squaw-Weed   ROOT   Deo. Nar.
Senecio aureus   HERB   Ton. Her. Acr. Deo. Nar. Emm.
Life Root. Golden Ragwort. Female
   Regulator. Blue Cohosh. Cocash Weed.
   Coughweed.

A female tonic and regulator.

Watervliet   1830, 1833, 1837, 1843, 1845, 1847, 1850, 1860
New Lebanon   1836, 1837, 1841, 1849, 1851, 1860
Mt. Lebanon   1866, 1872, 1873, 1874
Harvard   1851, 1853, 1857, 1860, 1873, 1880, 1885
New Gloucester   1864

Squill   BULB   Ton.
Urginea scilla
Scilla. Sea Onion.

Resembles digitalis in physiological action and is a poison in overdoses, causing death by heart paralysis. A fine rat poison.

Mt. Lebanon   1874

STARFLOWER   THE WHOLE HERB   Her. Sto. Ner. Ton.
Aster novae-angliae
Starwort. New England Aster.

As a tonic it acts similarly to Chamomile.

Watervliet   1837, 1843, 1845, 1847, 1850, 1860   Mt. Lebanon   1866, 1872
New Lebanon   1836, 1837, 1841, 1851, 1860   Union Village, Ohio   1850

STAR ROOT   THE ROOT   Ton.
Aletris farinosa
Star Grass. Ague Root. Colic Root.

This is of great utility in flatulent colic; a valuable bitter tonic.

Union Village, Ohio   1850

STEEPLEBUSH   LEAVES   Ast. Ton. A-sep. Feb.
Spiraea tomentosa   ROOT   Ast. Ton. A-sep. Feb.
Meadowsweet. Hardhack.

Useful as an astringent, and it is tonic in diarrhea.

New Lebanon   1841, 1851, 1860   Canterbury   1835, 1847
Mt. Lebanon   1866, 1872, 1874

STILLINGIA   ROOT   Cath. Alt.
Stillingia sylvatica
Queen's Root. Queen's Delight. Silver
   Leaf.

Invaluable in scrofula, syphilis, liver, cutaneous diseases, bronchitis, laryngitis, and lung complaints.

Mt. Lebanon   1874   New Gloucester   1864
Harvard   1857, 1860, 1868, 1873, 1880, 1885

STONE BRAKE   FLOWERS   Diu. Ton.
Eupatorium purpureum   ROOT   A-lith. Dia. Ast.
Queen of the Meadow. Gravel Root.
   Joe-Pye.

In decoctions the flowers are diuretic and tonic. The roots are astringent and useful as in diarrhea.

Harvard   1851, 1853, 1857, 1860, 1873, 1880, 1885
Canterbury   1847, 1848, 1854
New Gloucester   1864

STONE ROOT   ROOT AND PLANT   Diu. Sto. Stim.
Collinsonia canadensis
Horse Weed. Rich Weed. Ox Balm.
   Wound Wort.

Used in chronic catarrh of the bladder, fluor albus and debility of the stomach, lithic acid, and calculous deposits.

Watervliet   1830, 1833, 1837, 1843, 1845, 1847, 1850
New Lebanon   1836, 1837, 1841, 1851, 1860
Mt. Lebanon   1866, 1872, 1873, 1874
Union Village, Ohio   1850

STRAWBERRY   LEAVES   Ast. Feb. Ref.
Fragaria virginiana   VINES   Ast. Feb. Ref.

Useful in diarrhea, dysentery, intestinal debility, and night sweats. The fruit is used in calculous disorders and gout.

Watervliet   1860   Mt. Lebanon   1866, 1872, 1873, 1874
New Lebanon   1851, 1860   Union Village, Ohio   1847, 1850

SUMACH   BARK   Ton. Ast. A-sept.
Rhus glabra   BERRIES   Ast. Refrig. Diu.
Upland Sumach. Smooth Sumach.   LEAVES   Ton. Ast. A-sept. Diu.
   Pennsylvania Sumach.

Valuable in gonorrhea, leucorrhea, diarrhea, hectic fever, and scrofula. The berries are used in diabetes, bowel complaint, febrile diseases, canker, and sore mouth.

Watervliet   1860
New Lebanon   1851, 1860
Mt. Lebanon   1866, 1872, 1873, 1874
Harvard   1851, 1853, 1854, 1857, 1860, 1873, 1880, 1885
Canterbury   1835, 1847, 1848, 1854
Union Village, Ohio   1847, 1850
New Gloucester   1864

SUNFLOWER, GARDEN   SEED Exp. Ast. Diu.
Helianthus annus   LEAVES Ast.

Used in coughs and pulmonary affections, dysentery, and inflammation of the bladder and kidneys.

Watervliet 1860   Mt. Lebanon 1872, 1873, 1874

SUNFLOWER, WILD.   SEED Exp. Diu. Car. A-spas. Lax.
Helianthus divaricatus

Useful in treatment of bronchial and pulmonary affections.

Watervliet 1860   Mt. Lebanon 1866, 1874
New Lebanon 1851, 1860

SWEET CLOVER   HERB Emo. Dis.
Melilotus officinalis
King's Clover. Melilot. Yellow Sweet
    Clover.

The leaves and flowers boiled in lard are useful in all kinds of ulcers, inflammations, and burns.

Watervliet 1860   Mt. Lebanon 1866, 1874
New Lebanon 1851, 1860

SWEET FLAG   ROOT Carm. Stom. Stim. Aro.
Acorus calamus
Calamus. Sweet Rush.

Used in flatulent colic, dyspepsia, feeble digestion, and to aid the action of Peruvian bark in intermittents. Externally it is used to excite the discharges from blistered surfaces, indolent ulcers, and issues.

Watervliet 1830, 1833, 1837, 1843, 1845, 1847, 1850, 1860
New Lebanon 1836, 1837, 1841, 1851, 1860
Mt. Lebanon 1866, 1872, 1873, 1874
Harvard 1851, 1853, 1854, 1857, 1860, 1873, 1880, 1885
Canterbury 1835, 1847, 1848, 1854
Union Village, Ohio 1847, 1850
New Gloucester 1864

SWEET GALE   BUDS   Pec. Ast. Aro. Her.
Myrica gale   LEAVES   Pec. Ast. Aro. Her.
Meadow Fern. Bog Myrtle. Gale Fern.
   Sweet Willow.

This is a stimulant, alterative, depurative, and vulnerary.

Watervliet   1837, 1843, 1845, 1847, 1850, 1860
New Lebanon   1836, 1837, 1841, 1849, 1851, 1860
Mt. Lebanon   1866, 1872, 1874
Harvard   1853, 1854, 1857, 1860, 1873, 1880, 1885
Union Village, Ohio   1850
New Gloucester   1864

SWEET GUM   BARK   Pec.
Liquidambar styraciflua
Red Gum. Star-Leaved Gum.

Used as a household remedy for coughs resulting from colds. It is also useful when made into an ointment to rub on the throat.

Mt. Lebanon   1874

TAMARACK   BARK   Lax. Ton. Diu. Alt. Ape. Exp. Bal.
Larix americana
Hackmatack. American Larch.

Recommended in obstructions of the liver, rheumatism, jaundice, and cutaneous diseases.

CHS: "A beautiful tree in forests from Canada to Pennsylvania, April and May."

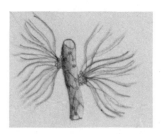

Watervliet   1860
New Lebanon   1841, 1851, 1860
Mt. Lebanon   1866, 1872, 1873, 1874
Harvard   1880, 1885
Union Village, Ohio   1850

TANSY

Tanacetum vulgare

Double Tansy. Sweet Tansy.

HERB Ton. Emm. Diaph. Ver. Sto. Sud. Aro.

Used in fevers, agues, hysterics, dropsy, worms, and as a fomentation in swellings, tumors, and inflammation.

Watervliet   1830, 1833, 1834, 1837, 1843, 1845, 1847, 1850, 1860

New Lebanon   1836, 1837, 1841, 1849, 1851, 1860

Mt. Lebanon   1866, 1872, 1873, 1874, 1888

Harvard   1851, 1853, 1854, 1857, 1860, 1868, 1873, 1880, 1885

Canterbury   1835, 1847, 1848, 1854

Union Village, Ohio   1847, 1850

New Gloucester   1864

THIMBLE WEED

Rudbeckia laciniata

Cone-Disk. Cone-Flower.

HERB Diu. Ton. Bal.

Valuable in Bright's disease, wasting of the kidneys, and urinary complaints generally.

CHS: "In the edges of swamps & ditches. Can. and U.S. Aug."

Watervliet   1837, 1843, 1845, 1847, 1850, 1860

New Lebanon   1837, 1841, 1851, 1860

Mt. Lebanon   1866, 1872, 1873, 1874

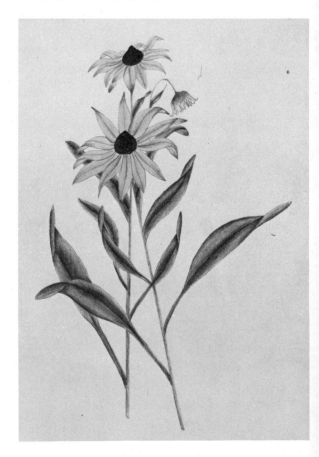

THISTLE ROOT   ROOT Ton. Ast. Diu.
Cirsium arvense
Canada Root. Canada Thistle. Cursed
   Thistle.

Boiled with milk for desentery and diarrhea.

Watervliet 1860   Mt. Lebanon   1866, 1872, 1873, 1874
New Lebanon   1851, 1860

THORN-APPLE   LEAVES (POISONOUS) A-spas. Nar. Sed.
Datura stramonium   Acr.
Apple. Peru. Jamestown Weed. Jimson   SEED (POISONOUS) A-spas. Nar. Acr.
   Weed. Stink Weed. Stramonium.

Used in epilepsy, ticdouloureux and nervous affections, and ophthalmic operations. The leaves
are smoked to relieve spasmodic asthma. The seeds are administered to prevent abortion. In large
doses it is an energetic narcotic poison. Its victims suffer the most intense agonies and die in
maniacal delirium. In medicinal doses it is reported to have been used as a substitute for opium.

Watervliet   1830, 1833, 1834, 1837, 1843, 1845, 1847, 1850, 1860
New Lebanon   1836, 1837, 1841, 1849, 1851, 1860
Mt. Lebanon   1866, 1872, 1874
Harvard   1851, 1853, 1854, 1857, 1860, 1868, 1873, 1880, 1885
Canterbury   1835, 1847, 1848, 1854
Union Village, Ohio   1847, 1850
New Gloucester   1864

THYME   HERB Sto. Aro. Ton.
Thymus serpyllum
American Wild. Mother of Thyme.
   Creeping Thyme.

Used in dyspepsia, weak stomach, hysteria, dysmenorrhea, flatulence, colic, headache, and to
produce perspiration.

Watervliet   1830, 1832, 1833, 1834, 1837, 1843, 1845, 1847, 1850, 1860
New Lebanon   1836, 1837, 1841, 1849, 1851, 1860
Mt. Lebanon   1866, 1872, 1874
Harvard   1851, 1853, 1854, 1857, 1860, 1868, 1873, 1880, 1885
Canterbury   1835, 1847, 1848, 1854
New Gloucester   1864

THYME, ENGLISH   HERB   Aro. Sto. Sti. Sud. Ton. Carm.
Thymus vulgaris   Emm. A-spas.
Common or Garden.

Used in dyspepsia, weak stomach, hysteria, dysmenorrhea, flatulence, colic, headache, and to produce perspiration.

Watervliet   1830, 1832, 1833, 1834, 1837   Mt. Lebanon   1873, 1874, 1888
New Lebanon   1836, 1837   Union Village, Ohio   1847, 1850

TILIA FLOWERS   FLOWERS   Sud. A-spas. Ner.
Tilia americana   LEAVES   Sud. A-spas. Ner.
Lime Tree. Linden.

The flowers and leaves are stomachic. A tea of linden, tilia flowers and leaves are admirable for promoting perspiration. It quiets coughs and relieves hoarseness resulting from colds.

New Lebanon   1851, 1860   Mt. Lebanon   1866, 1874

TOMATO
Hycopersicon esculentum

Extract of tomato was sold in several communities and was handled by the medical department because it was used in many preparations to make them more palatable.
"Tomato Pills: Take Wild Turnip, Lady Slipper and Caraway Seed, equal parts, ½ quantity castor oil and the same of rhubarb mixed with the extract of tomato."

New Lebanon   1849

TONQUA   BEAN   Aro. Nar. Ton.
Dipteryx odorata
Tonka Bean.

The fluid extract has been used in whooping cough with good results. Paralyzes the heart if used in large doses.

Mt. Lebanon   1847

TRILLIUM, PURPLE   THE ROOT   Ast. Ton.
Trilium purpureum
Bath Flower. Bethroot.

An astringent and, when boiled in milk, is of eminent benefit in cases of diarrhea. The root, made into a poultice, is very useful in stings of insects. The leaves boiled in lard are a good external application for skin affections.

New Lebanon   1841   Canterbury   1835, 1847
Mt. Lebanon   1874

TURKEY CORN   ROOT   Ton. Diu. Alt.
Dicentra canadensis
Corydalis. Turkey Pea. Stagger Weed.
   Squirrel Corn.

One of the best remedies in syphilitic diseases; also in scrofula and cutaneous affections.

New Lebanon   1851, 1860   Mt. Lebanon   1866, 1872, 1873, 1874

TURMERIC   ROOT   Aro. Ton. Lax. Stim.
Curcuma longa

(Webster's 2nd Ed. Turmeric—An East Indian herb (*Curcuma longa*) of the ginger family; also, its aromatic root stock, used as a condiment, yellow dye, and medicine.)

Mt. Lebanon   1874

TWINLEAF   ROOT   Stim. Diaph. Diu. Alt. A-spas.
Jeffersonia diphylla
Ground Squirrel Pea. Rheumatism Root.
   Helmet Pod.

Successfully used in chronic rheumatism, secondary syphilis, mercurial syphilis, dropsy, nervous affections, spasms, and cramps; also as gargle in diseases of the throat, scarlatina, and indolent ulcers.

Mt. Lebanon   1873   Union Village, Ohio   1850

UNICORN ROOT, FALSE   ROOT   Ton. Diu. Verm. Sto.
Chamaelirium luteum
Drooping Starwort. Starwort. Star Root.
   Helonias.

Invaluable as a uterine tonic, imparting tone and vigor to the reproductive organs; used in leucorrhea, amenorrhea, dysmenorrhea, and to remove the tendency to miscarriage.

Watervliet   1850, 1860   Mt. Lebanon   1866, 1872, 1873, 1874
New Lebanon   1851, 1860   Harvard   1880, 1885

Uva-Ursi   LEAVES   Ton. Diu. Ast. A-lith.
Arctostaphylos uva-ursi
Bearberry. Upland Cranberry. Mountain
  Cranberry. Mountain Box. Arbutus Uva
  Ursi.

Used in chronic affections of the kidneys and urinary passages, strangury, diabetes, fluor albus,
and excessive mucus discharges with the urine, lithic acid, etc.

Watervliet 1850, 1860	Canterbury 1835, 1847, 1848, 1854
New Lebanon 1851, 1860	Union Village, Ohio 1850
Mt. Lebanon 1866, 1872, 1873, 1874	New Gloucester 1864
Harvard 1851, 1853, 1854, 1857, 1860, 1868, 1873, 1880, 1885	

Valerian, American   ROOT   Sud. Ner. Ano. Sti.
Cyprepedium pubescens
Nerve Root. Yellow Moccasin Flower.
  Yellow Ladies' Slipper.

Used in cholera, nervous debility, hysteria, and low forms of fever where a nervous stimulant is
required.

Watervliet 1860	Mt. Lebanon 1866, 1872, 1874
New Lebanon 1851, 1860	Harvard 1854

Valerian, English   ROOT   Anti-spas. Ton. Sti. Sud. Sto.
Valerian officinalis
Great Wild Valerian. Vandal Root.

Used in cholera, nervous debility, hysteria, and low forms of fever where a nervous stimulant is
required.

Watervliet   1837, 1843, 1845, 1847, 1850, 1860
New Lebanon   1836, 1837, 1841, 1851, 1860
Mt. Lebanon   1866, 1872, 1874
Harvard   1851, 1853, 1854, 1857, 1860, 1868, 1873, 1880, 1885
Canterbury   1847, 1848, 1854
New Gloucester   1864

Valerian, Greek   ROOT   Sud. Ast. Feb.
Polemonium reptans

Used in cholera, nervous debility, hysteria, and low forms of fever where a nervous stimulant is
required.

Watervliet 1860	Union Village, Ohio 1850

Vervain

Verbena hastata

Wild Hyssop. Simpler's Joy. Erect
  Vervain. Blue Vervain.

HERB Ton. Eme. Exp. Sud.
ROOT Ton. Eme. Exp. Sud.

Used in intermittent fevers, colds,
obstructed menses, scrofula, gravel, and
worms.

CHS: "Frequently by roadsides and in low
grounds, mostly throughout the U.S. and
Can. July. Sept."

Watervliet   1830, 1833, 1837, 1843, 1845,
  1847, 1850, 1860

New Lebanon   1836, 1837, 1841, 1851, 1860

Mt. Lebanon   1866, 1872, 1874

Harvard   1851, 1853, 1854, 1857, 1860, 1868,
  1873, 1880, 1885

Canterbury   1835, 1847, 1848, 1854

Union Village, Ohio   1847, 1850

New Gloucester   1864

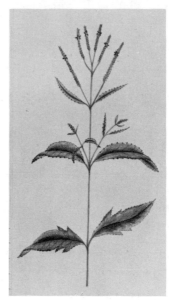

Violet

Viola pedata

Bird's-Foot Violet.

HERB Pec. Exp. Ton. Muc. Emol. Dem.
  Lax. Ape. Anti-syph. Sud.

Used in colds, cough, and sore throat.

CHS: "This is one of the most common
kinds of violet, found in low grassy woods
from Arctic Amer. to Florida. Apr. May."

Watervliet   1860
New Lebanon 1851, 1860
Mt. Lebanon   1866, 1872, 1873, 1874
Union Village, Ohio   1847, 1850

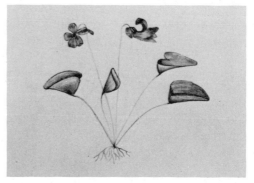

Violet, Canker

Viola rostrata

HERB Dem. Ton. Diu. Ape.

Said to be useful in pectoral and cutaneous diseases; also in syphilis.

Watervliet   1837, 1843, 1845, 1847, 1850, 1860
New Lebanon   1836, 1837, 1841, 1851, 1860
Mt. Lebanon   1866, 1872, 1873

VIRGIN'S BOWER   LEAVES   Sti. Ner.
Clematis virginiana
Travellers' Joy. Clematis.

Used in severe headache, cancerous ulcers, and as ointment in itch.

Watervliet   1837, 1843, 1845
New Lebanon   1837, 1841, 1851, 1860
Mt. Lebanon   1866, 1872, 1873, 1874
Union Village, Ohio   1850

WA-A-HOO   BARK   Ton. Lax. Alt. Diu. Cath. Exp.
Euonymus atropurpureus
Euonymous. Indian Arrow-Wood. Burning
   Bush. Spindle Tree.

Useful in intermittent fever, dyspepsia, torpid liver, constipation, dropsy, and pulmonary affections. (This is not recommended for home use.)

Groveland, N.Y.   1842   Mt. Lebanon   1866, 1872, 1873, 1874
Watervliet   1850   Harvard   1880, 1885
New Lebanon   1851, 1860   Union Village, Ohio   1850

WALNUT   BARK   Sty. Ton. Alt. Cath.
Juglans cinera   LEAVES Sty. Ton. Alt. Cath.
Hickory. Shagbarks. White Walnut. But-
   ternut Bark. Oil Nut.

Used in scrofula, debility, diarrhea, and as a gentle cathartic; as a wash for ulcers and sore eyes.

Watervliet   1860
New Lebanon   1851, 1860
Mt. Lebanon   1866, 1872, 1873, 1874

WATERCUP   HERB   Ton. Stim. Diu. Lax. Ner.
Sarracenia purpurea
Side-Saddle Flower. Pitcher Plant. Fly-
   trap. Huntsman's Cup. Small-Pox Plant.

Used in chlorosis, all uterine derangements, dyspepsia and gastric difficulties; said to be useful in smallpox.

New Lebanon   1851, 1860
Mt. Lebanon   1866, 1872, 1873, 1874

WATER HOARHOUND   HERB   Ton. Ast. Sed. Nar.
Lycopus europoeus
Water Bugle. Gipsy Wort.

This is a tonic and is mildly narcotic; has a quieting effect.

Groveland, N.Y.   1842
Mt. Lebanon   1872

WATERMELON   SEED   Muc. Diu. Dem. Ref.
Cucurbita vulgaris

Valuable in strangury, urinary affections, and dropsy.

Watervliet   1860
New Lebanon   1851, 1860
Mt. Lebanon   1866, 1872, 1873, 1874

WATER PEPPER   HERB   Exp. Sud. Ves. Anti-sep. Dia.
Polygonum hydropiper   Stim. Diu. Emm. Acr. Pec.
Smart Weed. Arsmart. Heartweed.

Used in amenorrhea, gravel, colds, coughs,
milk sickness, bowel complaints, and
erysipelas.

CHS: "The leaves are marked with a brown-
ish spot. Common around buildings and
fences, wet grounds. Leaves two to four
inches long. Stem leafy, one to two feet
high. June –Aug."

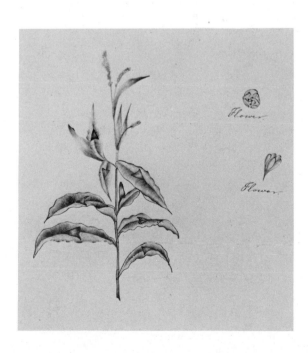

Groveland   1842

Watervliet   1837, 1843, 1845, 1847, 1850

New Lebanon   1836, 1837, 1841, 1849, 1851,
    1860

Mt. Lebanon   1866, 1872, 1873, 1874

Harvard   1851, 1853, 1854, 1857, 1860, 1868,
    1873, 1880, 1885

Canterbury   1835, 1847, 1848, 1854

Union Village, Ohio   1847, 1850

New Gloucester   1864

WHITE ROOT
Erigeron philadelphicus
White Weed. Ox Eye Daisy. White
   Daisy.

FLOWERS   Aro. Sto.
LEAVES   Aro. Sto.

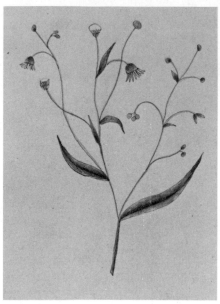

White root is chiefly employed as an insect
powder for fleas, etc. The fresh leaves or
flowers will destroy or drive them away.

CHS: "Woods and pastures throughout
North America. June to Aug."

Groveland   1842
New Lebanon   1836

WHITEWOOD
Liriodendron tulipifera
Tulip Tree. Cucumber Tree. Tulip Poplar.

BARK   A-per. Ton. Stim. Sto. Aro.

Useful in intermittent fever, low condition of the system, dyspepsia, diarrhea, and hysteria.

Watervliet   1830, 1833, 1837, 1843, 1845, 1847, 1850, 1860
New Lebanon   1837, 1841, 1851, 1860
Mt. Lebanon   1866, 1872, 1873, 1874
Harvard   1851, 1853, 1854, 1857, 1860, 1868, 1873, 1880, 1885
Canterbury   1835, 1847, 1848, 1854
New Gloucester   1864

WHORTLEBERRY
Vaccinium myrtillus
Bilberry. Blue Berry. Burren Myrtle.

BERRIES   Ast.
LEAVES   Ast.

The leaves are strongly astringent and somewhat bitter. They are of great value in diarrhea. A
mixture of equal parts of bilberry leaves, thyme, and strawberry leaves makes an excellent tea.

New Lebanon   1847

Wickup   HERB   Ast. A-sep. Eme.
Epilobium angustifolium   ROOT   Ast. A-sep. Eme.
Mare's Tail. Rose Bay. Willow-Herb.

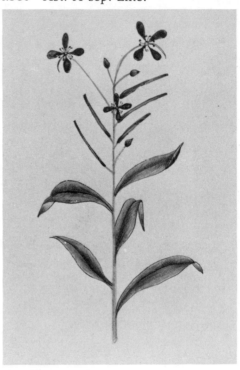

Used in dysentery, diarrhea, and where an astringent is required.

CHS: "In newly cleared lands, low waste grounds. Penn. to Arc. America. July. August."

New Lebanon   1851, 1860
Mt. Lebanon   1866, 1872, 1873

Wild Turnip   THE ROOT   Sti. Exp. Acr. Ton. Nar.
Arum triphyllum
Wake Robin. Jack-in-the-Pulpit. Dragon
   Root.

It is acrid, an expectorant and diaphoretic, and is violently irritating if improperly used by one unfamiliar with its peculiarities.

Groveland, N.Y.   1842   New Lebanon   1836, 1837, 1841, 1851, 1860
Watervliet   1837, 1843, 1845, 1847, 1850, 1860   Mt. Lebanon   1866, 1872, 1873, 1874

Wild Yam   ROOT   A-spas.
Dioscorea villosa
Colic Root.

Successfully used in bilious colic, spasms, cramps, flatulence, after-pains, and affections of the liver.

Mt. Lebanon   1873, 1874

WILLOW, PUSSY   BARK   Ton. Ast. Anthel. A-sep.
Salix discolor

Used in indigestion, in weak and relaxed condition of the bowels, diarrhea, worms, gangrene, and indolent ulcers. The buds are aphrodisiac.

Watervliet   1860
New Lebanon   1851, 1860
Mt. Lebanon   1866, 1872, 1873, 1874

WILLOW, ROSE   BARK   Ast. Ton.
Cornus Sericea
Red-Rod. Swamp Dogwood.

Bitter, astringent, detergent, and antiperiodic. Used occasionally as a substitute for quinine.

Watervliet   1830, 1833, 1837, 1843, 1845, 1847, 1850, 1860
New Lebanon   1836, 1837, 1841, 1849
Mt. Lebanon   1866, 1872, 1874
Union Village, Ohio   1850

WILLOW, WHITE   BARK   Ton. A-per. Ast.
Salix alba

Used in intermittent fever, debility of the digestive organs, hemorrhages, chronic mucus discharges, diarrhea, and dysentery. Exerts its virtues in the shape of an ointment.

Watervliet   1860
New Lebanon   1851, 1860
Mt. Lebanon   1866, 1872, 1873

WINTERGREEN   WHOLE PLANT   Diu. Sti. Sto. Emm.
Gaultheria procumbens
Tea Berry Plant. Checkerberry.
   Pipsissawa. Spicey Wintergreen.
   Box-Berry.

Increases flow of urine. Stimulates the stomach when used in small doses. Large doses are emetic.

CHS: "In woods, Can. and Northern States. Common, June. July."

Watervliet 1830, 1832, 1833, 1837, 1843, 1845, 1847, 1850, 1860

New Lebanon 1836, 1837, 1841, 1849, 1851, 1860

Mt. Lebanon 1866, 1872, 1874

Harvard 1851, 1853, 1854, 1857, 1860, 1868, 1873, 1880, 1885

Canterbury 1835, 1847, 1848, 1854

Union Village, Ohio 1850

New Gloucester 1864

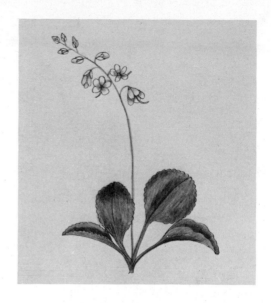

WITCH HAZEL

Hamamelis virginiana

Winter Bloom. Snapping Hazle. Snapping Hazle Nut. Spotted Alder.

Valuable in diarrhea, dysentery, and excessive mucus discharges; also as a wash in painful swellings, gargle for canker, and injection for fluor albus.

BARK Ton. Ast. Sed. Her.
LEAVES Ton. Ast. Sed.

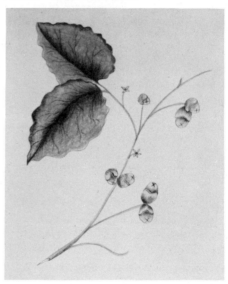

Watervliet 1837, 1843, 1845, 1847, 1850, 1860

New Lebanon 1836, 1837, 1841, 1851, 1860

Mt. Lebanon 1866, 1872, 1873, 1874

Harvard 1851, 1853, 1857, 1860, 1868, 1873, 1880, 1885

Canterbury 1835, 1847, 1848, 1854

Union Village, Ohio 1850

New Gloucester 1864

WORMSEED

Chenopodium ambrosioides

Oak Jerusalem Seed. Goose-Foot.

Valuable to expel worms from children.

SEED Anthel. A-spas. Ver. Sto. A-bil.

Watervliet 1847, 1850

New Lebanon 1851, 1860

Mt. Lebanon 1866, 1872, 1873, 1874

Harvard 1851, 1853, 1857, 1860, 1868, 1873, 1880

Canterbury 1835, 1847, 1848, 1854

Union Village, Ohio 1847, 1850

New Gloucester 1864

WORMWOOD, COMMON   HERB   Anthel. Ton. Nar. Sti. Ver. A-bil.
Artemisia absinthium   Sto.

Used in intermittent fever, jaundice, worms, to promote the appetite, and externally in bruises
and inflammations.

Watervliet   1830, 1832, 1833, 1834, 1837, 1843, 1845, 1847, 1850, 1860
New Lebanon   1836, 1837, 1841, 1851, 1860
Mt. Lebanon   1866, 1872, 1873, 1874, 1888
Harvard   1851, 1853, 1854, 1857, 1860, 1868, 1873, 1880, 1885
Canterbury   1835, 1847, 1848, 1854
Union Village, Ohio   1847, 1850
New Gloucester   1864

YARROW   HERB   Ton. Ast. Alt. Diur. Aro. Sto. Acr.
Achillea millefolium   Sti. Cath. Det.
Millefoil. Noble Yarrow. Lady's Mantle.

Used in hemorrhages, incontinence of urine,
diabetes, piles, dysentery, flatulency, and as
injection in leucorrhea.

CHS: "In fields and pastures. N.E. to Or.
and to the Arctic Sea. Flowers are white or
rose colored. July. Sept."

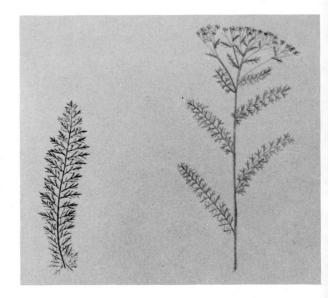

Watervliet   1830, 1833, 1837, 1843, 1845,
    1847, 1850, 1860
New Lebanon   1836, 1837, 1841, 1851, 1860
Mt. Lebanon   1866, 1872, 1873, 1874
Harvard   1851, 1853, 1854, 1860, 1868, 1873,
    1880, 1885
Canterbury   1835, 1847, 1848, 1854
Union Village, Ohio   1847, 1850
New Gloucester   1864

YELLOW JESSAMINE   ROOT   Feb.
Gelsemium sempervirens
Wild Jessamine. Woodbine.

A valuable febrifuge in all fevers, except congestive; also used in nervous irritability, headache,
and lockjaw.

Mt. Lebanon   1872, 1873, 1874

GLOSSARY

to modify its action or counteract a disagreeable effect

COSTIVENESS—constipation

CROUP—a spasmodic laryngitis in infants and children

CUTANEOUS—of or relating to the skin

D

DECOCTION—the act or process of boiling, usually in water, so as to extract the flavor or active principle; the extract thus obtained

DEMULCENT—a substance capable of soothing an inflamed or abraded mucous membrane or protecting it from irritation

DIAPHORETIC—an agent inducing sweating

DROPSY—an abnormal accumulation of watery fluid in body tissues or cavities

DYSENTERY—an often epidemic or endemic disease characterized by severe diarrhea, with passage of mucus and blood

DYSPEPSIA—a condition of disturbed digestion characterized by nausea, heartburn, pain, gas, and a sense of fullness due to local causes or to disease elsewhere in the body

E

EMETIC—an agent that induces vomiting

EMMENAGOGUE—an agent that promotes menstrual discharge

EMPIRIC—a member of an ancient sect of physicians who based their practice on experience alone, disregarding all theoretical and philosophical considerations

ERYSIPELAS—an acute febrile disease associated with intense local inflammation of the skin and subcutaneous tissues

F

FEBRIFUGE—an agent that mitigates or removes fever

FEBRILE—of or relating to fever

FLUX—a flowing or discharge of fluid from the body; usually an excessive or abnormal discharge from the bowels

FOMENTATION—the application of hot moist substances (as wet cloths) to the body for the purpose of easing pain

G

GLEET—a chronic inflammation of a bodily orifice in man or animals, usually accompanied by an abnormal discharge from the orifice

GONORRHEA—contagious inflammation of the genital mucus membrane

GOUT—a metabolic disease occurring in paroxysms and marked by a painful inflammation of the fibers and ligamentous parts of the joints

GRAVEL—a deposit of small calculous concretions in the kidneys and urinary bladder

GRIPING—causing a pinching spasmodic intestinal pain

I

INDOLENT—causing little or no pain; growing or progressing slowly; slow to heal

INFUSION—the introducing of a solution into a vein; the steeping or soaking, usually in water, of a substance (as a plant drug) in order to extract its virtues; the liquid extract obtained by the latter process

INSPISSATED—thickened by boiling

L

LEAD COLIC—intestinal colic associated with obstinate constipation due to chronic lead poisoning, called also painter's colic

LEUCORRHEA—a white, yellowish, or greenish white viscid discharge from the vagina

M

MATERIA MEDICA—material or substance used in the composition of medical remedies, a branch of medical science that treats of the sources, natures, properties, and preparation of the drugs used in medicine

MENORRHAGIA—abnormally profuse menstrual flow

MENSTRUUM—a substance that dissolves a solid or holds it in suspension

MORDANT—a chemical that serves to fix a dye in or on a substance by combining with the dye to form an insoluble compound

MUCILAGINOUS—relating to the secretion of mucilage, a gelatinous substance that swells in water without dissolving, and forms a slimy mass

N

NUX VOMICA—the poisonous seed of an Asiatic tree that contains several alkaloids but chiefly strychnine and brucine

O

OPHTHALMIA—an inflammation of the conjunctiva or of the eyeball

P

PARTURIENT—bringing forth or about to bring forth young

PHARMACOPOEIA—a book containing a selected list of drugs, chemicals, and medicinal preparations with descriptions of them, tests for their identity, purity, and strength, and formulas for making the preparations; especially one issued by official authority and recognized as a standard

PHTHISIS—a wasting or consumption of the tissue

POPULIN—a sweet crystalline glucoside found in aspen bark and leaves and poplar buds

POTHERB—an herb that is boiled for use as a vegetable

PROLAPSIS ANI—falling of the anus

PROLAPSIS UTERI—falling down of the uterus

Q

QUINSY—an acute infection of the throat, especially when discharging pus or mucus

R

RESINOID—plant material, soluble in organic solvents but not in water

RUBEFACIENT—a substance for external application that produces redness of the skin

S

SALICIN—a bitter, white crystalline beta-glucoside found in the bark and leaves of several willows and poplars; used as a tonic

SALT RHEUM—eczema

SCAB HEAD—a Shaker term for a scalp affliction

SCARLATINA—a term for scarlet fever

SCORBUTIC—of or relating to scurvy

SCROFULA—swelling of the lymph glands of the neck

SENEGA—the dried root of senega root containing an irritating saponin (a glycoside occurring in many plants which foams when in a water solution)

SPERMATORRHEA—abnormally frequent or excessive involuntary emission of semen without orgasm

STOMACHIC—relating to stomach; exciting action of stomach

STRANGURY—slow and painful discharge of urine drop by drop produced by spasmodic muscular contractions of the urethra and bladder

SYPHILIS—chronic, contagious, usually venereal disease caused by a spirochete

T

TETTER—any of various vesicular skin diseases (as ringworm eczema)

TIC DOULOUREUX—painful twitch; neuralgia

V

VERMIFUGE—serving to destroy or expel parasitic worms, especially of the intestine

VESICATION—an instance or the process of blistering; a blister

VOLATIZE—to make volatile, to cause to exhale or evaporate

VULNERARY—promoting healing of wounds

W

WEN—a cyst formed by obstruction of secreted material from a sebaceous gland

BIBLIOGRAPHY FOR THE HISTORY

Adrosko, Rita J. *Natural Dyes and Home Dyeing*. New York: Dover, 1971.

Andrews, Charles M. *The Colonial Period of American History*. New Haven: Yale University Press, 1934.

Andrews, Edward D. *The Community Industries of the Shakers*. New York State Museum Handbook, No. 15. Albany, N.Y.: University of the State of New York, 1933.

————. *The Hancock Shakers, 1780–1960*. New Haven: Carl Purington Rollins Press, Shaker Community, Inc., 1961.

————. *The People Called Shakers*. New York: Oxford University Press, 1953.

————, and Andrews, Faith. *Shaker Herbs and Herbalists*. New Haven: Carl Purington Rollins Press, Shaker Community, Inc.

Blinn, Henry Clay, ed. *The Life and Gospel Experience of Mother Ann Lee*. East Canterbury, N.H.: Shakers, 1901.

————. *The Manifesto, 1883–99*. Canterbury, N.H.

Bremer, Fredrika. *Homes of the New World*, vols. 1 and 2. Translated by Mary Howitt. New York: Harper & Brothers, 1853.

Briggs, Asa. *Victorian Cities*. New York: Harper & Row, 1963.

Brooklyn Botanical Garden. *Handbook on Herbs, Plants and Gardens*, vol. 14, no. 2, 1950.

Carter, Kate B. *Pioneer Medicines*. Salt Lake City: Daughters of Utah Pioneers, 1958.

Clark, Thomas D. *Pleasant Hill in Civil War*. Pleasant Hill, Ky: Pleasant Hill Press, 1972.

————, and Ham, F. Gerald. *Pleasant Hill and Its Shaker Community*. Pleasant Hill, Ky: Shakertown Press, 1968.

Clarkson, Rosetta E. *Herbs and Savory Seeds*. New York: Dover, 1972.

————. *Herbs, Their Culture and Uses*. New York: Macmillan, 1942.

————. *Magic Gardens*. New York: Macmillan, 1939.

Coleman, J. Winston, Jr., ed. *Kentucky, A Pictorial History*. Lexington, Ky.: University Press of Kentucky, 1971.

Coon, Nelson. *Using Plants for Healing*. Great Neck, N.Y.: Hearthside, 1963.

————. *Using Wayside Plants*. Great Neck, N.Y.: Hearthside, 1957.

Creevey, Caroline. *Flowers of Field, Hill and Swamp*. New York: Harper & Brothers, 1897.

Culpepper, Nicholas. *Culpepper's Complete Herbal*. London: W. Foulsham, n.d.

Desroche, Henri. *The American Shakers: From Neo-Christianity to Presocialism*. Translated by John K. Savacool. Amherst: University of Massachusetts Press, 1971.

Dioscorides. *The Greek Herbal*. Oxford: Oxford University Press, 1934.

Dixon, William Hepworth. *New America*. Philadelphia: Lippincott, 1867.

————. "Shakerism in the United States," *Westminster Review*, n.s. 3 (April 1861).

Doe, John E. *Beginning Again*. London: Hogarth Press, 1964.

Dwight, Timothy. *Travels in New England and New York*. New Haven: Timothy Dwight, 1822.

Earle, Alice Morse. *Old Time Gardens*. New York: Macmillan, 1901.

Elkins, Hervey. *Fifteen Years in the Senior Order of Shakers*. Hanover, N.H.: Dartmouth Press, 1853.

Evans, Elder Frederick W. *Autobiography of a Shaker*. New York: American News Co., 1888.

―――. *Compendium of the Origin, History, Principles, Rules & Regulations, Government, and Doctrines of the United Society of Believers in Christ's Second Appearing*. New York: Appleton, 1859.

―――, and Doolittle, Antoinette, eds. *Shaker and Shakeress, 1873–75*. Mt. Lebanon, N.Y.: n.d.

Felter, Harvey Wicker. *Genesis of American Materia Medica*. Cincinnati, 1927.

Fenton, William N. *Contacts Between Iroquois Herbalism and Colonial Medicine*. Washington, D.C.: Smithsonian Institution, 1941.

Freeman, Margaret B. *Herbs for the Medieval Household*. New York: Metropolitan Museum of Art, 1943.

Gibbons, Euell. *Stalking the Healthful Herbs*. New York: McKay, 1966.

Gray, Asa. *Manual of Botany*. 8th ed., rev. Merritt Lundon Fernald. New York: American Book Co., 1950.

Green, Calvin, and Wells, Seth Y. *A Summary View of the Millennial Church or United Society of Believers (Commonly Called Shakers)*. Albany, N.Y.: 1823.

Grieve, Maude. *Modern Herbal: The Medicinal, Culinary, Cosmetic and Economic Properties, Cultivation and Folklore of Herbs, Grasses, Fungi, Shrubs and Trees*. New York: Harcourt, 1931.

Gunther, Robert T. *The Greek Herbal of Dioscorides*. New York: Hafner, 1959.

Hedrick, Ulysses Prentiss. *A History of Agriculture in the State of New York*. New York: Hill & Wang, 1966.

Henkel, Alice. *American Medicinal Leaves and Herbs*. U.S.D.A. Bulletin no. 219. Washington, D.C.: Government Printing Office, 1911.

Holbrook, Stewart H. *The Golden Age of Quackery*. New York: Macmillan, 1959.

Holloway, Mark. *Heavens on Earth*. New York: Dover, 1966.

Holmes, Oliver Wendell. *Medical Essays*. Boston: Houghton Mifflin, 1861.

In Memoriam. Henry Clay Blinn 1824–1905. Concord, N.H.: Rumford Printing Co., 1905.

Jarvis, D. C., M.D. *Folk Medicine*. New York: Henry Holt, 1958.

Johnson, Theodore E., ed. *The Shaker Quarterly 1961*. Sabbathday Lake, Maine.

Kadans, Joseph M. *Encyclopedia of Medicinal Herbs*. New York: Arco, 1972.

Kreig, Margaret B. *Green Medicine*. Chicago: Apollo, 1971.

Lamson, David R. *Two Years' Experience Among the Shakers*. West Boylston, Mass., 1848.

Lassiter, William Lawrence. *Shaker Recipes for Cooks and Homemakers*. New York: Greenwich, 1959.

Leighton, Ann. *Early American Gardens: For Meate or Medicine*. Boston: Houghton Mifflin, 1970.

Leyel, Mrs. C. F. *Culpepper's English and Complete Herbal*. London: Culpepper House, 1947.

―――. *The Magic of Herbs*. London: Jonathan Cape, 1926.

―――. *The Truth About Herbs*. London: Andrew Dakers Limited, 1943.

Lockwood, Alice G. B. *Gardens of Colony and State Before 1840*. New York: Charles Scribner's Sons, 1931.

Lomas, G. Albert, ed. *The Shaker, 1871–72*. Watervliet, N.Y.

————. *The Shaker, 1876–77*. Watervliet, N.Y.

————. *The Shaker Manifesto, 1878–1882*. Watervliet, N.Y.

Lossing, Benson John. "The Shakers of Lebanon, New York," *Harper's New Monthly Magazine*, vol. 15, no. 86 (July 1857).

MacLean, John P. *A Bibliography of Shaker Literature with an Introductory Study of the Writings and Publications Pertaining to Ohio Believers*. Columbus, Ohio: Fred J. Heer, 1905.

McNemar, Richard. *The Kentucky Revival*. Albany, N.Y.: E. and E. Hosford, 1808.

Melcher, Marguerite F. *The Shaker Adventure*. Cleveland: The Press of Case Western Reserve University, 1960.

Meyer, Clarence. *American Folk Medicine*. New York: Crowell, 1918.

Meyer, Joseph E. *The Herbalist*. Hammond, Ind.: Indiana Botanic Gardens, 1934.

Millennial Laws, The. Orders and Rules of the Church at New Lebanon. Published by the Ministry and Elders, 1821.

Millennial Laws, The. Revised at New Lebanon, New York. Published by the Ministry and Elders, 1845.

Neal, Julia. *By Their Fruits, The Story of Shakerism in South Union, Kentucky*. Chapel Hill, N.C.: University of North Carolina Press, 1947.

————. *The Journal of Eldress Nancy*. Nashville: Parthenon Press, 1963.

Noyes, John Humphrey. *History of American Socialisms*. New York: Dover, 1966.

Old Herb Doctor, The: His Secrets and Treatments: Over 1,000 Recipes. Hammond, Ind.: Hammond Book Co., 1941.

Piercy, Caroline B. *The Valley of God's Pleasure*. New York: Stratford House, 1951.

Redford, Arthur. *The History of Local Government in Manchester, England*. 2 vols. New York: Longmans, Green and Co., 1939.

Robinson, Charles Edson. *A Concise History of the United Society of Believers Called Shakers*. East Canterbury, N.H. Shaker Village, 1893.

Sears, Clara Endicott, ed. *Gleanings from Old Shaker Journals*. Cambridge, Mass.: Houghton Mifflin, 1916.

Shaker Heights Then and Now. Publication Committee, Shaker Heights Board of Education. Cleveland, 1938.

Shimko, Phyllis. *Sarsaparilla Encyclopedia*. Aurora, Ore.: privately printed, 1969.

Sigerist, Dr. Henry E. *The Great Doctors*. New York: Dover, 1971.

Silliman, Benjamin. *Peculiarities of the Shakers, Described in a Series of Letters from Lebanon Springs in the Year 1832*. New York: J. K. Porter, 1832.

————. *Remarks Made on a Short Tour between Hartford and Quebec*. New Haven: S. Converse, 1820.

————. "Shakers," *Christian Monthly Spectator* 6 (1824).

Smith, J. E. A. *The History of Pittsfield—1880–1876*. Pittsfield, Mass.: Published by the author. n.d.

Taylor, Norman. *Plant Drugs That Changed the World*. New York: Dodd, Mead, 1965.

Testimonies of the Life, Character, Revelation and Doctrines of Mother Ann Lee. 2nd ed. Albany, N.Y.: Weed, Parsons and Co., 1888.

Webster, Helen Noyes. *Herbs. How to Grow Them and How to Use Them*. Newton: Charles T. Branford Co., 1939.

Wheelwright, Edith Grey. *The Physick Garden*. Boston: Houghton Mifflin, 1935.

BIBLIOGRAPHY FOR THE HERBAL COMPENDIUM

Bailey, Liberty Hyde, and Ethel Zoe, eds. *Hortus Second*. New York: Macmillan, 1940.

Barton, William C. P. *Vegetable Materia Medica of the United States*. Philadelphia: H. C. Carey and I. Lea, 1825.

Bigelow, Jacob, M.D. *Florula Bostoniensis*. 2d ed. Boston: Cummings, Hilliard and Co., 1824.

Cobb, Boughton. *A Field Guide to the Ferns and their Related Families*. Boston: Houghton Mifflin, 1956.

Eaton, Amos C. *Manual of Botany for North America*. Albany, N.Y., 1829.

Gray, Asa. *Manual of Botany*. 8th ed. rev. Merritt Lundon Fernald, ed. New York: American Book Co., 1950.

Grieve, Maud. *A Modern Herbal*. Ed. and introduction, Mrs. C. F. Leyel. London: Jonathan Cape, 1931.

House, Homer D. *Wild Flowers of New York*. Vols. 1, 2. Albany: New York State Museum, 1921.

Johnson, Laurence. *A Manual of the Medical Botany of North America*. New York: William Wood and Co., 1884.

Meyer, Joseph E. *The Herbalist*. Hammond, Ind.: Indiana Botanic Gardens, 1934.

Millspaugh, Charles F. *Medicinal Plants: An Illustrated and Descriptive Guide to Plants Indigenous to and Naturalized in the United States in Medicine (One Thousand Medicinal Plants)*. 2 vols. Philadelphia: John C. Yorston and Co., 1892.

Muhlenberg, Gothilf H. E. *General Catalog of the Plants of North America*. Lancaster, Pa., 1813.

Peterson, Roger Tory, and McKenny, Margaret. *Field Guide to Wildflowers*. Boston: Houghton Mifflin, 1968.

Petrides, George A. *A Field Guide to Trees and Shrubs*. Boston: Houghton Mifflin, 1958.

Rafinesque, C. S. *Atlantic Journal and Friend of Knowledge*. Philadelphia: printed for the author by H. Probasco, 1832–1833.

———. *A Life of Travels and Research in North America*. 1785–1840.

———. *Medical Flora and Manual of the Medical Botany of the United States*. Philadelphia: Atkinson & Alexandria. 1828.

———. *New Flora of North America*. Philadelphia, 1836.

Stearns, Samuel. *American Herbal or Materia Medica*. Walpole, N.H., 1801.

Torrey, John D. *Compendium of the Flora of the Northern and Middle United States*. New York, 1826.

Wherry, Edgar T. *Wild Flower Guide*. New York: Doubleday, 1948.

INDEX

Italic numbers refer to illustrations; **boldface** numbers, to Herbal Compendium entries.

Buckthorn Bark

Rhamnus Catharticus

UNITED SOCIETY, - AYER, MASS.

Essence Tanzy.

Es

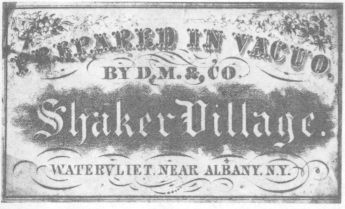

PREPARED IN VACUO
BY D. M. & CO.
Shaker Village.
WATERVLIET, NEAR ALBANY, N.Y.

SHAKER

Witch-Hazel

CLE
G

United So

SWE

ORDE

S. T. AT

HOREHOUND.
Marrubium vulgare.
D. M. & Co.
Watervliet, N. Y.

CATNIP,
Nepeta cataria.
D. M. & Co,
Watervliet, N. Y.

Not a Patent or a Proprietary Medicine, but made in
accordance with the following
FORMULA.
Take Opium, Camphor and Capsicum, each 8 lbs; Oil of
Peppermint, Sassafras and Spruce, each 2 lbs; Alcohol and
Cold Infus. of Witch Hazel, each 40 galls. Mix. *Note.*—Under
a law of Congress, passed Feb. 8, 1875, medicines put up with
published formula attached, are exempt from Int. Rev. Stamp.

DIRECTIONS.—*Internally,* for Cramps, Pain in the Stomach
and Bowels, Diarrhœa, Cholera Morbus and all internal Pains,
take 10 to 30 drops in sugar and water every half hour, until
relieved. *Externally,* Rub the painful and sore parts freely,
then lay on a cloth wet with the remedy and cover with cotton
batting to prevent evaporation.

To be shaken before used.

Sassafras Bark.

TANSY.

Tanacetum Crispum.

UNITED SOCIETY, AYER, MASS.

Essence Wormwood.

Essence Lavender.

WORM
Artemisia
D. M.
Watervlie

THESE HERBS
*Are guaranteed of the Finest Quality
and are always Fresh.*

MOTHERWORT
LEONORUS CARDIACA

RIKER-JAYNES DRUG STORES
BOSTON, MASS.
and other New England Cities.

MOTHERWORT

LB *EXTRACT OF*

THORN APPLE,

Datura Stramonium,

D. M.

PREPARED IN THE UNITED SOCIETY,
New-Lebanon, N. Y.

Jar   lb   oz.

S.
Salv
D. M
Wate

Hardha
Spiræ
D. M
WAT

Hea
Viola
D. M
Wate